Lippincott's Review Series

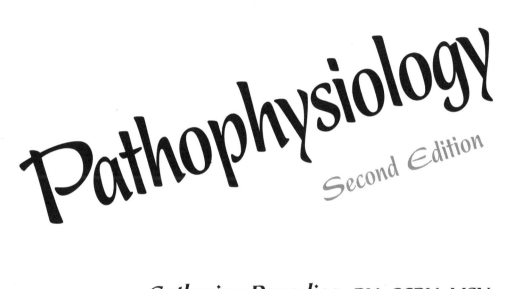

Pathophysiology

Second Edition

Catherine Paradiso, RN, CCRN, MSN

Senior Manager
Department of Clinical Practice
Meridian Health System
The Medical Center of Ocean County
Ocean County, New Jersey

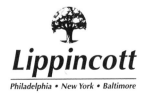

Lippincott

Philadelphia • New York • Baltimore

Senior Editor: Susan M. Glover, RN, MSN
Coordinating Editorial Assistant: Bridget Blatteau
Production Editor: Nicole Walz
Senior Production Manager: Helen Ewan
Production Service: Pine Tree Composition, Inc.
Printer/Binder: R.R. Donnelley & Sons Company
Cover Printer: Lehigh Press

Library of Congress Cataloging-in-Publication Data

Care has been taken to confirm the accuracy of the information presented and to
describe generally accepted practices. However, the authors, editors, and publisher
are not responsible for errors or omissions or for any consequences from application
of the information in this book and make no warranty, express or implied, with re-
spect to the contents of the publication.

The authors, editors and publisher have exerted every effort to ensure that drug
selection and dosage set forth in this text are in accordance with current recommendations and practice at the time of publication. However, in view of ongoing research, changes in government regulations, and the constant flow of information re-
lating to drug therapy and drug reactions, the reader is urged to check the package
insrt for each drug for any change in indications and dosage and for added warnings
and precautions. This is particularly important when the recommended agent is a
new or infrequently employed drug.

Some drugs and medical devices presented in this publication have Food and
Drug Administration (FDA) clearance for limited use in restricted research settings.
It is the responsibility of the health cre provider to ascertain the FDA status of each
drug or device planned for use in their clinical practice.

SMO0002422
1 01
£ 15.00
HPB
(Par)

Lippincott's
Review Series

Pathophysiology

0781718430

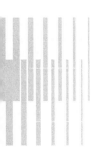

REVIEWERS

Judith H. Carlson, RN, MSN, GNP-C
Department Chair & Associate Professor
Nursing Department
St. Louis University
St. Louis, Missouri

Sharon R. Haymaker, PhD, CRNP
Associate Professor and Graduate Program Coordinator
School of Nursing
Bloomsburg University
Bloomsburg, Pennsylvania

Mary Ann Hensinger, RN, MSN
Nursing Instructor
MacQueen Gibbs Willis School of Nursing
Easton, Maryland

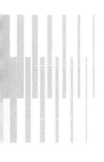

CONTRIBUTING AUTHORS

Donna Evertson-Bishop, RN, MS
Clinical Nurse Specialist
Women's Health
Meridan Health System
Jersey Shore Campus, New Jersey

Colleen A. DeBoer, RN, MSN, ANP-CS, OCN
Adult Nurse Practitioner
Memorial Sloan Kettering Cancer Center
New York, New York

Joan Harvey, RN, BSN
Nurse Clinician
Critical Care
Meridian Health System
Point Pleasant and Brick Campus, New Jersey

Genell Hilton, MS, CRNP, CCRN, CNRN
Family Nurse Practitioner
Maryland Primary Care
Arnold, Maryland

Maureen Howard, RN, MS, CCRN
Cardiovascular Clinical Specialist
Overlook Hospital
Summit, New Jersey

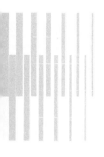

CONTRIBUTING AUTHORS
TO THE FIRST EDITION

Patricia Bartley-Daniele, RN, CCRN, MSN

Assistant Professor
Kingsborough Community College of the City
University of New York
Brooklyn, New York

Critical Care Nurse
Brookdale Hospital Medical Center
Brooklyn, New York
Chapter 15

Kathleen Beck-Lehman, MA, RN

Director of Perioperative Services
Meridian Health System
Mommouth County, New Jersey
Chapter 11

Carole Birdsall, RN, EdD

Associate Professor of Nursing
Hunter-Bellvue School of Nursing
Hunter College of the City University of
New York
New York, New York
Chapter 9

Mary Ellen Bonczek, RN, MPA

Chief Nurse Executive
Medical Center of Ocean County
Meridian Health System
Ocean County, New Jersey
Chapter 12

Joan Pasadino Bruno, RN C, MSN, CCRN

Clinical Nurse Specialist
Neonatal Intensive Care Unit
Beth Israel Medical Center
New York, New York
Chapter 18

Vidette Todaro Franceschi, RN, MSN

Medical-Surgical Clinical Nurse Specialist
Assistant Director of Nursing
Health Science Center at Brooklyn
State University of New York
Brooklyn, New York
Chapter 3

Genell Hilton, MS, RN, CCRN, CNRN

Nurse Education Specialist
Critical Care
Beth Israel Medical Center
New York, New York

Adjunct Faculty
School of Nursing
New York University
New York, New York
    Chapters 4, 5, 6, 7, 20

Maureen Howard, RN, MS, CCRN

Advance Medical-Surgical Instructor
School of Nursing
St. Vincent's Medical Center
Staten Island, New York

Co-director
Pulse-Cardiac Testing and Education Center
Staten Island, New York
    Chapter 2

Joanne Lavin, RN, EdD

Associate Professor
Kingsborough Community College of the City
University of New York
Brooklyn, New York

Consultant Supervision and Groups
Regents Hospital
Brooklyn, New York
    Test Consultant

Margaret Massoni, RN, MS, CS

Assistant Professor
Department of Nursing
College of Staten Island of the City
University of New York
Staten Island, New York
    Chapter 8

Shawn McCabe, RN, MSN, CCRN

Clinical Nurse Specialist/Trauma
University of Medicine and Dentistry
    of New Jersey
University Hospital
Newark, New Jersey
    Chapter 10

Martha Mulvey, MS, RN, CS

Clinical Nurse Specialist/Surgery
University of Medicine and Dentistry
    of New Jersey
University Hospital
Newark, New Jersey
    Chapter 17

Susan Neville, PhD, RN

Assistant Professor of Nursing
Hunter-Bellvue School of Nursing
Hunter College of the City University
    of New York
New York, New York
    Chapter 19

Lynda Olender-Russo, MA, RN, CS

Clinical Specialist
Brooklyn VA Medical Center
Brooklyn, New York

Adjunct Faculty
New York University
New York, New York
    Chapter 13

Dolores M. Donahue Shrimpton, RN, MA

Associate Professor
Kingsborough Community College of the City
    University of New York
Brooklyn, New York
    Chapter 16

Maureen Swick, RN, MSN, CNS, CNA, CCRN

Clinical Nurse Specialist for Critical Care
Medical Center of Ocean County
Point Pleasant, New Jersey
  Chapter 14

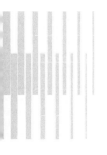

ACKNOWLEDGMENTS

This book and its companion, *Lippincott's Review Series: Fluids and Electrolytes,* were completed through the efforts of a team of people. I would like to thank them all for the dedication, commitment, and zeal they had for these projects. Their work is appreciated beyond words.

Rose Foltz, Developmental Editor. Thank you for devoting so much of your talent, expertise, and, most of all, your time to this project. Also, thank you for your kind and gentle patience. This book was enhanced through your efforts, and it is to the enormous benefit of the readers.

Cheryl Bryant, Manuscript Preparation. Thank you so very much for your commitment, time, patience, and, most of all, enthusiasm for these projects. Neither book would have been possible were it not for your work that many times was done in the wee hours of the morning.

Genell Hilton, contributor of five chapters, my colleague and friend whose work enabled the timely completion of this project. This book would never have been completed on time were it not for you. Your knowledge and professional work on this book is so very much appreciated. I look forward to further publishing endeavors.

David Reuss, Artist. Thank you for sharing your talent with me and the readers of these books. The energy you gave to these projects as well as time and commitment has made this a different kind of book.

Catherine

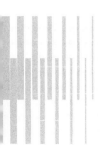

CONTENTS

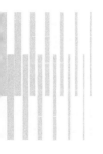

INTRODUCTION

Lippincott's Review Series is designed to help you in your study of the key subject areas in nursing. The series consists of nine books, one in each core nursing subject area:

Community and Home Health Nursing
Critical Care Nursing
Fluids and Electrolytes
Maternal-Newborn Nursing
Medical-Surgical Nursing

Mental Health
and Psychiatric Nursing
Pathophysiology
Pediatric Nursing
Pharmacology

Each book contains a comprehensive outline content review plus chapter study questions and a comprehensive examination, both with, answer key with rationales for correct and incorrect responses.

Lippincott's Review Series was planned and developed in response to your requests for outline review books that address each major subject area and also contain a self-test mechanism. These books meet the need for comprehensive subject review books that will also assist you in identifying your strong and weak areas of knowledge. Each book is a complete source for review and self-assessment of a single core subject—all nine together provide an excellent comprehensive review of entry-level nursing.

Each book is all-inclusive of the content addressed in major textbooks. The content outline review uses a consistent nursing process format throughout and addresses nursing care for well and ill clients. Also included are are necessary teaching and other concepts, including growth and development, nutrition, pharmacology, and body structures, functions, and pathophysiology. Special features of each book are Key Concepts and Nursing Alerts, which are identified by distinctive icons. Key Concepts ☼ are basic facts the nurse needs to know to perform the job with ease and efficiency. Nursing Alerts ✋ are fundamental guidelines the nurse can follow to ensure safe and effective care.

You can use the books in this series in several different ways. Overall, you can use them as subject reviews to augment general study throughout your basic nursing program and as a review to prepare for the National Council Licensure Examination (NCLEX-RN). How you use each book depends on your individual needs and preferences and on whether you review each chapter systematically or concentrate only on those chapters whose subject areas are particularly problematic or challenging. You may instead choose to use the comprehensive examination as a self-assessment opportunity to evaluate your knowledge base before you review the content outline. Likewise, you can use the study questions for pre- or post-testing after study, followed by the comprehensive examination as a means of evaluating your knowledge and competencies of an entire subject area.

Regardless of how you use the books, one of the strengths of the series is the self-assessment opportunity it offers in addition to guidance in studying and reviewing content. The chapter study questions and comprehensive examination questions have been carefully developed to cover all topics in the outline review.

Unlike the NCLEX examination that tests the cumulative knowledge needed for safe practice by an entry-level nurse, these practice tests systematically evaluate the knowledge base that serves as the building block for the entire nursing educational process. In this way, you can prepare for the NCLEX examination throughout your course of study. Good study habits throughout your educational program are not only the best way to ensure ongoing success, but also will prove the most beneficial way to prepare for the licensing examination.

Keep in mind that these books are not intended to replace formal learning. They cannot substitute for textbook reading, discussion with instructors, or class attendance. Every effort has been made to provide accurate and current information, but class attendance and interaction with an instructor will provide invaluable information not found in books. Used correctly, these books will help you increase understanding, improve comprehension, evaluate strengths and weaknesses in areas of knowledge, increase productive study time, and as a result help you improve your grades.

MONEY BACK GUARANTEE—Lippincott's Review Series will help you study more effectively during coursework throughout your educational program, and help you prepare for quizzes and tests, including the NCLEX exam. If you buy and use any of the nine volumes in Lippincott's Review Series and fail the NCLEX exam, simply send us verification of your exam results and your copy of the review book to the address below. We will promptly send you a check for our suggested list price.

Lippincott's Review Series
Marketing Department
Lippincott Williams & Wilkins
227 East Washington Square
Philadelphia, PA 19106-3780

Lippincott's Review Series

Pathophysiology

1 Respiratory Disorders

I.   Overview of pathophysiologic processes

A. Restrictive diseases

1. Restrictive diseases include any disorders that limit lung expansion and restrict chest wall movement throughout the respiratory cycle.

2. These disorders result in decreased lung volume, decreased pulmonary compliance, and increased work of breathing.
    a. Lung volume is the amount of air, measured in cubic centimeters, that is inhaled and exhaled with each breath.
    b. Pulmonary compliance is the ability of the lungs and thorax to expand and contract as air is inhaled and exhaled; this is sometimes referred to as *recoil*.
    c. Work of breathing is the effort required to expand and contract the lungs.
3. Atelectasis, pneumothorax, and pleural effusion are restrictive diseases. Pneumonia can also be classified as a restrictive disorder as well as a respiratory tract infection.

4. Restrictive diseases can be caused by parenchymal or lung disease (damage to actual lung tissue), neuromuscular alterations, chest wall disorders, musculoskeletal or neuromuscular disorders.

5. Musculoskeletal and neuromuscular disorders that can cause restriction include kyphosis, fractured ribs, muscular dystrophy, Guillain-Barré syndrome, and myasthenia gravis. These will be discussed in Chapter 6, Neuromuscular Disorders.

 6. **Other causes of restriction include obesity, pregnancy, abdominal distention, pain, or tight application of bandages.**

7. Risk factors for restrictive diseases include:
    a. Occupational hazards, such as inhalation of asbestos
    b. Trauma to the chest, such as rib fractures
    c. Surgeries that render patients unable to cough and deep breathe postoperatively
    d. Past or present history of musculoskeletal diseases

B. Obstructive diseases

1. **Obstructive diseases include any disorders in which an obstruction impedes airflow to the lungs.**

2. These diseases can be chronic or acute.
    a. Chronic diseases include asthma, bronchitis, and emphysema.
    b. Acute diseases include adult respiratory distress syndrome, acute respiratory failure, cystic fibrosis, and cancer.

 3. **Obstruction can be caused by edema of the airway or tongue, which can result from smoke inhalation, infection, or anaphylaxis.**

 4. **Obstruction also can result from impaired mucociliary transport caused by chemical damage or by chronic irritation from cigarette smoking.**
    a. The mucociliary system is composed of mucus-secreting goblet cells and cilia that help clear secretions and microorganisms from the airways.
    b. A change in the amount or character of respiratory secretions will cause the airways to fill with mucus and impede airflow.
    c. As elastic recoil decreases, an ineffective cough will result.
    d. Bronchoconstriction also will occur as a response mechanism.

5. Risk factors for obstructive disease include:
    a. Cigarette smoking (over time, it will damage parenchymal lung tissue causing loss of recoil)
    b. Prolonged exposure to pulmonary irritants

6. Acute obstructive diseases may occur secondary to these risk factors as well as from other causes.

C. Respiratory tract infections

 1. **Respiratory tract infections affect airway clearance and breathing patterns by changing the amount and character of secretions.**

2. Severe respiratory tract infections include tuberculosis and pneumonia.

3. *Pneumocystis carinii,* a virulent type of pneumonia, is associated with acquired immunodeficiency syndrome (AIDS).

4.   Risk factors for respiratory infections include:
a.   Exposure to infected persons
b.   Stress or other immunocompromised states that may allow microorganisms to invade and proliferate

D.   Pulmonary-related cardiac diseases

   1.   Certain cardiac diseases result from disorders of the pulmonary system.

2.   Pulmonary-related cardiac diseases, including cor pulmonale and pulmonary embolism, will be covered in Chapter 2, Cardiac Disorders.

II.   Physiologic responses to respiratory dysfunction

A.   Hypoxia
1.   Hypoxia refers to inadequate cellular oxygenation.
2.   It may result from:
a.   Insufficient oxygen intake
b.   Insufficient perfusion of oxygen in the pulmonary system or in the peripheral organs and tissues
c.   Inability of the blood to transport oxygen
d.   Insufficient oxygen-carrying capacity of the blood, which would occur with low levels of hemoglobin

B.   Cyanosis: a bluish discoloration of the skin indicating hypoxia; it results when oxygenation does not occur and carbon dioxide does not leave the blood.

C.   Dyspnea: difficult breathing. May occur as the need for oxygen exceeds the supply.

D.   Increased work of breathing: occurs when energy expenditure for respirations is excessive and great effort is required for breathing.

E.   Tachypnea: rapid breathing with respiratory rates higher than 24 to 26 breaths per minute.

F.   Cough
1.   An effective cough allows the body to expel excess mucus, keeping the airway clear.

   2.   An ineffective cough compromises airway clearance by preventing mucus from being expelled.

3.   Along with the mucociliary system, cough is a defense mechanism of the respiratory system.

G.   Adventitious breath sounds
1.   As fluid and mucus accumulate, abnormal breath sounds can be heard.

2.   Fluid is heard as rales (crackles); mucus is heard as rhonchi (gurgles).

H.   Clubbing of fingers
1.   Clubbing is an increase in the normal angle between the nail and its base (from 160 degrees to 180 degrees or more).

2. It usually is accompanied by a softening of the nail base.

I. Fatigue: feelings of tiredness and exhaustion that usually result when energy requirements for breathing become excessive

J. Pain

1. May or may not be present
2. Pain due to rib-cage injury, infection, or chest surgery may cause hypoventilation.

K. Hypoventilation

1. **Hypoventilation refers to a ventilation rate that is insufficient to meet the body's metabolic needs.**
2. It may result in respiratory acidosis because the acid (carbon dioxide) is not removed when ventilation is decreased.

L. Hyperventilation

1. **Hyperventilation refers to a ventilation rate that exceeds the body's metabolic needs.**
2. It may result in respiratory alkalosis because acids (carbon dioxide) are eliminated in excessive amounts, leaving excess base (bicarbonate) in the blood.

M. Respiratory acidosis

1. **This condition is commonly caused by hypoventilation, which reduces elimination of carbon dioxide (CO_2), leaving too much acid in the serum, revealing a low pH.**
2. The renal system tries to compensate by retaining HCO_3 to buffer the acid, moving the pH toward neutral; this occurs over a period of many hours to days.
3. Arterial blood gas (ABG) values reveal a low pH, a high CO_2, and a normal HCO_3 when renal compensatory mechanisms are not in place.

N. Respiratory alkalosis

1. **This condition is commonly caused by hyperventilation, which increases the removal of carbon dioxide, leaving too much base (HCO_3) in the serum, revealing a high pH.**
2. The renal system tries to compensate by increasing HCO_3 elimination in order to maintain the balance of HCO_3 to CO_2, thus moving the pH toward neutral; this occurs over a period of many hours to days.
3. ABG values reveal a high pH, a low CO_2, and a normal to high HCO_3 when renal compensatory mechanisms are not in place.
4. Table 1.1 illustrates arterial blood gas results reflecting acid–base disorders.

III. Atelectasis

A. Description

1. **Atelectasis refers to collapse of previously expanded lung tissue; a shrunken airless state of the alveoli.**
2. It can be primary or secondary.

TABLE 1-1
Acid–Base Imbalances: Arterial Blood Gas Analysis

DISORDER	pH	PaCO$_2$	HCO$_3$
Respiratory acidosis (uncompensated)	Below 7.35	Above 42	Normal
Respiratory acidosis (partially uncompensated)	Below 7.35	Above 42	Above 26 (Bicarbonate is retained to buffer the acid [CO$_2$] and move the pH to normal.)
Respiratory acidosis (fully compensated)	Normal	Above 42	Above 26
Respiratory alkalosis (uncompensated)	Above 7.45	Below 38	Normal
Respiratory alkalosis (partically compensated)	Above 7.45	Below 38	Below 22 (The kidneys eliminate bicarbonate to balance with the lowered acid levels, moving the pH toward normal.)
Respiratory alkalosis (fully compensated)	Normal	Below 38	Below 22
Metabolic acidosis (uncompensated)	Below 7.35	Normal	Below 22
Metabolic acidosis (partially compensated)	Below 7.35	Below 38	Below 22 (The respiratory system responds by hyperventilating, which eliminates the acid CO$_2$ in an attempt to eliminate extra acids and move the pH toward normal.)
Metabolic acidosis (fully compensated)	Normal	Below 38	Below 22
Metabolic alkalosis (uncompensated)	Above 7.45	Normal	Above 26
Metabolic alkalosis (partially compensated)	Above 7.45	Above 42	Above 26 (The respiratory system responds by hypoventilating to retain more acid so that the extra bicarbonate will be buffered, moving the pH toward normal.)
Metabolic alkalosis (fully compensated)	Normal	Above 42	Above 26

B. Etiology

1. Primary atelectasis is a condition in which lung tissue remains uninflated as a result of insufficient surfactant production.
   a. Surfactant is a lipoprotein that reduces the surface tension of the alveoli and prevents alveolar collapse.
   b. Primary atelectasis is present at birth and is typically found in premature and at-risk infants.
2. Secondary atelectasis is caused by airway obstruction, lung compression (such as occurs in pneumothorax or pleural effusion), or increased recoil of the lung due to diminished pulmonary surfactant.
   a. Airway obstruction can be caused by mucous plugs, tumors, or exudate.

b. The risk for secondary atelectasis increases after surgery because anesthesia, narcotic administration, and immobility promote retention of bronchial secretions, which may lead to bronchial obstruction.

C. **Pathophysiologic processes and manifestations**

1. Surfactant, which has a short half-life, must be constantly replenished by normal ventilation.

 2. Ineffective cough reflex diminishes tidal volume and decreases sigh mechanisms, leading to poor alveolar expansion.

 3. Increased viscosity of sputum leads to pooling of secretions in dependent areas.

4. Complete airway obstruction is followed by absorption of oxygen from dependent alveoli and collapse of that portion of the lung.

5. Severity of symptoms depends on the amount of lung tissue affected; most postoperative cases can be easily controlled, but if left untreated, the disease can progress from a small area to a larger area, eventually reducing that lung's ability to oxygenate.

 6. Symptoms can include:
   a. Crackles and gurgles from accumulation of secretions in the bases
   b. Diminished breath sounds from poor air entry at the site of collapse
   c. Progressive dyspnea and tachycardia resulting from decreased oxygen
   d. Progressive cough due to loss of secretions
   e. Hypoxemia

D. **Overview of nursing interventions**

1. Encourage the patient to cough and deep breathe.
2. Encourage the patient to perform incentive spirometry.
3. Administer antibiotics, as prescribed, to prevent or control infection.
4. Administer oxygen if necessary to improve delivery of oxygen to the alveolar level.
5. Provide adequate hydration.
6. Monitor breath sounds.
7. Monitor temperature for elevation.
8. Reposition frequently to prevent pooling of secretions and assist in lung expansion.

IV. **Pneumothorax**

A. **Description**

1. **Pneumothorax is the accumulation of air in the pleural space, which results in partial or complete lung collapse (Fig. 1-1).**

2. **Types include:**
   a. *Tension pneumothorax:* **Air can enter the pleural space but cannot leave it.**

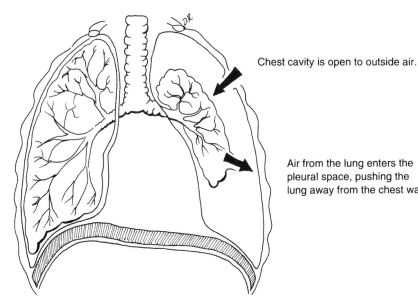

Chest cavity is open to outside air.

Air from the lung enters the pleural space, pushing the lung away from the chest wall.

FIGURE 1-1.
Pneumothorax.

    b.   *Secondary pneumothorax:* **Air enters the pleural space as a result of injury to the chest wall, respiratory structures, or esophagus.**

    c.   *Spontaneous pneumothorax:* **Air enters the pleural space when airfilled blebs (blisters) on the lung surface rupture.**

B.   **Etiology**

    1.   Tension pneumothorax results from unknown causes.

    2.   Secondary pneumothorax is caused by injury to the chest wall resulting from trauma (such as crushing injuries) or from punctures (such as stab wounds or gunshot wounds).

    3.   Spontaneous pneumothorax is caused by a ruptured bleb and is seen more commonly in smokers.

C.   **Pathophysiologic processes and manifestations**

    1.   **Severity of symptoms depends on the size of the injury and the amount of lung tissue left intact.**

    2.   Symptoms can include:

        a.   **Pleuritic pain (a sharp pain occurring during inhalation)**

        b.   **Increased respiratory rate**

        c.   **Dyspnea**

        d.   **Visible asymmetry of the chest, which results from rib fractures**

        e.   **Hyperresonant lung sounds**

        f.   **Decreased breath sounds over the area of pneumothorax**

        g.   **Trachea deviating to the injured side**

        h.   **Neck vein distention (resulting from greater amount of pressure in the thorax)**

          i.   Palpable subcutaneous emphysema (as air leaves the chest cavity and remains in the subcutaneous space)

          j.   Shifting of mediastinal structures to unaffected side of chest (caused by large pneumothorax)

          k.   Hypoxemia (seen on ABG) and clinical signs of shock, such as low blood pressure and tachycardia (caused by large pneumothorax)

    3.   In tension pneumothorax, the onset of symptoms is sudden and painful.

D.   **Overview of nursing interventions**

    1.   Monitor vital signs, checking for signs of shock (eg, low blood pressure and tachycardia).

    2.   Observe the patient's respirations (rate and depth); breathing pattern changes may indicate a worsening condition.

    3.   Position the patient in a semi-Fowler's position.

    4.   Monitor pulse oximetry.

    5.   Administer oxygen if necessary.

    6.   Administer analgesics as prescribed.

    7.   For a patient with chest tubes:

          a.   Maintain sterile dressing at chest tube insertion site.

          b.   Maintain patency and integrity of the closed chest drainage system and suction if ordered.

          c.   Evaluate amount of fluid and breath sounds to determine progress of closed chest drainage.

          d.   Assess for signs and symptoms of wound infection.

          e.   Assess for fear and anxiety and institute appropriate measures for alleviation and relief.

V.   **Pleural effusion**

A.   **Description**

    1.   **Pleural effusion refers to an abnormal accumulation of fluid in the pleural cavity, which occurs when fluid forms more quickly than it can be removed.**

    2.   Fluid may be transudate (hydrothorax), exudate (empyema), blood (hemothorax), or chyle, a milky fluid found in lymph fluid from the gastrointestinal tract (chylothorax).

    3.   Transudate fluid has a protein content that is less than 3.0 g/mL; exudate fluid has a protein content that is greater than 3.0 g/mL.

    4.   Lactate dehydrogenase, a measurable protein marker, is used to measure the protein content of pleural fluid samples.

B.   **Etiology**

    1.   *Hydrothorax* **is commonly caused by congestive heart failure; other causes include renal failure, nephrosis, liver failure, malignancy, and myxedema.**

    2.   *Empyema* typically results from infections, pulmonary infarction, malignancies, rheumatoid arthritis, and lupus erythematosus. It also can result from direct spread from adjacent bacterial pneumonia, rupture of a lung abscess, invasion from subphrenic infections, or trauma-related infections.

3. *Hemothorax* can be caused by chest injuries, chest surgery complications, malignancies, or rupture of a great vessel.
4. *Chylothorax* is caused by trauma, inflammation, or malignant infiltration that obstructs chyle transport from the thoracic duct into the central circulation.

C. **Pathophysiologic processes and manifestations**

1. Five mechanisms are associated with pleural effusion:
   a. *An increase in capillary pressure:* This occurs when the heart fails to pump blood back to the heart and fluid that has accumulated in the capillaries causes increased pressure in the area's blood vessels.
   b. *An increase in capillary permeability:* This occurs with conditions associated with inflammation.
   c. *A decrease in colloidal osmotic pressure:* This results as plasma proteins are diluted in plasma water, such as occurs in disease states that cause hypoalbuminemia (eg, liver disease and nephrotic syndrome).
   d. *An increase in intrapleural negative pressure*
   e. *An impairment in lymphatic drainage of the pleura*

2. **Pleural effusion results in a decreased lung volume on the affected side and a mediastinal shift toward the contralateral side. This places pressure on the other lung and causes a decreased lung volume on that side as well, making breath sounds diminished or absent.**

3. Emphysema is present in the pleural cavity.

4. **Characteristic signs of pleural effusion are diminished breath sounds and dullness or flatness to percussion.**

5. Other symptoms can include:
   a. Dyspnea (when 2000 mL or more of fluid accumulate)
   b. Pleuritic pain (when inflammation is present)
   c. Constant discomfort (large effusions)

6. The severity of hemothorax is determined by the volume of fluid:
   a. Minimal (300 to 500 mL)
   b. Moderate (500 to 1000 mL)
   c. Large (1000 mL or more)

7. Minimal hemothorax usually resolves in 10 to 14 days as small amounts of blood are naturally absorbed from the pleural space.

8. Moderate hemothorax fills about one third of the pleural cavity and may produce signs of lung compression and loss of intravascular volume.

9. Large hemothorax fills half or more of one side of the chest and requires immediate drainage.

10. Fibrothorax, the effusion of pleural surfaces by fibrin, hyalin, and connective tissue, may occur as a complication of moderate to large hemothorax; it results from the presence of fibrin containing blood and fluid.

D. **Overview of nursing interventions**

1. Observe the patient for signs of shock (eg, increased heart rate, decreased blood pressure).
2. Monitor respiratory status note changes in breath sounds or use of accessory muscles for breathing.

3. Administer analgesics as prescribed.
4. Position the patient for comfort and optimum respiratory function.
5. For moderate to large effusions when chest tubes are needed:
   a. Maintain fluid replacement therapy as ordered.
   b. Assist with insertion of chest tubes as ordered.
   c. Maintain patency of chest tubes.
   d. Prepare patient for surgery if bleeding cannot be stopped.
   e. Monitor pulse oximetry.

VI. Asthma

A. Description

1. **Asthma is an airflow obstruction caused by bronchoconstriction, which results from an allergic or hypersensitive reaction (Fig. 1-2).**
2. Asthma can be classified as extrinsic or intrinsic.

B. Etiology

1. *Extrinsic asthma* results from allergic reactions to inhalants, such as perfumes, flowers, dust, molds, and spores.
   a. It may be genetically transmitted.
   b. Onset usually occurs in childhood.
2. *Intrinsic asthma* results from unknown causes.

C. Pathophysiologic processes and manifestations

1. The immune system responds to presence of the allergens by causing bronchoconstriction.

2. **An increase in the size and number of goblet cells (cells that secrete mucus), submucosal goblet cells, and submucosal mucous glands accompanied by a thickening of the bronchial basement membrane causes an increase in viscosity and volume of mucus, which fills the airways.**

3. **The excessive accumulation of mucus and the basement membrane thickening impairs the transport of oxygen across the alveolar-capillary membrane, leading to hypoxia.**

4. Symptoms can include:
   a. Dyspnea
   b. Wheezing
   c. Chest tightness

D. Overview of nursing interventions

1. Administer bronchodilators (medications that enlarge bronchial tubes), steroids, and oxygen as ordered.
2. Administer antibiotics, as prescribed, to prevent secondary infection.
3. Provide inhalant therapy when indicated.
4. Provide bronchial hygiene when indicated.
5. Provide patient teaching, covering:
   a. Ways to prevent attacks, such as avoiding allergens
   b. Proper use of medication
   c. Anxiety control and breathing exercises.

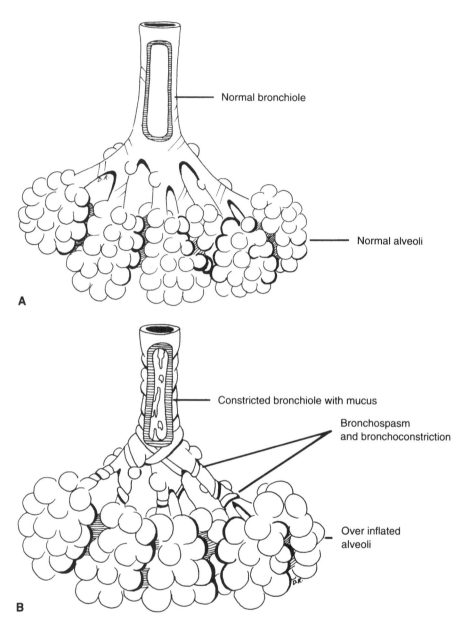

Normal bronchiole

Normal alveoli

A

Constricted bronchiole with mucus

Bronchospasm and bronchoconstriction

Over inflated alveoli

B

FIGURE 1-2.
(A) Normal airway and **(B)** asthma.

6. Monitor breath sounds
7. Monitor pulse oximetry.

VII. Bronchitis

A. Description

1. **Bronchitis is an inflammation of the bronchioles that impairs airflow; it may be acute or chronic.**
2. Acute bronchitis occurs when the bronchus becomes inflamed; chronic bronchitis results when inflammation occurs several times a year.
3. Chronic bronchitis can be diagnosed by the presence of a chronic productive cough that persists for 3 months a year for 2 consecutive years.

B. Etiology

1. **Bronchitis can be caused by exposure to pulmonary irritants, such as cigarette smoke and air pollutants.**
2. Bronchitis also can be caused by infections, including respiratory tract infections, pneumococcal infections, and influenza.

C. Pathophysiologic processes and manifestations

1. Enlargement and hyperactivity of mucus-secreting glands cause inflammation and narrowing of the airways, reducing ciliary efficiency (Fig. 1-3).

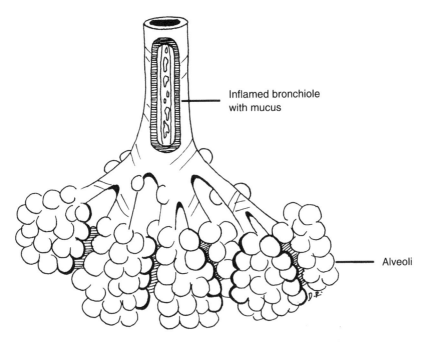

Inflamed bronchiole with mucus

Alveoli

FIGURE 1-3.
Bronchitis.

2. Infection may develop concurrently, further obstructing air passage through bronchial channels and leading to the development of pneumonia.
3. Inflammation occurs as bronchiole tissue is irritated.
4. Common findings include coughing and excessive sputum production.
5. Rhonchi can be heard over the airways; as the severity of symptoms increases, shortness of breath occurs.
6. Over many years, lung tissue damage leads to emphysema.

D. Overview of nursing interventions
1. Eliminate or minimize the patient's exposure to pulmonary irritants and to persons with respiratory tract infections or influenza.
2. Assess breath sounds.
3. Assess for signs and symptoms of worsening infectious process.
4. Clear airways with chest physical therapy and suctioning as appropriate.
5. Administer bronchodilators, as prescribed, to open the airways.
6. Encourage the patient to perform breathing exercises to maximize ventilation.
7. Provide patient teaching, covering:
    a. Adequate nutritional intake
    b. Medication therapy
    c. Avoidance of known irritants, ie, smoking and allergens

VIII. Emphysema

A. Description: airflow obstruction resulting from changes in lung tissue, characterized by acute exacerbations and remissions

B. Etiology
1. Emphysema results from cigarette smoking or long-term exposure to pulmonary irritants, such as air pollution.
2. It also can result from years of chronic bronchitis.

C. Pathophysiologic processes and manifestations
1. Chronic irritation leads to obstructive symptoms (eg, sputum production, cough, and CO_2 retention), which become progressively worse with age. CO_2 levels are higher in patients with emphysema, so their "normal" blood gas values look very different from the general population.
2. Chronic irritation also causes:
    a. Loss of alveolar elasticity, which makes exhalation difficult
    b. Reduced elasticity, which leads to hyperinflation of the lungs that worsens with time
    c. Destruction of alveolus, which leads to impaired membrane gas exchange
    d. Bronchoconstriction (Fig. 1-4)
3. Chronic inflammation causes a narrowing of the airways and production of excessive thick secretions.
4. Bronchial smooth muscle hyperactivity causes bronchoconstriction.

D. Overview of nursing interventions
1. Encourage the patient to avoid pulmonary irritants.
2. Administer fluids to liquefy secretions.

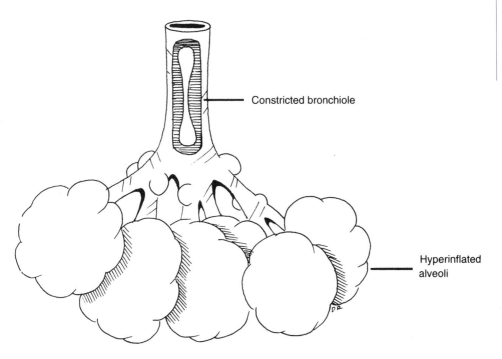

Constricted bronchiole

Hyperinflated alveoli

FIGURE 1-4.
Emphysema

3. Provide adequate nutrition.
4. Administer low-flow oxygen. Remember: CO_2 is the drive to breathe, so do not lower CO_2 levels in a patient with COPD or respiratory arrest will occur.
5. Administer antibiotics, as ordered, to prevent and control infection during acute exacerbations.
6. Administer steroids during an acute attack, as ordered, to reduce inflammation.

IX. Adult respiratory distress syndrome (ARDS)

A. **Description: a sequela of several diseases in which the lungs fill with water, making gas exchange impossible**
B. **Etiology**
   1. Adult respiratory distress syndrome results from unknown causes.
   2. The following conditions may lead to adult respiratory distress syndrome:
      a. Pneumonia
      b. Near drowning
      c. Reaction to drugs and inhaled gases
      d. Disseminated intravascular clotting
      e. Infection

  f.   Allergic reactions to inhalants
  g.   Diabetic ketoacidosis
  h.   Trauma
  i.   Burns
  j.   Shock

C.   Pathophysiologic processes and manifestations

  1.   Increased permeability of the alveolar-capillary membrane permits fluid and protein to move from the vascular compartment into the pulmonary interstitium and alveoli, causing noncardiac pulmonary edema.
  2.   Plasma protein inactivates surfactant, causing injury to the surfactant-producing alveolar cells.
  3.   Alveolar surface tension markedly increases.
  4.   Increased pressure from excessive fluid, coupled with increased surface tension, causes alveolar collapse, making the lungs stiff and difficult to inflate.
  5.   Lung compliance decreases and work of breathing increases.
  6.   Alveolar ducts and alveoli become lined with hyaline membranes, compromising the diffusion of respiratory gases.
  7.   These changes make gas exchange impossible and are manifested by:
       a.   Crackles and gurgles, which are present as fluid and mucus accumulate
       b.   Accumulation of fluid, which makes diffusion of gases across alveolar-capillary membrane difficult
       c.   Impaired diffusion, which causes hypoxemia to persist despite increased inspired oxygen
       d.   Respiratory distress
       e.   Extensive bilateral consolidation of lung tissue, which is visible on x-ray
  8.   ABG analysis will reveal a decreasing PO_2 and high PCO_2 while high-flow oxygen is being administered, indicating that the pathology is at the gas exchange area of the alveolus and capillary.

D.   Overview of nursing interventions

  1.   Monitor fluid intake.
  2.   Administer steroids, as ordered, to reduce inflammation.
  3.   Assess for complications, such as pneumothorax.
  4.   Institute mechanical ventilation with the addition of positive expiratory-end pressure (PEEP) as ordered.
  5.   Provide care necessary for the patient on mechanical ventilation. Monitor airway pressures for increases. When on PEEP, monitor BP closely especially during the time period immediately following the application. Assess for complications related to PEEP (decreased BP, pneumothorax).
  6.   Protect the airway from injury.
  7.   Relieve anxiety by reassuring the patient about his or her status.
  8.   Monitor breath sounds.

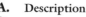 **X.   Acute respiratory failure (ARF)**

A.   Description

  1.   Acute respiratory failure, a disease sequela, occurs when the lungs are

unable to adequately oxygenate the blood or prevent carbon dioxide retention.

 2. ARF occurs when PO_2 level is 50 mm Hg or less and when PCO_2 level is 50 mm Hg or above.

3. ARF can develop in persons with normal lungs or may occur in patients with chronic disease of the lungs or chest wall.

B. Etiology

1. ARF can be caused by an infection, such as pneumonia.

2. It also may be caused by exacerbation of COPD.

C. Pathophysiologic processes and manifestations

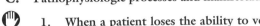 1. When a patient loses the ability to ventilate *or* perfuse at the alveolar-capillary level, oxygen absorption and carbon dioxide elimination will not occur.

2. When a disease that affects gas exchange (eg, pulmonary edema) is the primary cause of ARF, hypoxia and hypercapnia result. ABG studies reveal $PO_2 < 55$ to 60 mm Hg and a $PCO_2 > 40$ mm Hg.

3. Impaired oxygen perfusion and carbon dioxide removal result in hypoxemia and hypercapnia.

    a. As hypoxia progresses, stupor, coma, bradycardia, and hypotension result.

    b. Hypercapnia results in vasodilation and may sedate the central nervous system (CNS).

4. Impaired oxygen perfusion also leads to:

    a. Tachycardia

    b. Diaphoresis

    c. Mild increases in blood pressure

    d. Restlessness

    e. Agitation

    f. Cool skin

D. Overview of nursing interventions

1. Institute mechanical ventilation to facilitate oxygenation.

2. Provide care necessary for the patient on mechanical ventilation such as maintenance of artificial airway, nutrition, hydration.

3. Monitor breath sounds and pulse oximetry and/or ABGs.

4. Assess mental status.

5. Assess for complications, such as pneumothorax.

6. Administer antibiotics, as prescribed, to treat respiratory infections.

7. Monitor secretions for signs of infections or worsening of symptoms.

8. Obtain cultures prior to the administration of antibiotics.

9. Monitor temperature.

10. Use closed system suction if available. Otherwise use proper technique when suctioning.

11. Administer bronchodilators, as prescribed, to open constricted airways.

XI. Cystic fibrosis

A. Description: chronic obstructive disease characterized by exocrine secretion of thick, tenacious, and copious mucus in the respiratory, gastrointestinal, and reproductive tracts

B. Etiology: cystic fibrosis is genetically transmitted.

C. Pathophysiologic processes and manifestations

1. **Bronchial obstruction results in ineffective airway clearance, which causes mucus stasis.**

2. **Mucus stasis leads to infection, commonly with such organisms as *Pseudomonas aeruginosa* or *Staphylococcus.***

3. Permanent parenchymal damage results as bronchial walls are destroyed and the bronchioles become dilated.

4. Obstruction of gastrointestinal ducts leads to nutritional deficiencies.

5. As the disease progresses, normal lung tissue is replaced by connective tissue.

6. Cor pulmonale eventually results from chronic excessive workload.

D. Overview of nursing interventions

1. Liquefy secretions with increased fluid intake and administration of mucolytics, as ordered.

2. Monitor fluid and electrolyte balance.

3. Maintain adequate nutritional status.

4. Clear airways with postural drainage. Position to maximize respiratory function.

5. Monitor for signs and symptoms of infection (elevated temperatures, change in sputum color/consistency).

6. Administer antibiotics to control infection, as prescribed.

7. Monitor pulse oximetry and ABGs.

8. Administer oxygen to improve oxygenation.

9. Institute mechanical ventilation if the patient's condition deteriorates.

XII. Tuberculosis

A. Description

1. **Tuberculosis is an infection caused by the bacillus *Mycobacterium tuberculosis.***

2. This bacillus usually affects the lungs, but it can also invade other structures.

B. Etiology and incidence

1. **Tuberculosis is caused by inhalation of *M. tuberculosis* bacilli spread from droplets.**

2. Tuberculosis, once a major health problem, had been controlled for many years; however, incidence is increasing due to the large number of immunocompromised patients acquiring it as an opportunistic infection and the evolution of a multidrug-resistant form of the bacillus.

C. **Pathophysiologic processes and manifestations**
1. Inhaled bacilli multiply in the lungs, causing inflammation; some bacilli may leave the lungs and multiply in other body systems.
2. Pulmonary macrophages and white cells migrate to the infected area, surrounding and isolating the bacilli and producing a lesion called a tubercle.
3. Scar tissue grows around the tubercle, preventing further multiplication.
4. The bacilli within the tubercle become inactive, forming a cheeselike substance called caseation necrosis.
5. The isolated bacilli can remain dormant for life. However, if the patient's immune response becomes impaired, live bacilli will escape into the bronchial tree and cause the patient to become contagious again.
6. **Administration of steroids can result in immunosuppression, which can reactivate the disease in its contagious form.**
7. Patients may be asymptomatic, or the symptoms may have a more insidious onset.
8. **Characteristic signs of tuberculosis are:**
   a. **Cough producing purulent sputum**
   b. **Night sweats**
   c. **Hemoptysis (blood in the sputum)**
9. Other symptoms can include:
   a. Low-grade fever
   b. Fatigue
   c. Lethargy
   d. Weight loss
   e. Anorexia
   f. Chest pain

D. **Overview of nursing interventions**
1. Provide routine screening through use of skin test, sputum culture, or chest x-ray.
2. Administer antimycobacterial medications as ordered:
   a. Antimycobacterial therapy is used for patients with active tuberculosis.
   b. It is also used as a prophylactic for those exposed to active tuberculosis.
   c. Two different medications are usually prescribed to prevent the emergence of drug-resistant organisms.
4. Isolate contagious patients in negative pressure rooms.
5. Maintain strict isolation techniques for visitors as well as hospital staff.
6. Ensure adequate hydration.
7. Maintain adequate nutritional status.
8. Clear airways by suctioning or positioning in semi-Fowler's or Fowler's position.
9. Administer oxygen therapy to improve oxygenation.
10. Institute respiratory therapy as prescribed/Monitor pulse oximetry.
11. Obtain frequent sputum cultures.
12. Provide patient teaching, covering:
    a. Recurrence and spread of the disease
    b. Proper use of prescribed medications

XIII. Pneumonia

A. Description: acute infection of the lung varying in severity and causing fluid accumulation.

B. Etiology: causative organisms include bacteria, viruses, fungi, and protozoa

C. Pathophysiologic processes and manifestations

 1. Organisms may enter the respiratory tract through inspiration or aspiration of oral secretions; *Staphylococcus* and *Gram-negative* bacilli may reach the lungs through circulation in the bloodstream.

 2. Normal pulmonary defense mechanisms (cough reflex, mucociliary transport, pulmonary macrophagus) usually protect against infection. However, in susceptible hosts, these defenses are either suppressed or overwhelmed by the invading organism.

 3. The invading organism multiplies and releases damaging toxins, causing inflammation and edema of the lung parenchyma; this results in accumulation of cellular debris and exudate.

 4. Lung tissue fills with exudate and fluid, changing from an airless state to a consolidated state.

5. In viral pneumonia, the ciliated epithelial cells become damaged.

 6. Severity of symptoms depends on the extent of pneumonia present (eg, partial lobe, full lobe [lobar pneumonia], or diffuse [bronchopneumonia]).

7. Symptoms can include:
   a. Fever
   b. Chills
   c. Malaise
   d. Cough
   e. Pleuritic pain
   f. Increased tactile fremitus on palpitation
   g. Rales and rhonchi on auscultation
   h. Dyspnea

D. Overview of nursing interventions

1. Administer antibiotics specific for the causative organism, as prescribed and confirmed by culture and sensitivity.
2. Control fever with acetaminophen as ordered.
3. Assess vital signs, monitor respiratory status.
4. Monitor pulse oximetry.
5. Monitor exercise tolerance.
6. Monitor breath sounds note changes in sputum production.
7. Encourage adequate fluid intake.
8. Provide bronchial hygiene.
9. Maintain adequate nutritional status.
10. Perform chest physiotherapy as indicated.
11. Administer oxygen therapy as ordered.
12. Attempt to prevent pneumonia in susceptible hosts. For example:

    a. Frequent positioning, deep breathing and coughing exercises in the post-op patient

    b. Chest PT

    c. Avoid contact with persons who have respiratory infections, crowds, malls and shopping centers

XIV. *Pneumocystis carinii* pneumonia (PCP)

A. Definition: the most common pulmonary infection occurring in persons afflicted with AIDS

B. Etiology

  1. The protozoa *Pneumocystis carinii* is the causative organism; it grows only in an immunocompromised host.

  2. Immunocompromise can occur in human immunodeficiency virus (HIV) infection; it also can result from:

    a. Cancer chemotherapy treatment

    b. Immunosuppressant therapies (eg, drugs used to prevent organ rejection in transplant recipients)

C. Pathophysiologic processes and manifestations

  1. The protozoa *Pneumocystis carinii* proliferates, causing the infection and infiltration that occur with other pneuomonias.

  2. As the infection progresses, fever, cough, dyspnea are present and fluid fills the lung.

  3. Inflammation at the alveolar level occurs, reducing the capacity for diffusion to occur.

  4. This reduction in diffusion causes hypoxemia.

  5. Hypoxemia may be so severe that ARF may occur.

D. Overview of nursing interventions

  1. Administer Bactrim®, the drug of choice, as prescribed.

  2. Administer fluids to provide hydration.

  3. Administer antipyretics, as ordered.

  4. Provide adequate nutrition.

  5. Follow interventions as stated above for pneumonia.

XV. Lung cancer

A. Description

  1. Lung cancer refers to malignant tumor growth within the bronchial tissue or lung parenchyma.

  2. Types of cancers include:

    a. *Squamous cell,* which constitutes 35 to 50% of all lung cancers

    b. *Adenocarcinoma,* which constitutes 15 to 35% of all lung cancers

    c. *Small cell (oat cell),* which constitutes 20 to 25% of all lung cancers

    d. *Large cell,* which constitutes 10 to 15% of all lung cancers

B. Etiology and incidence

  1. Predisposing factors include:

   a. **Chronic exposure to pulmonary irritants, such as cigarette smoke, asbestos, or air pollutants**
   b. **Family history of lung cancer**
   2. Lung cancers tend to have a poor prognosis, unless the cancer is very well defined and easily removed by surgery.
C. Pathophysiologic processes and manifestations
   1. As the lung tissue experiences irritation, it undergoes a series of changes and eventually gives rise to a tumor.
   2. Symptoms depend on the size of the tumor and the area affected.
   3. Symptoms can include:
       a. Cough
       b. Wheezing
       c. Shortness of breath
       d. Hemoptysis
       e. Chest pain (commonly occurs with tumors of the pleura and mediastinum)
       f. Hoarseness
       g. Dysphagia (in larger tumors compressing the esophagus)
       h. Weight loss
   4. Metastases can occur, especially when the original tumor is near areas of lymph drainage.
   5. Some tumors may secrete hormones, usually antidiuretic hormone (ADH) or adrenocorticotropin hormone (ACTH), causing metabolic abnormalities associated with excesses of these hormones (eg, when a tumor secretes ADH, the kidney will reabsorb water; when a tumor secretes ACTH, the adrenal glands will secrete steroids).
D. Overview of nursing interventions
   1. Prepare the patient for surgery if the tumor is small enough to be removed.
   2. Prepare the patient for planned treatments, including chemotherapy or radiation.
   3. Control pain with analgesics, as prescribed.
   4. Maintain adequate oxygenation by providing rest periods and possibly administering oxygen.
   5. Maintain adequate nutritional status.
   6. Provide emotional support to the patient and family.
   7. Involve case management and social services to arrange home health care and assist with financial resources for treatment services and emotional support services as necessary.

Bibliography

Aherns, T. S. (1993). Changing perspectives in the assessment of oxygenation. *Critical Care Nurse,* 13(4):78–83.

Bullock, B. L., & Rosendahl, P. P. (1992). *Pathophysiology: Adaptations and alterations in function* (3rd ed.). Philadelphia: J. B. Lippincott.

Groer, M., & Shekleton, M. (1989). *Basic pathophysiology: A holistic approach* (3rd ed.). St. Louis: Mosby.

Grossbach, I. (1994). COPD patient in acute respiratory failure. *Critical Care Nurse,* 14(3): 32–38.

Hamner J. (1995). Challenging diagnosis: Adult respiratory syndrome. *Critical Care Nurse,* 15(5): 46–53.

Kohlman, V. C., Lindsey, A., & West, C. (1993). *Pathophysiological phenomena in nursing* (2nd ed.). Philadelphia: W. B. Saunders.

McCance, K. L., & Huether, S. E. (1994). *Pathophysiology: The biologic basis for disease in adults and children* (2nd ed.). St. Louis: Mosby–Year Book.

Porth, C. M. (1994). *Pathophysiology: Concepts of altered health states* (4th ed.). Philadelphia: J. B. Lippincott.

Price, S. A., & Wilson, L. M. (1992). *Pathophysiology: Clinical concepts of disease processes* (4th ed.). St. Louis: Mosby–Year Book.

Ulrich, S. P., Canale, S. W., & Wendell, S. A. (1990). *Nursing care planning guides* (2nd ed.). Philadelphia: W. B. Saunders.

STUDY QUESTIONS

1. Which of the following symptoms is a physiologic response to respiratory dysfunction?
   a. jaw pain
   b. flushing
   c. left arm pain
   d. fatigue

2. Diseases that limit lung expansion are known as:
   a. obstructive diseases
   b. restrictive diseases
   c. infectious diseases
   d. asthmatic diseases

3. Respiratory acidosis is a sequela of:
   a. hyperventilation
   b. hypoventilation
   c. hypocapnia
   d. tachypnea

4. The pathophysiologic processes and symptoms in atelectasis results from:
   a. inadequate expansion
   b. excessive cough
   c. accelerating hypoxemia
   d. high fever

5. Steroids are given to treat ARDS in order to:
   a. reduce infection
   b. improve pain
   c. improve oxygenation
   d. reduce inflammation

6. A nurse caring for an asthmatic would expect to administer bronchodilators because of:
   a. an increased cough reflex
   b. a decreased cough reflex
   c. decreased sputum production
   d. the bronchoconstriction present in asthma

7. In emphysema, the nurse expects to identify:
   a. difficulty exhaling
   b. decreased mucus

   c. increased cilia
   d. bronchodilation

8. Adult respiratory distress syndrome (ARDS) differs from acute respiratory failure (ARF) in that:
   a. both are acute conditions that turn chronic
   b. ARDS cannot be caused by allergic reactions
   c. ARDS is related to water in the lungs
   d. ARF does not cause hypoxia

9. Exocrine secretion of thick, tenacious mucus in the respiratory tract is characteristic of which of the following disorders?
   a. tuberculosis
   b. asthma
   c. bronchitis
   d. cystic fibrosis

10. Administration of which of the following medications may result in reactivation of dormant tuberculosis bacilli?
    a. rifampin
    b. prednisone
    c. isoniazid (INH)
    d. insulin

11. In emphysema, the nurse administers low-flow oxygen because:
    a. high-flow oxygen removes respiratory drive
    b. low-flow oxygen increases energy
    c. low-flow oxygen improves nutrition
    d. high-flow oxygen decreases pulmonary capacity

12. Respiratory alkalosis is a sequelae of:
    a. hypoventilation
    b. hyperventilation
    c. tachycardia
    d. bradycardia

ANSWER KEY

Question	Correct answer	Correct answer rationale	Incorrect answer rationales
1.	d	Fatigue is almost always a symptom of respiratory disorders. It occurs from an increase in energy requirements needed to breathe and deliver oxygen to the tissues.	a, b, and c. These symptoms are more likely associated with cardiac disease, not respiratory disease.
2.	b	Restrictive diseases limit lung expansion.	a. Obstructive diseases impede airflow to the lung. c. Infectious diseases involve pathogenic organism invasion. d. This response is incorrect.
3.	b	Respiratory acidosis results from hypoventilation, because the acid (carbon dioxide) is not removed when ventilation is decreased.	a. Hyperventilation results in respiratory alkalosis. c. Hypocapnia refers to decreased CO_2 in the blood. d. Tachypnea refers to a respiratory rate greater than 24 to 26 breaths per minute.
4.	a	Atelectasis is a collapse of a portion of the lung that results when expansion of the lung is inadequate.	b, c, and d. These are symptoms of respiratory disorders.
5.	b	Steroids are administered to reduce inflammation associated with emphysema which narrows the airways and challenges oxygenation.	a. This choice is incorrect because steroids do not decrease the likelihood of infection. In fact they increase the chances of infection. b. This choice is incorrect because pain is not necessarily associated with emphysema, and steroids are not given for pain in this situation. c. This choice is incorrect because oxygenation will be improved only because of reduced inflammation.
6.	d	Symptoms of asthma are caused by bronchoconstriction, therefore a bronchodilator is one of the treatments of choice.	a, b, and c. These choices are incorrect because the cough reflex is not pertinent to the administration of bronchodilators. Sputum production is increased, not decreased, in emphysema.

Question	Correct answer	Correct answer rationale	Incorrect answer rationales
7.	a	Chronic irritation found in emphysema causes loss of alveolar elasticity and alveolar destruction. This makes exhalation difficult because the alveoli do not recoil after inhalation. This causes air to stay in the alveoli, and exhalation is difficult for the person.	b. This choice is incorrect because in emphysema, excessive, thick secretions are produced. c and d. These choices are incorrect because a nurse does not examine, nor can a nurse find, cilia. Bronchoconstriction rather than bronchodilation is present.
8.	c	ARDS is a sequela of several diseases in which the lungs fill with water, making gas exchange impossible.	a. Both ARDS and ARF are acute disorders requiring immediate management. b. ARDS may be related to allergic reaction to inhalants. d. ARF results in hypoxia.
9.	d	Cystic fibrosis is a chronic obstructive disease characterized by exocrine secretion of thick, tenacious, copious mucus.	a. Tuberculosis is an infectious disease characterized by night sweats and hemoptysis. b and c. Asthma and bronchitis are obstructive diseases characterized by bronchoconstriction.
10.	b	Administration of prednisone, a steroid, can result in immunosuppression, which can reactivate the disease.	a and c. These are antitubercular drugs. d. This drug is used to treat diabetes.
11.	a	Higher flows of oxygen lower carbon dioxide levels, which is the person's drive to breathe.	b. This choice is incorrect because the opposite is true, which is described above. c. This choice is incorrect because oxygen flows are not related to nutrition d. This choice is incorrect because pulmonary capacity is not related to oxygen flow as administered by a nurse.
12.	b	Hyperventilation causes respiratory alkalosis because the acid (carbon dioxide) is eliminated through rapid breathing.	a. This choice is incorrect because hypoventilation causes respiratory alkalosis c and d. These choices are incorrect because changes in heart rate do not result in changes in arterial blood gases.

2 Cardiac Disorders

I.   **Overview of pathophysiologic processes**

    A. Ischemic diseases

        1. Ischemic diseases include disorders in which impaired coronary circulation causes an imbalance between coronary blood flow and myocardial oxygen needs.

        2. These disorders begin with anginal chest pain; about 25% of patients (especially the elderly and diabetic patient) will complain of dyspnea when experiencing myocardial ischemia.

        3. If left untreated, ischemic diseases can lead to myocardial infarction (MI); experts now believe that 95% of all heart attacks are caused by plaque rupture.

        4. Angina pectoris is classified as an ischemic disorder; as this process continues, MI can develop, resulting in irreversible cell death.

5. Risk factors for ischemic diseases include:
   a. Family history of heart disease
   b. High-fat diet
   c. Sedentary lifestyle
   d. History of hypertension or diabetes
   e. Smoking

B. **Cardiac failure**

1. Cardiac failure refers to the inability of the heart to pump enough blood to meet the metabolic needs of body tissues.
2. It can occur when the heart is diseased or when the heart is normal but is placed under excessive demands.
3. Sympathetic stimulation occurs as an unwanted compensatory mechanism and causes increased afterload, increased myocardial workload, and decreased renal blood flow. New selective beta blockers are being used to decrease this response.
4. An estimated 2.3 million Americans have heart failure; the incidence has increased due to the increased rate of survival from MI.

5. **Cardiac failure becomes cardiogenic shock as tissue perfusion ceases; this results in pulmonary edema—a life-threatening complication.**
6. Cor pulmonale may be present as right-sided cardiomegaly evolves due to obstructive respiratory disease.

7. **Pulmonary embolism is a life-threatening complication.**
8. Cardiac arrest is the worst-case scenario that can result from MI or cardiogenic shock.
9. The major risk factor for cardiac failure includes any history of heart disease.

C. **Valvular heart disease**

1. Valvular heart disease occurs when the heart valves are unable to fully open (stenotic) or fully close (regurgitant).
2. Stenotic valvular disease decreases the forward flow of blood from one chamber to another.
3. Regurgitant valvular disease causes some blood to flow backward into the chamber it came from.

4. Risk factors for valvular heart disease include:
   a. Congenital valve defects
   b. Valvular damage (eg, endocarditis from intravenous drug abuse and rheumatic disease)

D. **Electrophysiologic disorders**

1. The specialized cells of the heart have electrophysiologic properties.
   a. *Automaticity:* Ability to generate spontaneous action potential without stimulus
   b. *Rhythmicity:* Regular generation of an action potential by the heart's conduction system
   c. *Conductivity:* Ability to conduct electrical impulses
   d. *Refractoriness:* Inability of the cardiac muscle to respond to a second stimulus that might occur after a contraction

2. An alteration in any of these properties can produce a *dysrhythmia,* or abnormal heart rhythm, which interferes with the heart's pumping ability.

3. **Risk factors for electrophysiologic disorders include:**
    a. **Ischemic disorders**
    b. **Ingestion of certain drugs (eg, all cardiac drugs and antihistamines)**
    c. **Electrolyte disorders**

E. Infectious disorders

1. Infectious cardiac disorders can alter the structure and function of the heart, rendering contractions ineffective.
2. These kinds of disorders can be caused by viruses, bacteria, or inflammation.
3. Pericarditis, infective endocarditis, and myocarditis are classified as infectious cardiac disorders.
4. Risk factors for infectious cardiac disorders include:
    a. Immunosuppression
    b. Intravenous drug use

F. Cardiomyopathies

1. Cardiomyopathies are a group of heart diseases that affect only the heart muscle and not other structures, such as the coronary arteries.
2. These disorders can be primary or secondary to other diseases.
    a. Primary cardiomyopathies result from unknown causes.
    b. Secondary cardiomyopathies result from infections, nutritional deficits, connective tissue diseases, and muscle-wasting states.
3. Cardiomyopathies can be classified as hypertrophic, congestive, or restrictive.

4. **Risk factors for cardiomyopathies include:**
    a. **Severe nutritional deficits (eg, anorexia)**
    b. **Connective tissue diseases (eg, scleroderma)**
    c. **Cardiac infectious diseases (eg, myocarditis)**

II.   Physiologic responses to cardiac dysfunction

A. Chest pain

1. Dullness, heaviness, or a sensation of pressure in the chest is associated with myocardial ischemia, which results from insufficient blood supply to the muscle cells of the heart.
2. Chest pain commonly occurs when the myocardial need for oxygen is greater than the supply.

B. Dyspnea

1. Dyspnea, or difficult breathing, can occur as the myocardial need for oxygen increases.
2. It may be a sign of early congestive heart failure due to alveolar swelling.

C. Syncope

1. Syncope is a transient loss of consciousness, which results from insufficient blood flow to the brain.

    2. It can occur as a result of decreased cardiac output due to cardiac rhythm disturbances, valvular disease, and carotid hypersensitivity.

D. Palpitations
    1. Palpitations are described as a fluttering, racing, pounding, or skipping heartbeat.
    2. These can occur with rhythm disturbances such as sinus tachycardia, atrial fibrillation, and premature beats.

E. Abnormal heart sounds: Sounds produced by turbulent blood flow from one chamber to another (S3, S4) or across heart valves (murmurs) (Table 2-1).

F. Crackles: Sound (rales) produced by air passing through an accumulation of fluid in the alveoli cells; this occurs when pressure in the vascular space is high.

G. Edema
    1. Edema is an accumulation of excess fluid in the body tissues that occurs when pressure in the vascular space is high.
    2. The extent and the depth of the edema indicate the severity of the condition.

H. Electrocardiographic changes

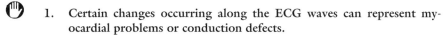   **1. Certain changes occurring along the ECG waves can represent myocardial problems or conduction defects.**

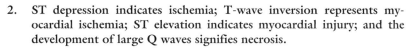   **2. ST depression indicates ischemia; T-wave inversion represents myocardial ischemia; ST elevation indicates myocardial injury; and the development of large Q waves signifies necrosis.**

  I. Dysrhythmias
    1. Dysrhythmias are disturbances in the heart rate or rhythm that result from either an alteration in the cardiac cells' automaticity or conductivity. Ischemia or injury to cardiac cells typically causes dysrhythmias. Electrolyte disorders, hypoxia, or medications can also cause dysrhythmias.

TABLE 2-1
Abnormal Heart Sounds

SOUND	TIMING	CAUSE	BEST AUSCULTATION
S1	beginning of systole	normal closure of the mitral and tricuspid valves	diaphragm
S2	beginning of diastole	normal closure of the aortic and pulmonic valves	diaphragm
S3	early diastole	left ventricular dysfunction as with CHF	bell
S4	late diastole	ventricular resistance to filling as with MI	bell
Murmur	systolic	aortic or pulmonic stenosis mitral or tricuspid regurgitation	either
Murmur	diastolic	mitral or tricuspid stenosis aortic or pulmonic regurgitation	either

2.   Dysrhythmias can be insignificant or life-threatening.

J.   **Abnormal cardiac enzymes: Necrosis of the myocardial cells results in the release of enzymes into the blood; these include creatine phosphokinase (CPK), creatine phosphokinase-myoglobin (CPK-MB), and lactic dehydrogenase (LDH).**

K.   Decreased cardiac output

1.   Cardiac output is stroke volume (volume of blood ejected with each cardiac contraction) times heart rate.

2.   Decreased cardiac output can produce tachycardia, weak peripheral pulses, altered level of consciousness, oliguria, shortness of breath, and cool, pale skin.

L.   Hyperlipidemia: An abnormal accumulation of lipid in the blood; commonly occurs with a high-fat diet, but can also be familial.

III.   **Angina pectoris**

A.   Description

1.   Angina pectoris is substernal or retrosternal chest pain associated with temporary or reversible myocardial ischemia.

2.   It is the first phase of cardiac ischemic disorders that commonly occurs with coronary artery disease.

3.   There are three types of angina pectoris.

a.   *Stable angina* has a predictable pattern; it is uncomplicated, occurs on exertion, and is relieved by rest.

b.   *Unstable angina* (also known as crescendo angina) occurs when attacks accelerate in frequency, intensity, and duration; it is more severe than stable angina, indicating a worse degree of ischemia.

c.   *Variant (also known as Prinzmetal's) angina* occurs spontaneously with no relationship to activity or cold weather; a high incidence of MI is associated with this type of angina, because ST segment elevation occurs with this condition and is also present in infarction.

B.   Etiology

1.   Angina pectoris is caused by inadequate oxygen supply to the myocardium due to decreased blood flow through the coronary arteries (Fig. 2-1).

2.   Decreased blood flow commonly results from the progressive development of atherosclerosis within the coronary arteries, which narrows the arterial lumen.

a.   Nonmodifiable risk factors for atherosclerosis include advancing age, male gender, postmenopausal status, African-American race, and family history.

b.   Modifiable risk factors for atherosclerosis include cigarette smoking, hypertension, hyperlipidemia, diabetes, obesity, stress, and inactivity.

3.   Other causes of decreased blood flow include vasoconstriction from spasm or drugs, low blood pressure, low blood volume, and dysrhythmias.

4.   Angina may be precipitated when the oxygen needs of the myocardium ex-

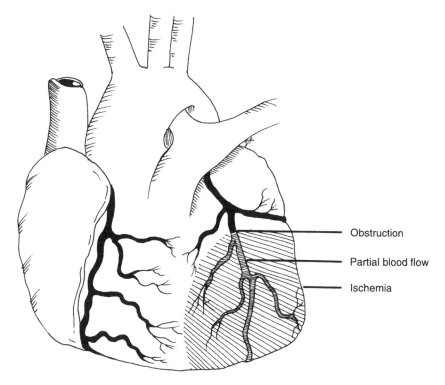

FIGURE 2-1.
Angina pectoris.

ceed the oxygen supply (eg, during exertion or emotionally stressful situations, in cold weather, after eating heavy meals, or after ingesting cocaine).

C. Pathophysiologic processes and manifestations

1. An imbalance between coronary muscle demand and supply causes pain.
2. Chest pain can be described as retrosternal dullness, heaviness, or pressure that may radiate to the arms or neck. The pain may last for 30 seconds to 30 minutes and may be accompanied by shortness of breath.
3. A 12-lead ECG may demonstrate T-wave inversion; cardiac enzymes will be normal.
4. Unstable angina is characterized by a change in frequency, duration, or intensity of pain.
5. Variant or Prinzmetal angina occurs at rest and results from coronary artery spasm; this may occur without atherosclerosis.

D. Overview of nursing interventions

1. Assess patient for risk factors to determine presence of atherosclerosis.
2. Institute exercise stress testing to identify ST abnormalities, as ordered.
3. Prepare patient for coronary angiography, as ordered, to obtain a definitive diagnosis by identifying the location and degree of lesions.
4. Prepare patient for possible surgical interventions such as percutaneous

transluminar coronary angioplasty (PTCA) with or without stenting; athrectomy, coronary artery bypass graft (CABG) surgery.

5. Administer nitrates, as prescribed, to vasodilate the coronary arteries and allow more blood flow to the myocardium.
6. Administer β-adrenergic blocking agents, as prescribed, to decrease the oxygen requirements of the heart by decreasing the heart rate and blood pressure.
7. Administer aspirin (ASA) to decrease platelet aggregation.
8. Administer oxygen, as ordered, to improve oxygen supply.
9. Institute measures to decrease myocardial oxygen demand, such as sedation and rest.
10. Provide patient teaching to identify and reduce risk factors.

IV. Myocardial infarction (MI)

A. Description: ischemic myocardial cell necrosis
B. Etiology: causes of MI include coronary artery obstruction due to the progressive development of atherosclerosis; coronary artery spasm; embolism; plaque rupture (Fig. 2-2).

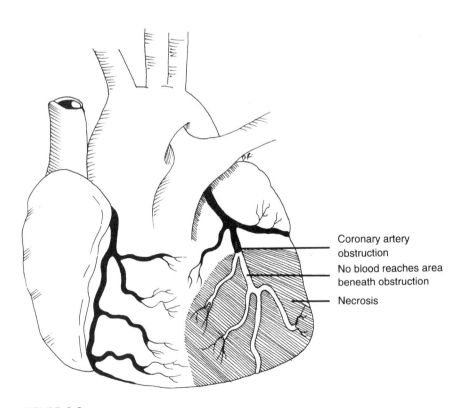

Coronary artery obstruction

No blood reaches area beneath obstruction

Necrosis

FIGURE 2-2.
Myocardial infarction.

C. **Pathophysiologic processes and manifestations**

1. The severity of the disease depends on the size of the damaged area and the effect of the damage on cardiac output.
2. While cell death is occurring, the heart is using oxygen and glycogen stores; as a result, lactic acid accumulates.
3. As areas of the heart become necrotic, changes will occur in the ECG reading in the respective leads.

4. **Symptoms can include:**
   a. **Chest pain (described as substernal, crushing with radiation to the arm, neck, jaw, or back; pain is unrelieved by nitroglycerine)**
   b. **Dyspnea**
   c. **Changes in heart rate**
   d. **Nausea**
   e. **Vomiting**
   f. **Fever (up to 101°F over the first 24 to 48 hours)**
   g. **Increased WBC count and sedimentation rate**
5. Twelve-lead ECG may show ST elevation as the MI is evolving or Q waves when the MI is complete.
6. After the onset of MI, enzyme elevation occurs.
   a. CPK-MB elevates in 2 to 4 hours.
   b. CPK enzymes, with the cardiac-specific CPK-MB fraction, peak in 12 to 18 hours.
   c. Serum glutamic-oxaloacetic transaminase (SGOT) peaks in 24 to 36 hours.
   d. LDH peaks in 48 to 72 hours.

D. **Overview of nursing interventions**

1. Establish perfusion as soon as possible, because the heart cells can sustain ischemia for only about 20 minutes before cell death occurs.
2. Administer morphine sulfate or nitrates, as prescribed, to relieve chest pain.
3. Administer thrombolytic agents such as streptokinase, tissue plasminogen activator (TPA), or Retaplase® (RPA), as prescribed, to limit infarct size.
4. Provide supplemental oxygen via nasal cannula.
5. Monitor vital signs every 1 to 2 hours.
6. Monitor cardiac rhythm for dysrhythmias, such as premature ventricular contractions (PVCs), ventricular tachycardia, second-degree type-II atrioventricular (AV) block, and complete heart block.
7. Monitor for signs of congestive heart failure.
8. Maintain intravenous line for emergency access.
9. Maintain bedrest, with the patient in semi-Fowler's position, for the first 24 hours.
10. Administer medications (eg, digitalis, antiarrhythmics, vasodilators, vasopressors, anticoagulants, diuretics, potassium, Colace, and sedatives) to limit the potential of complications, as ordered.
11. Institute measures to decrease the oxygen demand (eg, provide a calm and restful environment, encourage the patient to rest, control pain).
12. Prepare patient for possible surgical interventions such as percutaneous

transluminar coronary angioplasty (PTCA) with or without stenting; athrectomy, coronary artery bypass graft (CABG) surgery.

13.   Provide patient teaching to identify and reduce risk factors.

V.   Congestive heart failure (CHF)

A.   Description

1.   CHF is a condition in which body tissues become congested due to the heart's inability to pump a sufficient amount of blood to meet the tissues' metabolic needs.

2.   CHF can be classified as left-sided or right-sided, but it commonly involves both sides.

B.   Etiology

1.   Causes of CHF include:

   a.   **Disorders in which cardiac output is decreased (eg, MI or any of the myopathies), with fluid accumulation in the body tissues accompanied by increasing right and left ventricular pressure.**

   b.   **Inadequate emptying of blood from the ventricles due to decreased contractility, valvular disease, congenital defects, hypertension, hypervolemia, and anemia. Inadequate emptying allows blood to accumulate in the vessels, organs, or chamber located behind the failing ventricle.**

2.   Typically, right-sided heart failure is a sequela of left-sided heart failure.

C.   Pathophysiologic processes and manifestations

1.   Impaired left ventricular function allows pressure to build in the left ventricle, back up into the left atrium, and accumulate within the pulmonary circulation.

2.   Resultant manifestations of left-sided failure are respiratory in nature and can include:

   a.   Dyspnea
   b.   Orthopnea
   c.   Productive cough
   d.   Frothy sputum
   e.   Crackles
   f.   Pallor
   g.   Elevated pulmonary capillary wedge pressure (PCWP) and central venous pressure (CVP)

3.   Impaired right ventricular function allows pressure to build in the right ventricle, back up into the right atrium, and accumulate within the venous circulation.

4.   **Resultant manifestations of right-sided failure are venous in nature and can include:**

   a.   **Jugular vein distention (JVD)**
   b.   **Edema**
   c.   **Ascites**
   d.   **Hepatomegaly**
   e.   **Fatigue**

      f.   Elevated CVP
5. Compensatory mechanisms include tachycardia, ventricular hypertrophy, and left heart dilation.

D.   **Overview of nursing interventions**
1. Administer supplemental oxygen, as prescribed.
2. Monitor pulse oximetry and ABGs closely.
3. Position the patient in high Fowler's to promote optimal lung expansion.
4. Administer medications to improve cardiac output, as prescribed (eg, digitalis to increase contractility, Lasix to promote diuresis, and ACE inhibitors to decrease preload and afterload).
5. Monitor vital signs frequently.
6. Monitor intake and output and daily weights.
7. Monitor electrolyte levels and assess for imbalances.
8. Provide the patient with a quiet environment, limit activities, assist with activities of daily living (ADLs), and coordinate nursing care to conserve the patient's energy and prevent fatigue.
9. Prepare the patient for echocardiography or transesophageal echocardiography (TEE).
10. Educate the patient regarding preventive measures to avoid reoccurrence, especially in the areas of diet, daily weights and sodium restriction.

VI.   Cardiogenic shock

A.   **Description: insufficient tissue perfusion due to the heart's inability to pump enough blood**

B.   **Etiology**

1. Causes of cardiogenic shock include:
    a.   **Myocardial infarction**
    b.   **Congestive heart failure**
    c.   **Cardiomyopathy**
    d.   **Pulmonary edema**
    e.   **Cardiac tamponade**
2. It may also result from ineffective pumping due to cardiac dysrhythmias and from acute disruption of valvular function.

C.   **Pathophysiologic processes and manifestations**
1. The effects of inadequate tissue perfusion on the body's organs result in systemic symptoms.
2. Decreased cerebral perfusion causes restlessness, lethargy, confusion, and altered level of consciousness.
3. Respiratory manifestations include increased respiratory rate as the need for oxygen increases; as circulation through the lungs decreases, cough, crackles, low PAO_2, and increasing $PACO_2$ result.
4. Cardiovascular manifestations include:
    a.   Rapid, weak pulse
    b.   Normal initial blood pressure, then hypotension
    c.   Elevated CVP readings (normal CVP is approximately 4 to 10 cm)
    d.   Elevated PCWP readings (normal PCWP is 4 to 13 mm Hg)

5. As perfusion to the periphery decreases, the skin becomes cool and pale.
6. Reduced renal perfusion results in oliguria.

D. Overview of nursing interventions

1. Administer medications to improve cardiac output (eg, inotropic drugs, preload and afterload reducers, diuretics, and sedatives), as prescribed.
2. Monitor PCWP to determine left ventricular function.
3. Prepare the patient for insertion of an intraaortic balloon pump, if indicated.
4. Monitor oxygenation status including respiratory rate, lung sounds, pulse oximetry, and ABGs.
5. Institute ventilator support, if indicated.
6. Monitor vital signs closely.
7. Maintain strict intake and output measurements; measure urine output hourly.
8. Promote rest and provide comfort measures.

VII. Acute pulmonary edema

A. Description: a medical emergency in which fluid accumulates in the interstitial spaces and alveoli of the lung, interfering with gas exchange and resulting in severe hypoxia (Fig. 2-3).

B. Etiology

1. A common cause of acute pulmonary edema is inadequate contractility of the left ventricle, as in CHF. Pumping is impaired to the extent that the pulmonary capillary pressure far exceeds the capillary osmotic pressure, causing fluid to move rapidly from the capillaries to the interstitial tissue and the alveoli.
2. Acute pulmonary edema also can result from other causes of increased pulmonary capillary permeability, such as exposure to toxic gases, infectious processes, drug reactions, and rapid infusion of intravenous fluid or blood.

C. Pathophysiologic processes and manifestations

1. When cardiac output drops, the heart is not able to circulate fluid. Blood then pools in the pulmonary circulation.
2. Acute pulmonary edema may occur at night, after a person has been reclining for some time. Dependent lower extremity edema fluid returns to the vascular compartment and is redistributed to the pulmonary circulation, because the heart is unable to pump the fluid effectively.

3. **Manifestations include respiratory alterations, such as:**
    a. **Dyspnea**
    b. **Orthopnea**
    c. **Air hunger**
    d. **Tachypnea**
    e. **Wheezes**
    f. **Crackles**
    g. **Productive cough with frothy or blood-tinged sputum (due to rapid fluid shifts that rupture capillaries)**
4. Signs and symptoms resulting from decreased cardiac output, which can occur at any time, include:

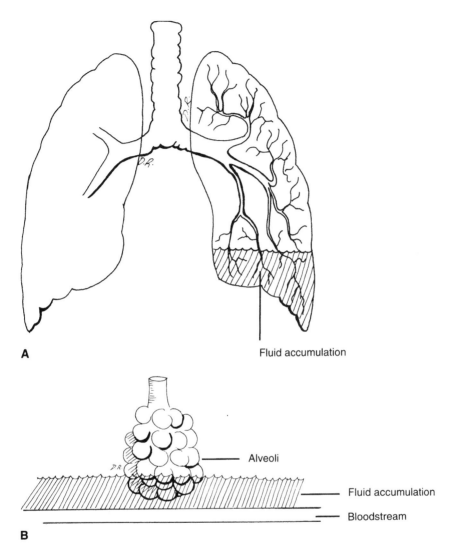

FIGURE 2-3.
(A) Acute pulmonary edema. **(B)** Excessive interstitial fluid accumulation prevents the exchange of gas back and forth between the alveoli and blood.

     a. Restlessness
     b. Anxiety
     c. Confusion
     d. Weak, rapid pulse
     e. Pallor
     f. Cyanosis

5. PCWP will be elevated as fluid accumulation causes increased pressure in the vessels of the lungs.

D.   Overview of nursing interventions

1.   Administer supplemental oxygen to maintain gas exchange, as ordered.
2.   Institute ventilatory support, if indicated.
3.   Reduce fluid volume in the pulmonary circulation by positioning the patient in high Fowler's, using rotating tourniquets, and administering morphine, diuretics, aminophylline, and vasodilators, as prescribed.
4.   Administer digitalis, as prescribed, to improve left ventricular contractility.
5.   Monitor vital signs and electrolyte status.
6.   Provide a calm, restful, and supportive environment.
7.   Educate the patient to prevent recurrent episodes.

VIII.   Cor pulmonale

A.   Description: right-sided disorder of the heart resulting from pulmonary disease

B.   Etiology: occurs secondary to chronic obstructive lung disease or any disorder that causes long-term pressure increases in the lungs

C.   Pathophysiologic processes and manifestations

1.   Lung disease increases the pressure on the pulmonary vessels; this pressure is known as pulmonary vascular resistance (PVR).
2.   Increased vascular pressure backs up to the right ventricle, the chamber that supplies the lung, causing increased pressure.
3.   This pressure rise causes hypertrophy of the heart muscle in the right ventricle, because the right ventricle must work harder to move blood through the lungs.
4.   As the disease progresses, symptoms of right-sided heart failure (eg, edema in the liver and legs) may develop.
5.   If a second disease develops (eg, MI, pneumonia, or infection), heart failure may occur.
6.   Right ventricular hypertrophy is noted on the chest x-ray and ECG.
7.   Other manifestations may include:
     a.   Chest pain
     b.   Louder-than-normal pulmonary component of S2 (the second heart sound)
     c.   Pulmonic valve murmur
     d.   Tricuspid valve murmur (may accompany right ventricular failure)

D.   Overview of nursing interventions

1.   Reduce cardiac workload by allowing the patient to rest and providing a calm environment.
2.   Institute measures to reverse underlying lung disease.
3.   Undertake the same interventions if heart failure is present.

IX.   Pulmonary embolism

A.   Description: partial occlusion of the pulmonary circulation by a blood clot (embolus)

B. Etiology

1. Any conditions that produce or accelerate blood clotting can cause embolism development; such conditions include:

   a. Venous stasis (resulting from immobility, obesity, pregnancy, old age, sickle cell disease, CHF)

   b. Hypercoagulability (resulting from certain medications [birth control pills] or metabolic conditions [infection])

   c. Vessel trauma (may result in clot release)

2. Emboli may also occur from substances other than blood.

   a. Fat emboli may result from administration of lipids or release of fat from the bone marrow (due to long-bone trauma).

   b. Emboli from amniotic fluid may travel from the uterus to the bloodstream during childbirth.

   c. Air emboli may enter the bloodstream during hemodialysis or insertion of a central line.

C. Pathophysiologic processes and manifestations

1. A clot forms in a vessel, and part or all of it breaks away and travels to the lung.

2. The clot obstructs blood flow to the lung, causing cell necrosis (pulmonary infarction) to the area usually supplied with blood.

3. Massive occlusion occurs when a major artery is obstructed.

4. Embolism with infarction refers to the condition in which a portion of the lung has died from hypoxia (Fig. 2-4).

5. Embolism without infarction refers to the condition in which there is a clot in the lung, but cell death has not occurred.

6. Multiple emboli refers to the condition in which there is more than one clot in the lung.

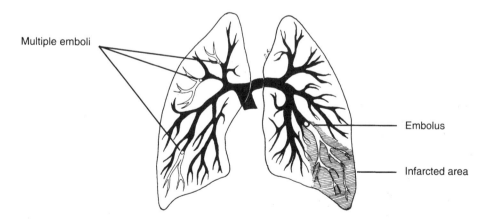

FIGURE 2-4.
Pulmonary embolism and infarction. Pulmonary embolism obstructs blood flow to a part of the lung, causing necrosis.

7. Symptoms vary depending on the size and position of the embolism; most common symptoms include:
   a. Dyspnea
   b. Pleural pain
   c. Hemoptysis
   d. Fever
   e. Leukocytosis
8. Shock, hypotension, tachypnea, tachycardia, and chest pain are signs of more massive embolic occlusion and usually result in death; the larger the vessel occluded, the larger the area affected.

D. **Overview of nursing interventions**
1. Administer anticoagulants to prevent further clot formation; the body's fibrinolytic system will destroy the original clot.
2. Prevent the development of additional emboli by analyzing the patient's risk factors.

X. Cardiac arrest

A. **Description: cessation of breathing and circulation due to the loss of cardiac pump function; this is a medical emergency.**

B. **Etiology**
1. The most common causes of cardiac arrest are ventricular tachycardia and ventricular fibrillation due to congenital heart disease, MI, heart failure, drug effects, electrical shock, hypoxia, hemorrhage, or mechanical ventricular irritation.
2. Severe bradyarrhythmias due to electrolyte imbalances, near drowning, or hypothermia may also lead to cardiac arrest.

C. **Pathophysiologic processes and manifestations**
1. Manifestations are absence of pulse and absence of breathing in an unconscious victim.
2. The victim's skin will appear ashen gray.

D. **Overview of nursing interventions**
1. Identify this medical emergency promptly in order to restore heart function.
2. Initiate cardiopulmonary resuscitation (CPR) 4 to 6 minutes after the cardiac arrest to avoid irreversible brain damage. (Keep in mind that patients with cardiac arrest due to hypothermia may be revived after longer periods of time.)
3. Undertake advanced cardiac life support, including defibrillation or cardioversion, oxygenation and ventilation, intravenous catheter insertion, drug therapy, dysrhythmia identification, acid–base balance, and blood pressure support.

XI. Valvular disease

A. **Description**
1. Valvular disease refers to dysfunction of the heart valves.

2.   The two types of dysfunctions are:
- a.   Narrowing of the valve opening (stenosis)
- b.   Failure of a valve to close properly (regurgitation)
3.   Valvular disease typically involves the mitral and aortic valves, although any of the heart valves may be affected.

B.   Etiology
1.   The most common cause of valvular disease is rheumatic heart disease; inflammatory changes resulting from it cause scar tissue to form on the valves, causing shortening and deformation of the valve structure.
2.   Other causes of valvular disease include:
- a.   Papillary muscle rupture
- b.   Infective endocarditis
- c.   Atherosclerosis
- d.   Congenital valve defects

C.   Pathophysiologic processes and manifestations
1.   The significance of valvular disease is determined by the degree of cardiac dysfunction.
2.   *Mitral valve stenosis* leads to left atrial hypertrophy, increased left atrial pressure, and, eventually, increased pulmonary pressures. It can cause atrial fibrillation with thrombus formation and CHF.

   3.   **Common symptoms of mitral valve stenosis include:**
- a.   **Palpitations**
- b.   **Chest pain**
- c.   **Weakness**
- d.   **Fatigue**
4.   *Mitral valve regurgitation* leads to left atrial and left ventricular hypertrophy. It can cause atrial fibrillation, systemic embolization, elevated left-sided heart pressures, and CHF. Patients with this disorder can remain asymptomatic for 10 to 20 years, despite severe regurgitation.
5.   *Aortic valve stenosis* leads to left ventricular hypertrophy. It can cause CHF, pulmonary edema, atrial fibrillation, vertigo, and syncope. Exertional dyspnea is a common symptom.
6.   *Aortic valve regurgitation* leads to left ventricular hypertrophy and a widening pulse pressure. It can cause left heart failure, dysrhythmias, and throbbing peripheral pulses.
7.   *Tricuspid stenosis* leads to right atrial enlargement. It can cause right-sided heart failure and a decrease in right ventricular cardiac output.
8.   *Tricuspid regurgitation* leads to venous overload and a decreased cardiac output.
9.   *Pulmonic stenosis* leads to right ventricular hypertrophy and systemic congestion and can cause right-sided heart failure.
10.   *Pulmonic regurgitation* leads to backflow of blood into the right ventricle and can cause right-sided heart failure.
11.   *Mitral valve prolapse* leads to a bulging of the valve leaflet into the left atrium during ventricular systole. It has recently been associated with autonomic dysfunction.

   12.   **Manifestations of mitral valve prolapse can include:**

        a.   Chest pain
        b.   Weakness
        c.   Dyspnea on exertion
        d.   Palpitations
        e.   Exercise intolerance
        f.   Dysrhythmias
        g.   **Midsystolic click (may be present)**

13. Murmur will be present in all forms of valvular disease.
    a. For mitral and tricuspid stenosis and aortic and pulmonic regurgitation, it will be diastolic in origin.
    b. For aortic and pulmonic stenosis and mitral and tricuspid regurgitation, it will be systolic in origin.
14. Chamber hypertrophy will be evident on ECG and echocardiogram.
15. Signs and symptoms of CHF also may occur.

D. **Overview of nursing interventions**
   1. Institute interventions associated with CHF (see Section V, D).
   2. Prepare patient for surgery to replace or repair the defective valve (eg, valvular replacement, percutaneous balloon valvuloplasty, or mitral commissurotomy); afterward, provide appropriate postoperative care.
   3. Administer β-blockers, as ordered, to manage mitral valve prolapse.
   4. Provide patient teaching regarding the disease process and treatment plan.

XII.   Dysrhythmias

A. **Description**
   1. Dysrhythmias are disturbances in heart rate or rhythm that develop from disturbances in automaticity, excitability, refractoriness, or conductivity.
   2. Dysrhythmias can be insignificant or life-threatening and can occur in the atria, in the ventricles, or in both.
   3. Types of dysrhythmias include:
      a. Bradycardic rhythms (abnormally slow heart rates)
      b. Tachycardic rhythms (rapid heart rates)
      c. Atrial dysrhythmias (originate in the atria)
      d. Ventricular dysrhythmias (originate in the ventricle)
      e. Junctional dysrhythmias (originate in the AV node)

B. **Etiology**
   1. *Bradycardic rhythms* can result from:
      a. Ischemia of the conduction system (as seen with MI)
      b. Increased parasympathetic tone (as seen with the Valsalva maneuver)
      c. Hypothermia
      d. Drug effects (such as digitalis toxicity)
   2. *Tachycardic rhythms* can result from:
      a. Ischemic response (as seen with an MI)
      b. Normal response to pain
      c. Fever
      d. Exertion
      e. Anxiety
      f. Hypotension
      g. Decreased cardiac output

       h.   Drug effects (such as digitalis toxicity and stimulant ingestion)

  3.   *Atrial dysrhythmias* result from prolonged pressure exerted on atrial cells as seen with CHF and valvular heart disease.

  4.   *Ventricular dysrhythmias* result from ventricular cell ischemia (as seen with acute MI), electrolyte imbalances (eg, hypokalemia, hypoxia, acidosis), and digitalis toxicity.

  5.   *Junctional dysrhythmias* result from malfunction of the SA and AV node, displacing the pacemaker downward into the nodal tissue; this can result from ischemia or medications.

C. **Pathophysiologic processes and manifestations**

  1.   Dysrhythmias interfere with the heart's pumping ability.

  2.   Bradycardic rhythms impair blood flow to vital organs by decreasing total cardiac output.

  3.   Tachycardic rhythms shorten diastolic filling time and subsequently decrease stroke volume and overall cardiac output.

  4.   Atrial dysrhythmias reduce the overall cardiac output by 20%.

  5.   Ventricular dysrhythmias can dramatically reduce diastolic filling to a point where cardiac output is severely diminished or nonexistent, producing absence of pulse and blood pressure.

  6.   Junctional dysrhythmias may be tachycardiac or bradycardiac.

  7.   Manifestations of dysrhythmias include dizziness and syncope, if cardiac output drops.

D. **Overview of nursing interventions**

  1.   Administer antidysrhythmic medications, as prescribed, according to the type of dysrhythmia; medications may include:

      a.   Sympathomimetics (atropine, isoproterenol) for bradycardiac rhythms

      b.   β-blockers (propranolol), cardiac glycosides (digitalis), or calcium channel blockers (verapamil) for tachycardiac rhythms

      c.   Digitalis, quinidine or Pronestyl, and anticoagulants (heparin and Coumadin) for atrial dysrhythmias

      d.   Lidocaine, procainamide, quinidine, phenytoin, amiodarone, and disopyramide phosphate for ventricular dysrhythmias such as PVCs and ventricular tachycardia with a pulse

      e.   Bretylium® tosylate for ventricular fibrillation

  2.   Prepare the patient for electrical interventions, such as a pacemaker (temporary or permanent), cardioversion, or defibrillation, depending on each situation.

  3.   Prepare the patient for possible electrophysiology studies and signal average electrocardiography (SAECG)

  4.   Institute measures to address the underlying cause (eg, treat infection, reduce stimulants, withhold digitalis, relieve anxiety, replace electrolytes, or provide oxygen).

  5.   Provide patient education regarding diagnosis and therapy.

XIII. Pericarditis

A. **Description**

  1.   Pericarditis refers to inflammation of the pericardium.

    2. It may be acute, chronic, or constrictive:

        a. *Acute pericarditis* is associated with a fibrous exudate and is usually self-limiting.

        b. *Chronic pericarditis* is characterized by an increase in inflammatory exudate that continues beyond an anticipated period of time.

        c. *Constrictive pericarditis* is characterized by scar tissue that forms between the visceral and parietal layers of the pericardium.

B. **Etiology**

    1. Pericarditis is commonly associated with increased capillary permeability, which allows plasma proteins to invade the pericardial space.

    2. Causes of *acute pericarditis* include idiopathic and viral syndromes, uremia, bacterial infections, MI, postpericardiotomy syndrome, rheumatic fever, and physical and chemical agents.

    3. *Chronic pericarditis* is associated with rheumatic fever, congenital heart conditions, hypertension, lupus, rheumatoid arthritis, scleroderma, myxedema, and acute and chronic renal failure. Pericarditis with effusion commonly occurs in persons being maintained on hemodialysis.

    4. *Constrictive pericarditis* is associated with longstanding pyrogenic infections or postviral infections.

C. **Pathophysiologic processes and manifestations**

    1. The inflammatory process of *acute pericarditis* occurs in response to stimulation of the immune system, which, after insult to the pericardium from infection or radiation therapy, causes inflammation and exudate formation on the pericardial sac.

    2. Inflammation produces chest pain, a pericardial friction rub, and ST elevation on 12-lead ECG.

    3. Chest pain worsens with deep breathing, coughing, swallowing, and changing position.

    4. This type of pericarditis is typically preceded by fever, malaise, and flulike symptoms.

    5. *Chronic pericarditis* produces minimal signs and symptoms; this type of pericarditis is typically identified by routine chest film.

    6. In *constrictive pericarditis,* fibrous scarring and calcification cause obliteration of the pericardial cavity as the layers adhere, encasing the heart in a rigid way.

    7. Pericardial effusion (accumulation of fluid in the pericardial cavity) can develop in all forms of pericarditis. It may also occur in hypoproteinemic states as well as in hypervolemia.

    8. Cardiac tamponade is cardiac compression that results from an excessive accumulation of fluid or blood in the pericardial space. It can occur as the result of effusion, trauma, rupture, or dissecting aneurysm. It also can follow pericarditis and pericardial effusion if they are not treated.

    9. Rapid accumulation of fluid in the pericardial space results in increased CVP, decreased cardiac output, pulsus paradoxus, tachycardia, narrowed pulse pressure, and muffled heart sounds.

    10. Symptoms of pericarditis worsen with effusion and tamponade. Such symptoms include pulsus paradoxus, distant heart sounds, and low voltage on the ECG. A pericardial friction rub is the hallmark sign of pericarditis, but disappears in pericardial effusion.

11. An early sign of tamponade is ascites without peripheral edema; Kussmaul's sign and neck vein distention also occur.

D. Overview of nursing interventions

1. Prepare the patient for echocardiography, radiation-scanning procedures, or computerized tomography to identify the location and extent of inflammation or effusion.
2. Obtain aspiration and laboratory analysis of the pericardial fluid to identify the causative agent, as ordered.
3. Administer the appropriate antibiotic, if warranted.
4. Administer anti-inflammatory medications to reduce inflammation, as ordered.
5. Prepare the patient in severe cardiac tamponade for pericardiocentesis to remove fluid from the pericardial sac.
6. Monitor vital signs frequently.
7. Provide support and reassurance.
8. Provide patient teaching covering:
   a. Disease process
   b. Causative factors
   c. Preventive measures

 XIV. **Infective endocarditis**

A. Description

1. Infective endocarditis refers to an inflammation or infection of the endocardium or the heart valves.
2. It can be classified as either acute or subacute.
   a. *Acute infective endocarditis* commonly affects persons with normal hearts.
   b. *Subacute infective endocarditis* mainly affects persons with damaged hearts.

B. Etiology and incidence

1. *Acute infective endocarditis* is caused by *Staphylococcus aureus* and β-hemolytic *Streptococcus*. Infection occurs when the organism invades the bloodstream. It is unclear what causes the infecting organism to localize on normal heart valves.
2. *Subacute infective endocarditis* is caused by organisms normally present in the body (eg, *Streptococcus viridans,* nonhemolytic and microaerohilic streptococci). These organisms become engrafted on the damaged valves.
3. Other causative organisms include *Escherichia coli, Klebsiella, Proteus, Pseudomonas, Salmonella, Candida,* and *Histoplasma.*
4. Predisposing conditions include congenital heart disease, rheumatic heart disease, mitral valve prolapse, and cardiac defects; however, 50 to 60% of acute infective endocarditis cases occur without previous cardiac deformities.

C. Pathophysiologic processes and manifestations

1. Usually, the heart valve has already sustained some damage when microbial colonization occurs.

2. Microbes that are in the blood adhere to the damaged surface and proliferate.
3. Initial damage to the valves (also known as endothelium) exposes the basement membrane, which, in turn, attracts platelets; clot formation subsequently occurs.
4. Sloughing of disease, with erosion of valve leaflets or myocardial damage, can produce congestive heart failure.
5. Irregular vegetation on the heart valves can cause brain, kidney, spleen, or mesenteric embolization.

6. Manifestations of *acute infective endocarditis* **may include:**
    a. **Sudden fever**
    b. **Septicemia**
    c. **Valvular insufficiency**
    d. **Heart failure**
    e. **Stroke**
    f. **Splenic infarction**
7. Manifestations of *subacute infective endocarditis* may include:
    a. Chronic low-grade fever
    b. Anemia
    c. Weight loss
    d. Splenomegaly
    e. Heart murmur
8. Peripheral manifestations may include petechiae, splinter hemorrhages, Roth's spots, and Osler's nodes. Allergic vasculitis is thought to be responsible for producing peripheral manifestations.
9. Blood cultures are positive; leukocytosis and an elevated sedimentation rate are usually present.
10. ECG may reveal conduction abnormalities.
11. Transesophageal echocardiography may identify the presence and location of lesions.

D. Overview of nursing interventions
1. Institute appropriate testing to identify the pathogen, as ordered.
2. Minimize the organism's effect on the heart by using appropriate antibiotic therapy, as prescribed, for 4 to 6 weeks.
3. Institute broad-spectrum antibiotic therapy, as ordered, while awaiting bacteriologic confirmation (eg, intravenous high-dose penicillin with gentamicin, streptomycin, or vancomycin).
4. Provide supportive therapy to prevent and manage heart failure.
5. Prepare the patient for valve replacement surgery if medical intervention fails.
6. Prevent the disease by administering antibiotics prophylactically before the patient undergoes any procedure that may cause bacteremia.

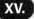 **Myocarditis**

A. Description: focal or diffuse inflammation of the myocardium; may be viral (most common) or bacterial (rare)
B. Etiology
1. Viral myocarditis may be caused by the coxsackie virus.

2. Bacterial myocarditis is associated with rheumatic fever and the diphtheria toxin.

3. Other causes include hypersensitivity reactions, autoimmune responses, chemical and physical agents, and radiation therapy.

C. **Pathophysiologic processes and manifestations**

1. Myocarditis can be asymptomatic or can produce symptoms of heart failure.

 2. **Manifestations of viral myocarditis may include:**
    a. **Tachycardia**
    b. **Dyspnea**
    c. **Low-grade fever**
    d. **Malaise**
    e. **History of upper respiratory infection**

3. In young adults, sudden death has occurred; in adults, viral myocarditis is likely to be benign and self-limiting.

4. Laboratory analysis reveals leukocytosis and elevated serum glutamic-oxaloacetic transaminase (SGOT), serum glutamic pyruvic transaminase (SGPT), and lactic dehydrogenase (LDH).

 5. **ECG abnormalities include ventricular dysrhythmias, AV blocks, ST elevation, T-wave inversion, and transient Q waves. Because the whole heart is affected, all 12 leads will show abnormalities.**

6. Manifestations of right and left heart failure can occur with advanced disease.

D. **Overview of nursing interventions**

1. Obtain viral antigen detection or serologic testing, as ordered, to aid in diagnosis.

2. Prepare the patient for myocardial biopsy, which may also aid diagnosis.

3. Administer appropriate antibiotics for bacterial myocarditis, as ordered.

4. Institute measures to decrease cardiac workload, such as bedrest.

5. For the patient with heart failure:
    a. Administer digitalis, diuretics, and oxygen therapy, as ordered.
    b. Restrict sodium.
    c. Encourage activities that improve oxygen supply and decrease oxygen demand.

6. Administer antiarrhythmics, with caution, for dysrhythmias; administer anticoagulants for thromboembolic events, as prescribed.

7. Use immunosuppressive therapy, as prescribed, to resolve inflammation.

XVI. Hypertrophic cardiomyopathy

A. **Description**

1. Hypertrophic cardiomyopathy refers to a condition of hypertrophy of the ventricular muscle mass, with a subsequent small left ventricular volume.

2. With this condition, abnormal patterning of fibers produces uncoordinated ventricular contraction and impaired relaxation.

B. **Etiology**

1. Hypertrophic cardiomyopathy results from unknown causes.

2. It commonly is familial and is inherited as an autosomal dominant trait.

C.   Pathophysiologic processes and manifestations

1.   Manifestations can be absent to incapacitating.
2.   Elevations in left ventricular end diastolic pressure are due to impaired ventricular filling and increased ventricular wall thickness; resulting manifestations include chest pain, dyspnea, fatigue, and syncope that increases with exertion.
3.   Ventricular and atrial dysrhythmias may occur. Sudden death may occur and can be common in certain families.
4.   Hypertrophic cardiomyopathy can be definitively identified with angiocardiography.
5.   Technetium scan confirms decreased left ventricular volume, and thallium defines the mass and configuration.
6.   ECG reveals changes associated with left ventricular hypertrophy.

D.   Overview of nursing interventions

1.   Administer β-blockers, vasodilators, and nitrates, as prescribed, to provide symptomatic relief of chest pain, dyspnea, and tachycardia.
2.   Administer antiarrhythmic medications (amiodarone), as prescribed.
3.   Prepare the patient for pacemaker therapy, if necessary.
4.   Educate the patient regarding the disease process, family screening, and possible lifestyle changes.

Bibliography

Berne, R. M. & Levy, M. N. (1998). *Physiology* (4th ed.). St. Louis: C. V. Mosby.

Brunner, L. S., & Suddarth, D. S. (1996). *Textbook of medical-surgical nursing* (8th ed.). Philadelphia: J. B. Lippincott.

Civetta, J. M., Taylor, R. W. & Kirby, R. R. (1997). *Critical care* (3rd ed.). Philadelphia: Lippincott-Raven Publishers.

Guyton, A. C. (1995). *Textbook of medical physiology* (9th ed.). Philadelphia: W. B. Saunders.

Polaski, A. L. & Tatro, S. E. (1996). *Core principles and practice of medical-surgical nursing.* Philadelphia: W. B. Saunders.

STUDY QUESTIONS

1. Which of the following findings would suggest a diagnosis of angina?
   a. elevated cardiac enzymes and ST elevation on ECG
   b. ST changes on ECG and a pericardial friction rub
   c. normal cardiac enzymes and T-wave inversions on ECG
   d. abnormal heart sound and elevated sedimentation rate

2. Prolonged ischemia to myocardial cells that eventually leads to necrosis results in:
   a. leukocytosis
   b. decreased CK–MB levels
   c. ST elevation on ECG
   d. abnormal ABGs

3. For the last 6 months, Ms. Kennedy, age 65, has been taking Isordil (a nitrate drug) to prevent the occurrence of chest pain. Today she reports that the pain occurs when she walks up the two flights of stairs in her home. These findings suggest:
   a. unstable angina
   b. chronic stable angina
   c. Prinzmetal's angina
   d. angina decubitus

4. The treatment for symptomatic bradycardia includes:
   a. digitalis and lidocaine
   b. atropine and temporary pacing
   c. cardioversion and verapamil
   d. Lasix and carotid sinus massage

5. The emergent treatment for ventricular tachycardia with a pulse includes:
   a. lidocaine and cardioversion
   b. bretylium and Lasix
   c. digitalis and temporary pacing
   d. verapamil and carotid sinus massage

6. Which of the following results in sinus bradycardia?
   a. hypothermia
   b. hypotension
   c. fever
   d. ischemia

7. Which of the following conditions is most likely to be predominantly familial?
   a. subacute endocarditis
   b. acute pericarditis
   c. hypertrophic cardiomyopathy
   d. dilated cardiomyopathy

8. When providing patient teaching for a person susceptible to the development of infective endocarditis, the nurse should include information on the use of:
   a. prophylactic antibiotic therapy
   b. prophylactic immunosuppressive therapy
   c. diuretics for weight gain
   d. face masks with ill family members

9. On auscultation, a mitral valve prolapse often produces:
   a. diastolic murmur
   b. pericardial friction rub
   c. nonejection click
   d. S3

10. Leftsided heart failure is manifested by:
    a. peripheral edema and JVD
    b. hepatomegaly
    c. dyspnea and tachycardia
    d. chest pain and bradycardia

11. A nurse caring for a patient with mitral valve regurgitation and atrial fibrillation should be most concerned about:
    a. possible embolization
    b. elevated right sided pressures
    c. right atrial hypertrophy
    d. right ventricular hypertrophy

12. A nurse caring for cardiac patients knows that sudden development of a ventricular dysrhythmia can mean:
    a. V node malfunction
    b. ventricular ischemia
    c. valvular disease
    d. increased cardiac output

13. A nurse is auscultating the lungs of a patient with cardiomyopathy. She hears crackles. This is significant because:
    a. the lungs are not perfusing
    b. the heart is overcontracting
    c. cardiogenic shock may be occurring
    d. blood pressure may be rising

14. The nurse should know that the valsalva maneuver can cause:
    a. ventricular tachycardia
    b. atrial fibrillation
    c. junctional rhythm
    d. bradycardia

ANSWER KEY

Question	Correct answer	Correct answer rationale	Incorrect answer rationales
1.	c	In angina, the 12-lead ECG may demonstrate T-wave inversion; cardiac enzymes will be normal.	a. Indicates MI. b. Indicates pericarditis. d. Indicates endocarditis.
2.	c	In necrosis, the ST segment will be elevated on the ECG.	a. Leukocytosis is part of the inflammatory response following MI. b. Increased CK–MB levels result from MI. d. Abnormal ABGs are not a result of prolonged ischemia.
3.	a	Unstable angina is characterized by a change in frequency, duration, or intensity of pain.	b. There would be no pain with normal activity. c. Prinzmetal's angina occurs at rest. d. There is no such entity.
4.	b	Sympathomimetic administration (atropine and Isuprel) as well as pacemaker insertion are treatment modalities for symptomatic bradycardia.	a. Digitalis is used to treat atrial dysrhythmia; lidocaine is used to treat ventricular tachycardia. c. Verapamil is used to treat tachycardia. d. Lasix is a diuretic used to treat CHF.
5.	a	These are first-line treatment modalities for ventricular tachycardia with a pulse.	b. Bretylium is used to treat ventricular fibrillation. c. Digitalis is used in atrial dysrhythmia. d. Verapamil is used to manage tachycardiac rhythms.
6.	a	Hypothermia results in sinus bradycardia.	b, c, and d. All of these can result in tachycardiac rhythms.
7.	c	Hypertrophic cardiomyopathy is familial and is inherited as an autosomal dominant trait.	a and b. These are inflammatory diseases. d. Cardiomyopathies are classified as hypertrophic, congestive, or restrictive.
8.	a	Prevention of infective endocarditis involves the use of prophylactic antibiotics before the patient undergoes any procedure that may cause bacteremia.	b. Prophylactic immunosuppressive therapy would further increase the patient's susceptibility to infective endocarditis. c. Using diuretics for weight gain is an inappropriate action. d. This will not prevent endocarditis.

Question	Correct answer	Correct answer rationale	Incorrect answer rationales
9.	c	A nonejection click is a manifestation of mitral valve prolapse.	a. A diastolic murmur is found in mitral and tricuspid stenosis. b. A friction rub is a symptom of pericarditis. d. An S3 is a sound produced by turbulent blood flow from one chamber to another.
10.	c	Manifestations of left-sided heart failure are respiratory in nature.	a and b. These are symptoms of right-sided heart failure. d. Chest pain and bradycardia are not common manifestations of heart failure.
11.	a	Embolization can cause severe damage, such as stroke or infarction. This is then the most important of all of the possible choices.	b. This choice is incorrect because it is left-sided pressures that increase in the presence of mitral valve regurgitation. c. This choice is incorrect because the left atrium is hypertrophied in this condition. d. This choice is incorrect because the left ventricle is hypertrophied in this condition.
12.	b	Ventricular ischemia can result in arrythmia.	a. This choice is incorrect because AV node malfunction would be caused by AV node ischemia. b. This choice is incorrect because valvular disease would be more likely to cause an atrial dysrhythmia. d. This choice is incorrect because an increased cardiac output would not cause arrythmia.
13.	c	The heart will not pump adequately in cardiogenic shock. The decrease in cardiac output leads to accumulation of fluid in the lungs. Crackles can be heard as fluid is present, and this fluid will impede the transport of oxygen across the alveolar capillary membrane.	a, b, and d. These choices are not correct because they are not sequelae of cardiomyopathy and are not connected to the presence of crackles.
14.	d	The valsalva maneuver will cause stimulation to the Vagus nerve, which in turn causes bradycardia.	a, b, and c. These choices are incorrect. The valsalva maneuver will not cause these dysrhythmias.

3

Vascular Disorders

I. Overview of pathophysiologic processes

A. Arterial diseases

1. Arterial diseases affect those vessels that transport blood and oxygen to body tissues.

2. Diseased arteries cause ischemia, or inadequate delivery of oxygen to the tissues.

3. When any body part loses its oxygen supply, necrosis (cell death) occurs, resulting in pain and loss of function.

4. Arterial disease can affect any artery; it is particularly dangerous when the arteries that supply the major organs (eg, heart, brain, and kidneys) are affected.

5. Arteriosclerosis (atherosclerosis), aneurysm formation, arteriosclerosis obliterans, Raynaud's phenomenon and disease, arterial embolism, thromboangiitis obliterans, and diabetic arteriosclerotic disease are classified as arterial disorders. Hypertension can be classified as a disease of the heart or great vessels.

6. Risk factors for arterial disorders include:
    a. High-fat and high-cholesterol diet
    b. Genetic predisposition

B. Venous diseases

1. Venous diseases affect those vessels that bring blood from the peripheral tissues back to the heart to receive oxygen.

2. Venous diseases lead to pooling of blood in the extremities, resulting in interstitial edema.

3. Ulceration and thrombus formation may result from venous disorders.
4. Venous thrombosis (thrombophlebitis), varicose veins, and venous stasis ulcers are venous diseases (Fig. 3-1).
5. Risk factors for venous disease include:
   a. Genetic predisposition
   b. Obesity, pregnancy, and other conditions that can impair blood return from the extremities

C. Lymphatic diseases
   1. Lymphatic diseases affect those vessels that return fluids from the tissues.

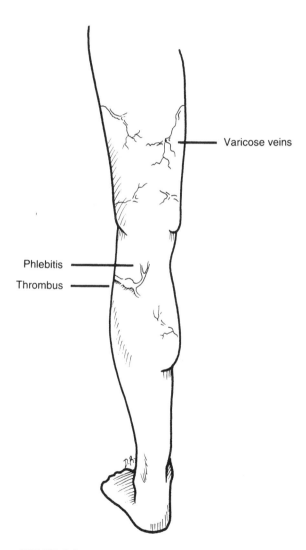

FIGURE 3-1.
Venous disorders of the leg.

    2.   Lymph vessel damage results in interstitial edema as tissue fluids back up.

    3.   Lymphedema and acute lymphangitis are diseases of the lymph vessels.

    4.   Risk factors for lymphatic disease include:

        a.   Tumor formation (lymph disease may result from mechanical obstruction)

        b.   History of lymph cancer or lymph node dissection

        c.   Overwhelming or prolonged infection or inflammation in the area.

II. Physiologic responses to vascular dysfunction

A. Arterial responses

    1.   *Ischemia*

        a.   Ischemia refers to reduced oxygenation to a body part, which can occur when vessels are so diseased that they are unable to transport oxygen-rich blood.

        b.   It results in pain to the affected part.

    2.   *Paresthesia:* decreased sensation in the extremities, described as tingling or numbing.

    3.   *Pain*

        a.   Pain occurs in the feet and leg muscles and may be described as burning, throbbing, or cramping.

        b.   Usually, it is brought on by exercise but may also occur with elevation of lower extremities.

    4.   *Intermittent claudication*

        a.   Pain in exercising muscles; most commonly occurs in the calf but may occur anywhere in the lower extremity.

        b.   It is directly related to decreased blood supply during activity and recedes with rest.

    5.   *Temperature changes:* Extremities are cold due to decreased blood supply.

    6.   *Skin color changes:* Skin is pale, especially on elevation; dependent rubor, or redness, occurs as blood rushes downward in the extremity.

    7.   *Reactive hyperemia:* Reduced blood flow to an extremity results in arteriolar dilatation; when the blood supply is restored, the affected area becomes warm and red from the congestion.

    8.   *Pulse changes*

        a.   Peripheral pulses may be diminished or absent.

        b.   A notable difference in the strength or character of pulses from one side of the body to the other may exist.

    9.   *Prolonged capillary refill:* 3 seconds or more is required for filling.

   10.   *Ulcers:* Open lesions occurring on the feet resulting from diminished distal perfusion. Figure 3-2 illustrates stasis ulcer.

B. Venous responses

    1.   *Pain*

        a.   Pain occurs in the feet and leg muscles and is described as aching or throbbing.

        b.   It results from venous stasis and usually increases as the day progresses, especially with prolonged dependent positioning (eg, sitting or standing).

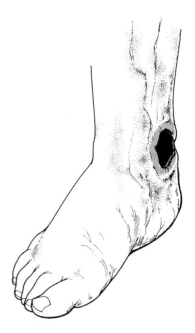

FIGURE 3-2.
Stasis dermatitis with a stasis ulcer from long-term venous stasis. (Bullock, B. L. (1996) *Pathophysiology: Adaptations and Alterations in Function* (4th ed.). Philadelphia: Lippincott-Raven.

  2. *Temperature changes:* Skin will be warm to the touch because blood can enter but not leave the affected area.
  3. *Skin color changes:* Skin may be reddened or cyanotic.
  4. *Edema:* pooling of fluid resulting in swelling or enlargement of affected parts.
  5. *Venous stasis ulcers:* skin breakdown due to increased pressure resulting from chronic pooling of blood.
  6. *Decreased mobility:* may result from edema.

C. Lymph responses
  1. *Edema:* occurs as tissue fluids back up.
  2. *Pain and discomfort:* caused by edema.

III. Arteriosclerosis (Atherosclerosis)

A. Description
  1. Arteriosclerosis is a general term describing arterial disorders in which degenerative changes in arteries result in decreased blood flow.
  2. Atherosclerosis is the most common form of arteriosclerosis; in this condition, excessive lipid accumulation leads to degenerative changes in the intima of arteries.

B. Etiology and incidence
  1. The cause of arteriosclerosis is unknown; however, certain risk factors are believed to contribute to the development of the disorder.

  2. **Major risk factors include:**
    a. **Hypertension (most significant factor)**

   b.   Cigarette smoking (because nicotine has a direct vasoconstrict-ing effect)
   c.   Elevated serum cholesterol (because fat causes obstructive plaques)
   d.   Obesity (because the heart must pump harder and therefore ex-erts more tension on the vessels)
   e.   Diabetes mellitus (because high serum glucose causes damage to the vessel wall, worsening over time)
3. Other presumed risk factors include increasing age, physical inactivity, and a family history of arteriosclerosis.
4. Incidence is higher in men than in women.

C. **Pathophysiologic processes and manifestations**
   1. Pathophysiologic changes are generalized and may involve large and small arteries or arterioles.
   2. Lipids deposit on the intima of the arteries, possibly resulting from years of a high-fat diet.
   3. Calcification, thrombosis, and fibrosis contribute to the development of a *plaque* or *atheroma*, which occludes blood flow; however, not every dis-eased vessel will have plaque formation.
   4. Affected vessels develop hypertrophy and the arterial walls lose their elastic-ity, making blood transport difficult. As a result, organs perfused by dam-aged vessels will display symptoms of varying severity; the worse the pathol-ogy, the more severe the symptoms.
   5. Areas affected vary from one person to another, as does the degree of pathology. Symptoms depend on the organ involved.
   6. The most commonly affected areas are:
      a.   *Heart:* Coronary artery disease is caused by atherosclerosis of the coronary arteries and can lead to angina, myocardial infarction (MI), and death.
      b.   *Brain:* Cerebroarteriosclerosis can lead to transient ischemic attacks (TIAs), cerebrovascular accidents (CVAs), and death.
      c.   *Kidneys:* Renal arterial stenosis can cause chronic renal failure.
      d.   *Extremities:* Arterial occlusive disease can lead to gangrene of the digits and intermittent claudication.
   7. Some degree of arterial fibrosis, thickening, and loss of elasticity accom-pany the normal aging process. These involutional changes are expected as a person ages; however, combined with other risk factors, these changes may lead to more serious disease.

D. **Overview of nursing interventions**
   1. Institute measures aimed at preventing the disease.
   3. Teach patient how to minimize his or her risk of developing disease.
   4. Provide education and referrals to help the patient stop smoking.
   3. Teach the patient to maintain a proper diet to control obesity and hyper-tension.
   4. Provide stress-reduction techniques.
   5. Educate the patient about diabetes control, if indicated.
   6. Teach the patient how to relieve symptoms (ie, elevate extremity).
   7. Teach the patient how to recognize worsening of disease and when to seek help.

IV.   **Hypertension**

A.   Description

1.   Hypertension refers to excessive tension exerted by blood on arterial walls, which results in an intermittent (labile) or sustained elevation in blood pressure.

2.   The elevation may be in either systolic or diastolic pressure, or in both pressures. Usually, a sustained systolic pressure over 140 mm Hg or a diastolic pressure greater than 90 mm Hg indicates hypertension.

3.   Types include primary hypertension, secondary hypertension, hypertensive crisis, and isolated systolic hypertension.

4.   *Primary hypertension* (essential or idiopathic hypertension) appears to be a familial disease of unknown etiology, although numerous risk factors have been identified.

5.   *Secondary hypertension* (nonessential hypertension) develops secondary to another disease.

6.   *Hypertensive crisis* is a sudden acute elevation in arterial blood pressure that can be life threatening.

   a.   Hypertensive urgency refers to a severe elevation in blood pressure that is producing no organ damage and therefore remains asymptomatic.

   b.   Hypertensive emergency is a life-threatening, severe elevation in blood pressure accompanied by signs and symptoms of deterioration.

7.   *Isolated systolic hypertension* refers to an elevation in systolic blood pressure greater than 140 mm Hg without a concurrent elevation in diastolic blood pressure. This disorder primarily affects elderly persons.

B.   Etiology and incidence

1.   Primary hypertension results from unknown causes, although several risk factors have been identified (see Display 3-1); it accounts for 80% of hypertension cases.

2.   *Secondary hypertension* results from preexisting diseases and accounts for approximately 10% of hypertension cases; diseases that can trigger its development include:

DISPLAY 3-1
Risk Factors for Primary Hypertension

- Age (incidence is higher in adults between ages 30 and 70)
- Genetic predisposition (incidence is higher in African Americans)
- Family history
- Obesity
- Sendentary lifestyle
- Cigarette smoking (nicotine directly affects blood vessels)
- Stress (increased epinephrine secretion increases cardiac oxygen demand, heart rate, and vessel diameter)
- Excessive ingestion of sodium or saturated fats

      a.   Renal diseases (eg, renal vascular disorders, chronic glomerulonephritis, pyelonephritis, polycystic renal disease, and obstructive uropathy); renal disease may cause accelerated renin release, which, in turn, elevates blood pressure

      b.   Cushing's syndrome, which causes accumulation of extracellular sodium and water

      c.   Primary aldosteronism, which causes accumulation of extracellular sodium and water

      d.   Hypothyroidism and hyperthyroidism, which cause alterations in cardiac output

      e.   Coarctation of the aorta, which affects blood pressure because blood cannot leave the heart easily

  3.   Other possible causes of *secondary hypertension* include excessive alcohol ingestion and prolonged use of oral contraceptives.

  4.   *Hypertensive crisis* is usually associated with acute processes such as ischemic chest pain, pulmonary edema, or intracerebral hemorrhage. Some illnesses are the result of hypertension, and others have hypertension as a sequela, such as renal disease.

  5.   *Isolated systolic hypertension* is believed to result from a combination of factors common to the elderly, including decreased cardiac output and increased peripheral and renal vascular resistance. In addition, older adults are more likely to have some form of occlusive atherosclerotic disease.

C.   **Pathophysiologic processes and manifestations**

  1.   **Arterial blood pressure is equal to cardiac output times peripheral resistance.**

  2.   **Elevations in blood pressure are a direct result of increased peripheral vascular resistance (such as vasoconstriction), increased cardiac output (increased heart rate or stroke volume), or a combination of both.**

  3.   The renin-angiotensin-aldosterone system is responsible for producing vasoconstriction whenever blood flow to the kidneys decreases. This is accomplished by renin secretion and angiotensin formation.

  4.   Angiotensin formation results in increased aldosterone secretion by affecting the adrenal cortex.

  5.   Aldosterone secretion causes water and sodium retention in the kidneys, resulting in increased extracellular fluid volume.

  6.   Increased extracellular volume consequently leads to increased cardiac output and an increase in arterial pressure.

  7.   The sympathetic nervous system also controls blood pressure by releasing norepinephrine from the postganglionic nerve fibers.

  8.   The release of norepinephrine in situations associated with a stress response causes vasoconstriction.

  9.   Primary hypertension usually begins with intermittent elevations in diastolic blood pressure and progresses to sustained blood pressure elevation; usually, there are no symptoms.

 10.   Manifestations of coronary artery disease, CVAs, and renal failure occur commonly as a result of longstanding hypertension.

 11.   Risk factors that worsen this process include:

      a.   Age (blood vessels stiffen and become more resistant).

      b.   Obesity (making it harder for the heart to pump through the denser tissue).

      c.   Diabetes (blood vessels undergo changes from diabetes).

      d.   Water retention (causes excessive fluid for the heart to circulate).

      e.   Medications (some medications cause hypertension as a side effect.

      f.   Genetics (hypertension may be hereditary).

D. **Overview of nursing interventions**

1. Administer antihypertensive medications, as ordered, to control blood pressure.
2. Administer intravenous antihypertensives, as prescribed, to control hypertensive emergency.
   a. Monitor the patient for signs of deterioration.
   b. Assess and report effectiveness of therapy.
3. Instruct the patient on the importance of complying with medication therapy; explain possible side effects, including vertigo and impotence.
4. Teach the patient or significant other about blood pressure measurement techniques.
5. Instruct the patient to limit dietary sodium because it enhances water retention, which increases intravascular volume resulting in elevated blood pressure.
6. Emphasize the importance of reporting any effects that may indicate the development of complications, including:
   a. Visual disturbances such as blurring or loss of acuity (may signify retinal hemorrhage)
   b. Decreased urine output (may indicate renal insufficiency)
   c. Weakness or paresthesia (may result from TIA or CVA)
7. Teach the patient how to identify and modify risk factors when possible. Age, genetics, and preexisting disease are not modifiable risk factors.

V. Aneurysm

A. **Definition**

1. An aneurysm is an abnormal dilatation of a blood vessel wall; it may occur in any vessel.
2. Types of aneurysms include fusiform (involving all three layers of the vessel wall) and saccular, which can rupture (Fig. 3-3).

B. **Etiology**

1. Causes include atherosclerosis (which may cause plaque formation and erode the blood vessel wall) and arteriosclerosis and hypertension (which may cause pressure on the arterial walls).
2. Saccular aneurysms may be caused by trauma; at the site where the arterial wall is dissected, a clot may form (false aneurysm) or blood may collect at the aneurysm site (saccular aneurysm).
3. A dissecting aneurysm occurs when the layers of the artery separate from each other. Figure 3-4 illustrates dissection of an aneurysm in the aorta.
4. Rupture occurs when the vessel bursts under pressure. It is more likely to occur when intra-abdominal pressure increases (such as on lifting) or if hypertension is present in the vessels.

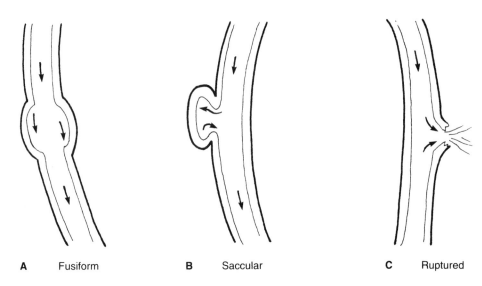

| **A** Fusiform | **B** Saccular | **C** Ruptured |

FIGURE 3-3.
Aneurysm types. Outpouching of aneurysms assumes several forms. A ruptured aneurysm can cause fatal bleeding.

C. Pathophysiologic processes and manifestations

1. As contraction occurs, pressure is exerted on the arterial wall.
2. Hypertension increases this pressure over time, leading to the development of a weakness in the vessel wall that manifests as an aneurysm.
3. The vessel wall also may be eroded by plaque formation, which occurs over time.

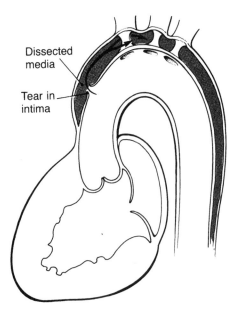

Dissected media

Tear in intima

FIGURE 3-4.
Consequences of dissection from the ascending aorta across the arch of the aorta. (Bullock, B. L. (1996) *Pathophysiology: Adaptations and Alterations in Function* (4th ed.). Philadelphia: Lippincott-Raven.)

4. The aorta is the most commonly affected vessel (see Chapter 5 for information on cerebral aneurysms). Figure 3-5 shows a fusiform aneurysm in the aorta.
5. Symptoms vary depending on the affected vessel; severity of symptoms also depends on the size of the aneurysm.
6. Symptoms may include:
   a. Pain in the abdomen or in the extremities (may occur if the limbs are deprived of blood and, therefore, oxygen)
   b. Shortness of breath (due to pressure on internal organs)
7. A dangerous complication is dissected or ruptured aneurysm, which results in blood volume loss and possible death.

D. **Overview of nursing interventions**
1. Prepare the patient for surgery, the only treatment; afterward, provide appropriate postoperative care.
2. Administer fluid replacement therapy for a patient with a dissected aneurysm.
3. Provide appropriate care for a patient who has surgery for aneurysm repair. The needs will depend on the location and length of the surgery. For example, a person with a cerebral aneurysm will have a different treatment course and possible postoperative complications than a person with an abdominal aneurysm.
4. Be alert when caring for a patient needing aneurysm repairs.

VI. Arteriosclerosis obliterans (peripheral arteriosclerotic disease)

A. **Description: a condition in which the blood supply to the extremities is occluded by atherosclerotic plaques (atheroma)**
B. **Etiology**
1. Arteriosclerosis obliterans results from unknown causes, although there are a number of predisposing risk factors.

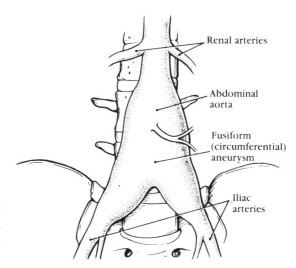

Renal arteries

Abdominal aorta

Fusiform (circumferential) aneurysm

Iliac arteries

FIGURE 3-5.
Fusiform aneurysm of the aorta. (Bullock, B. L. (1996) *Pathophysiology: Adaptations and Alterations in Function* (4th ed.). Philadelphia: Lippincott-Raven.)

2. Risk factors for arteriosclerosis obliterans are the same as those for arteriosclerosis (see Section III, B).

C. **Pathophysiologic processes and manifestations**

1. Peripheral atherosclerotic disease is characterized by progressive changes in the intima of the arteries; these changes lead to arterial narrowing, occlusion, and chronic ischemia of affected areas. Changes in the arteries with consequent endothelial damage predominantly result from lipid accumulation.

2. Symptoms are directly related to the gradual, covert development of ischemia:

   a. Intermittent claudication results from insufficient oxygenation of active or exercising muscle tissue.

   b. Pulses may be diminished or absent due to the decreased blood flow.

   c. Pain, beginning in the most distal aspects of the extremity, may occur at rest as occlusive disease progresses; in femoropopliteal disease, pain occurs in the calf.

   d. Affected extremities may have poor hair and nail growth, along with dry skin.

   e. Aortoiliac disease can result in pain or claudication in the hips, buttocks, and calves; in males, impotence may occur depending on the location and severity of occlusion.

   f. Extremities will become pale after 1 or 2 minutes elevation, and rubor will ensue with dependent positioning.

D. **Overview of nursing interventions**

1. Instruct the patient to increase activity, walking a total of 60 minutes a day with rest stops whenever claudication occurs; doing so will increase the distance the patient can walk before pain develops as well as improve stamina and collateral circulation.

2. Instruct the patient to eliminate all forms of tobacco use because nicotine is a powerful vasoconstrictor and will further reduce perfusion.

3. Teach the patient proper foot care and the importance of daily inspections for injury because the extremities may lose sensation and poor perfusion hinders healing.

4. Administer analgesics, as prescribed, to provide pain relief in advanced stages of the disease.

VII. **Raynaud's disease and phenomenon**

A. **Description**

1. Raynaud's disease and Raynaud's phenomenon are characterized by episodes of arteriospasm with resultant ischemia in the extremities, particularly the digits of the hands.

2. The clinical findings of the disease and the phenomenon are the same, but the etiologies are different.

B. **Etiology and incidence**

1. Raynaud's disease is idiopathic, although it appears to be hereditary; it occurs most commonly in women, usually those between ages 18 and 40.

2. Raynaud's phenomenon occurs secondary to other disorders including:

     a. Occlusive arterial diseases (eg, arteriosclerosis obliterans and thromboangiitis obliterans)

     b. Connective tissue diseases (eg, systemic scleroderma, lupus erythematosus, and dermatomyositis)

     c. Primary pulmonary hypertension

     d. Hypothyroidism

     e. Neurologic diseases (eg, central or peripheral neuropathy and carpal tunnel syndrome)

  3. Environmental risk factors include exposure to chemical irritants and vibratory tools.

  4. Incidence is higher in the northern climates and during the winter months.

C. Pathophysiologic processes and manifestations

  1. Vasospasm occurs intermittently, precipitated by cold exposure or emotional stress.

  2. Attacks may be short (lasting a few minutes) or can continue for hours.

  3. Episodes are manifested by color changes of the affected areas.

     a. Biphasic changes: Cyanosis and then reactive hyperemia occurs.

     b. Triphasic changes: Pallor and then cyanosis may occur when the vasospasm results in arterial occlusion; reactive hyperemia occurs in response to the ischemic changes (hypoxia-induced vasodilatation).

  4. Pain, if experienced, is directly related to ischemia.

  5. Paresthesia often occurs.

  6. Peripheral pulses may be normal or diminished during an episode.

  7. Small ulcerations on the most distal aspects of the digits may develop; these can be painful.

  8. For Raynaud's disease, a history of symptoms for 2 years is necessary for diagnosis.

  9. Longstanding disease may lead to changes in appearance of the affected digits, with the skin becoming shiny and firm with a loss of subcutaneous tissue (sclerodactyly).

  10. With Raynaud's phenomenon, manifestations of the underlying disease also are apparent.

D. Overview of nursing interventions

  1. Assess the patient to determine the degree of digital involvement, noting color changes and breaks in skin integrity.

  2. Instruct the patient to keep extremities warm by wearing appropriate clothing and avoiding contact with cold substances; if rewarming is necessary, tell the patient to rewarm extremities slowly.

  3. Instruct the patient to avoid use of tobacco, because nicotine stimulates vasoconstriction.

  4. Teach the patient to use relaxation techniques to reduce the occurrence of attacks (because muscle relaxation may promote vascular relaxation).

  5. Administer pain medications, as prescribed, for severe disease.

  6. Institute interventions for Raynaud's phenomenon based on the underlying cause.

VIII. **Arterial embolism**

A. Description

 1. **Arterial embolism refers to a sudden arterial occlusion caused by emboli, which results in acute ischemia to the affected body parts.**

2. Emboli may be composed of gas, solid material (such as a blood clot), liquid, or fat.

B. Etiology

1. Many arterial emboli stem from thrombus formation in the cardiac chambers. These are likely to form if the chambers do not completely empty of blood, which is the case in some cardiac disorders.

2. Arteriosclerotic conditions may predispose patients to emboli formation.

3. Blood vessel pathology may lead to development of thrombus, which break off to form emboli.

4. Surgery involving manipulation of blood vessels, such as in the pelvic area, can lead to emboli.

 5. **Other surgeries, such as liposuction, can lead to development of fat emboli.**

6. **An air embolism can occur if air enters the body through a normally sealed area, such as a central line catheter.**

C. Pathophysiologic processes and manifestations

1. Arterial emboli occlude the vessel leading to ischemia of the affected body part and possibly infarction.

2. Pain may or may not be present, depending on the degree of occlusion and the site affected.

3. The occlusion may lead to paresthesia or paralysis of affected parts as the blood supply is reduced.

D. Overview of nursing interventions

1. Assess the location and extent of the occlusion to determine appropriate interventions.

2. Assess cardiopulmonary status because emboli may lodge in the cardiac or pulmonary vasculature—a life-threatening condition.

3. Assess the affected body part, and report all changes in color, temperature, and pulse.

4. Administer anticoagulant therapy, as ordered, to decrease incidence of additional emboli formation and expansion. The patient should have full knowledge of how to care for himself or herself while on coumadin.

5. Protect the affected extremity and keep it below the horizontal plane.

6. Administer analgesics, as ordered, for pain relief.

7. Prepare the patient for surgery, which is likely if the occlusion is located in a large artery; afterward, provide appropriate postoperative care.

IX. **Thromboangiitis obliterans (Buerger's disease)**

A. Description

1. Thromboangiitis obliterans is characterized by inflammatory changes in both arteries and veins, resulting in destruction of small and medium vessels.
2. Usually, vessels in the lower extremities are involved, but the upper extremities may be also be affected.

B. **Etiology and incidence**
1. Thromboangiitis obliterans results from unknown causes, although theories exist that it is related to an autoimmune disorder.
2. It affects male cigarette smokers between ages 20 and 40; there is a small incidence (5%) in females. There is no documented evidence that it occurs in nonsmokers.

C. **Pathophysiologic processes and manifestations**
1. Panarteritis (inflammation of all arteries) or panphlebitis (inflammation of all veins) occurs, leading to obstruction from swelling.
2. Thrombophlebitis may either precede the disorder or occur concomitantly.
3. Gangrene of the extremities commonly occurs.
4. Cessation of smoking will limit the effects of the disorder.
5. Occasionally, the coronary, mesenteric, and cerebral arteries are involved.
6. Other symptoms may include:
   a. Pain and tenderness in the affected extremity
   b. Shiny, red skin on the affected extremity
   c. Cyanosis
   d. Thickened nails

D. **Overview of nursing interventions**
1. Instruct the patient to stop smoking cigarettes to prevent serious complications.
2. Administer vasodilators, as ordered, to alleviate vasospasms.
 3. **Teach the patient how to manage side effects of these medications.**

X. **Diabetic arteriosclerotic disease**

A. **Description**
1. Diabetes mellitus usually precipitates vascular disease; classifications include large vessel and microvascular disease.
 2. **Three types of vascular disease are commonly associated with diabetes.**
   a. **Atherosclerosis (occurs commonly and is usually more severe)**
   b. **Peripheral vascular disease (occurs commonly)**
   c. **Diabetic microangiopathy (a change in small blood vessels distinguished by diffuse thickening of the capillary basement membranes in all organs and microaneurysm formation)**
3. Over time, the damage done to blood vessels effect major organs such as the heart, retina, brain, kidneys.

B. **Etiology: diabetic arteriosclerotic disease results from unknown causes**

C. **Pathophysiologic processes and manifestations**
1. Pathophysiologic processes and manifestations are the same as those for arteriosclerosis and arteriosclerosis obliterans (see Sections III,C).

2. Diabetic retinopathy can result from microangiopathy and can lead to blindness.
3. In nonproliferative retinopathy, manifestations include increased capillary permeability, microaneurysms and retinal hemorrhage, and edema (noted on ophthalmologic exam).
4. In proliferative retinopathy, a more advanced disease, neovascularization in the retina extends into the vitreous, and retinal hemorrhaging occurs.
5. Manifestations of advanced retinopathy include:
    a. Changes in vision due to macular edema
    b. Retinal detachment
6. Changes in the diabetic kidney, known as diabetic nephropathy, are described in Chapter 14, Section IX, C.
7. The arteriosclerosis, atherosclerosis, and microangiopathy effect the blood supply to the heart and brain. This can result in coronary artery disease and eventual transient ischemic attacks (TIAs) or cerebral vascular accident.

D.   Overview of nursing interventions

1. **Control blood glucose levels (the most important intervention).**
2. Undertake interventions to manage arteriosclerosis, hypertension, and arteriosclerosis obliterans (see Sections III, D; IV, D and VID).
3. Explain to the patient with retinopathy the importance of annual ophthalmologic exams.
4. Instruct the patient to report any vision changes such as blurring, black spots, or sudden vision loss.

5. **Make sure the patient understands the relationship between present glucose control and future complications.**

XI.   Venous thrombosis (thrombophlebitis)

A.   Description

1. Venous thrombosis refers to inflammation of a vein precipitating thrombus (blood clot) formation; it almost always occurs in the veins of the extremities, although it may occur in the neck veins or occasionally in the trunk.
2. Types of venous thrombosis include:
    a. *Deep vein thrombosis* (DVT), a stationary clot that forms in the deeper veins of the legs
    b. *Superficial thrombophlebitis,* an inflammation of a more superficial vein closer to the surface; this condition is accompanied by formation of a stationary clot within the vein.
3. Phlebothrombosis refers to thrombus formation without venous inflammation.
4. Phlebitis refers to inflammation of one or more veins without resultant clot formation.

B.   Etiology

1. **Three factors known as Virchow's triad are associated with venous thrombosis, which occurs when two of the three factors are present. These factors are:**
    a. **Trauma to the vessel wall, especially the endothelium**

  b. **Any state that results in venous stasis**
  c. **Changes in blood constituents or hypercoagulability, such as occurs with infection**
 2. Thrombophlebitis can become septic when caused by intravenous lines, access procedures, and intravenous drug abuse.
 3. A number of risk factors are associated with the development of venous thrombosis (see Display 3-2).

C. Pathophysiologic processes and manifestations

 1. **Thrombi formation is believed to occur when both venous stasis and hypercoagulability exist. Stagnated blood will accumulate in the pocket areas of the vessel valves, resulting in hypercoagulability (because activated coagulation factors are not removed from the blood).**
 2. Traces of thrombin activate the clotting mechanisms of platelet aggregation and conversion of fibrinogen to fibrin.
 3. Trauma or damage to the vessel walls from injury or phlebitis may cause platelet adhesion to the vein wall.
 4. DVT and phlebitis are acute diseases that may result in pulmonary embolism (as pieces of the clot break off and travel to the lung) or chronic venous insufficiency.
 5. Signs and symptoms of pulmonary embolism include:
  a. Sudden chest pain
  b. Dyspnea
  c. Decreased blood oxygen (PO_2)
  d. Agitation
  e. Cyanosis
  f. Tachycardia
 6. Manifestations of chronic venous insufficiency include:
  a. Chronic venous occlusion with resultant venous pooling and stasis
  b. Shifting of fluids from the intravascular to the interstitial compartments (especially in the ankles) as a result of dependent positioning

---

DISPLAY 3-2
Major Risk Factors Associated with Venous Thrombus

- Prolonged bed rest
- Surgery
- Advanced age
- Immobility
- Heart failure
- Pregnancy
- Use of oral contraceptives
- Obesity
- Malignancy
- Varicose veins
- Polycythemia
- Dehydration

        c.   Edematous, discolored extremity

        d.   Formation of venous stasis ulcers

 7. **The affected area will be red, swollen, hot, and tender; a positive Homans' sign (calf pain on dorsiflexion of the foot) will be present.**

D. Overview of nursing interventions

    1. For DVT:

        a.   Assess respiratory and circulatory functions frequently to prevent complications such as pulmonary embolism.

        b.   Administer anticoagulant therapy, as prescribed; monitor prothrombin time (PT) and partial thromboplastin time (PTT).

        c.   Administer thrombolytic therapy, as prescribed; monitor clotting profiles and observe for signs of hemorrhage.

        d.   Avoid manipulation (eg, massage) of affected extremities so as not to dislodge the clot.

        e.   Elevate the extremity to promote venous return.

        f.   Observe the extremity for edema, measuring the circumference 10 to 20 cm above and below the knee.

        g.   Instruct the patient to avoid aspirin while on anticoagulant medications to prevent excessive bleeding.

    2. For superficial thrombophlebitis:

        a.   Apply warm compresses over the affected site.

        b.   Elevate the extremity.

        c.   Administer anti-inflammatory agents (eg, aspirin or ibuprofen), as prescribed.

 3. **For chronic venous insufficiency, educate the patient about the prevention of phlebitis, thrombosis, and venous stasis ulcers, including:**

        a.   **Use of antiembolism stockings**

        b.   **Avoiding excessive constriction**

        c.   **Elevating lower extremities above the heart level when lying down**

        d.   **Avoiding venous pooling from sitting or standing for long periods**

XII. **Varicose veins**

A. **Description: dilated tortuous veins occurring most commonly in the lower extremities and lower trunk; may be primary or secondary**

B. **Etiology and incidence**

    1. Primary varicose veins appear without provocation in young persons and occur in the lower extremities; causative factors include a familial tendency and undetected valvular or vein wall defects.

    2. Incidence of primary varicose veins is higher in women than in men.

    3. Secondary varicose veins occur from damaged venous valves, most likely due to extrinsic factors such as:

        a.   Pregnancy

        b.   Thrombosis

     c.   Aging

     d.   Trauma

C. Pathophysiologic processes and manifestations

    1. The damaged valves or vein walls cause reversed flow, resulting in venous dilatation.

    2. **The actual site of damage-causing varicosity remains unknown; possible sites include the saphenofemoral junction and the perforator veins of the lower extremities.**

    3. The patient may experience discomfort; if the disease is extreme, it can be disfiguring and lead to an altered body image.

D. Overview of nursing interventions

    1. Aim interventions at relieving discomfort and improving appearance to diminish feelings of inadequacy.

    2. Encourage the patient to wear support stockings to reduce discomfort and avoid elastic bandages or any type of constricting clothing.

    3. Prepare the patient for surgery if pain is unrelieved or chronic phlebitis develops or for cosmetic purposes; afterward, provide appropriate postoperative care.

    4. Prepare the patient for sclerotherapy, if indicated, which involves injecting a solution that destroys the vein by fibrosis; afterward:

       a.   Instruct the patient about the importance of wearing compression bandages for at least 3 weeks.

       b.   Encourage walking to promote venous drainage.

XIII. Venous stasis ulcers

A. **Description: a lesion that usually develops on a lower extremity as a result of chronic venous hypertension**

B. Etiology

    1. Venous stasis ulcers usually result from chronic venous insufficiency.

    2. Other causes include any condition resulting in venous stasis or vein occlusion, such as trauma to the vessels, DVT, or obstruction.

    3. Incidence is increasing among the elderly.

C. Pathophysiologic processes and manifestations

    1. As venous stasis occurs, interstitial fluid shifts from the intravascular compartments, causing edema.

    2. Edema eventually leads to skin breakdown and ulcer formation.

    3. The affected area will usually be inflamed; drainage may be present and aching or pain may occur.

    4. Tissue necrosis and infection can also occur.

D. Overview of nursing interventions

    1. Assess the affected site for signs of infection, noting the color of drainage and the surrounding skin.

    2. Obtain specimen for culture and sensitivity if signs of infection exist.

    3. **Keep ulcer clean; use cleansing agents as prescribed to flush out necrotic tissue.**

4. Prepare the patient for surgical debridement if there is sloughing.
5. Use appropriate dressings (eg, sterile, nonadhesive, or absorbent).
6. Use bandages or stocking for compression, possibly in combination with dressings.

XIV. Lymphedema

A. Description: excessive accumulation of lymph fluid due to damaged or obstructed lymph vessels, with subsequent subcutaneous tissue swelling; may be primary or secondary

B. Etiology
1. Primary lymphedema results from unknown causes; possible causes include:
   a. Aplasia (absence of lymph vessels)
   b. Hypoplasia (less than the normal amount of lymph vessels)
   c. Hyperplasia (more than the normal amount of lymph vessels)
2. Types include:
   a. Congenital lymphedema
   b. Lymphedema praecox (occurs during puberty and is the most common type)
   c. Lymphedema tardia (occurs late in life, during the postmenopausal period)
3. Incidence of primary lymphedema is higher in women.
4. Secondary lymphedema results from another disease process; diseases that may lead to it include:
   a. Neoplasms
   b. Infections, such as dermatophytosis of the foot
   c. Mosquito-transmitted filariasis
   d. When lymph vessels are removed during surgery (eg, mastectomy).

 5. **Other causes of secondary lymphedema include procedures that obliterate lymph tissue, such as high-dose radiation therapy and surgical removal of lymph nodes.**

C. Pathophysiologic processes and manifestations
1. The lymph vessels or lymph nodes become obstructed either from swelling (eg, varicose veins) or from a mechanical obstruction (eg, tumor).
2. The increased quantity of lymph backs up and causes swelling in the affected extremity.
3. When the extremity is in the dependent position, swelling becomes more evident.
4. Edema may be soft and nonpitting as the process begins.
5. As the process continues, edema becomes firm.

D. Overview of nursing interventions
1. For primary lymphedema, institute palliative interventions to relieve swelling and discomfort.
2. For secondary lymphedema, assess the patient to determine the underlying cause.
3. Encourage the patient to exercise, which may move fluid from the lymph system into the circulation.

    4. Elevate the extremity to help move the fluid.

    5. Administer diuretics, as prescribed.

XV. **Acute lymphangitis**

A. Description

    1. Acute lymphangitis is an acute inflammation of one or more lymphatic vessels.

    2. If the nodes along the affected lymph vessels become involved, this is called lymphadenitis.

B. Etiology: causative organism is usually *Streptococcus pyogenes,* which enters the lymphatic system via a wound or from cellulitis on an extremity

C. Pathophysiologic processes and manifestations

    1. The organism travels from a peripheral site toward regional lymph nodes, resulting in enlargement and inflammation of lymph vessels.

    2. Red, warm, and sometimes discomforting streaks form in the inflamed area and extend to regional lymph nodes. The nodes become enlarged, red, and tender.

    3. Affected lymph nodes are usually in the groin, cervical area, and axillae.

    4. Common symptoms include hyperthermia with chills, headache, and tachycardia.

    5. Laboratory results will usually show leukocytosis.

    6. Rarely, the infection progresses to necrosis, ulceration, or suppurative cellulitis.

D. Overview of nursing interventions

    1. Monitor the infection site closely; report signs of worsening immediately.

    2. Administer antibiotics, analgesics, or antipyretics, as prescribed.

    3. Explain to the patient the importance of complying with the medication regimen.

Bibliography

Bullock, B. (1996). *Pathophysiology: Adaptations and alterations in function* (4th ed.). Philadelphia, Lippincott.

Carpenito, L. J. (1991). *Nursing care plans and documentation: Nursing diagnoses and collaborative problems.* New York: J. B. Lippincott.

Clayton, T. (1989). *Taber's cyclopedic medical dictionary* (16th ed.). Philadelphia: F. A. Davis.

Ganong, William F. (1997). *Review of Medical Physiology* (18th ed.). Stamford, CT: Appleton and Lange.

Guyton, Arthur C., & Hall, John E. (1996). *Textbook of medical physiology* (9th ed.). Philadelphia: W. B. Saunders.

Hurst, J. W. (ed.). (1991). *Current therapy in cardiovascular disease* (3rd ed.). Philadelphia: B. C. Decker.

Kinney, M., Packa, D., & Dunbar, S. (1993). *AACN's clinical reference for critical care nursing* (3rd ed.). St. Louis: C. V. Mosby.

McCance, K. L., & Huether, S. E.(1994). *Pathophysiology: The biologic basis for disease in adults and children* (2nd ed.). St. Louis: Mosby–Year Book.

Porth, C. (1994). *Pathophysiology: Concepts of altered health states* (4th ed.). Philadelphia: Lippincott.

Silver, M. D. (ed.) (1991). *Cardiovascular pathology,* Vol I (2nd ed.). New York: Churchill Livingstone.

Tierney, L., McPhee, S., Papadakis, M., & Schroeder, S. eds. (1993). *Current medical diagnosis and treatment.* Norwalk, CT: Appleton & Lange.

STUDY QUESTIONS

1. Which of the following factors is not a predisposing factor for arteriosclerosis?
   a. diabetes mellitus
   b. heredity
   c. hypertension
   d. anemia

2. Mr. Johnstone, age 60, has been hospitalized for chronic renal failure. He is a heavy smoker and has been under treatment for hypertension, high cholesterol, and obesity. The most likely contributing factor for his renal failure might be:
   a. neurologic dysfunction
   b. cystitis
   c. renal arterial stenosis
   d. gastritis

3. Secondary hypertension may result from:
   a. glomerulonephritis
   b. sedentary lifestyle
   c. stress
   d. hereditary factors

4. Blood pressure elevations directly result from:
   a. increased cardiac output or increased peripheral resistance
   b. venous stasis
   c. decreased peripheral resistance
   d. diminished blood flow

5. Teaching for a patient with hypertension should include:
   a. diet and fluid restrictions
   b. activity restrictions and diet
   c. diet, medication regimen, and blood pressure measurement
   d. infection prevention, and signs and symptoms of internal bleeding

6. A postoperative surgical patient develops pain, redness, and edema in the calf. These symptoms may potentially indicate which of the following conditions?
   a. arterial embolism
   b. varicose veins
   c. thrombophlebitis
   d. lymphedema

7. When assessing a postoperative patient with thrombophlebitis for signs of pulmonary embolism, the nurse would:
   a. observe the extremities for edema
   b. observe for sudden onset of chest pain, dyspnea, and cyanosis
   c. assess the extremity for rash or hyperthermia
   d. monitor the pulse in the extremity

8. When developing a teaching plan for a patient with thrombophlebitis, which of the following instructions would the nurse not include?
   a. wear antiembolic stockings
   b. avoid venous pooling from sitting or standing for long periods
   c. keep extremity below the horizontal plane
   d. avoid excessive constriction

9. Venous stasis ulcers are caused by:
   a. arterial hypotension
   b. chronic venous hypertension
   c. thrombophlebitis
   d. Raynaud's phenomenon

10. The etiology of thromboangiitis obliterans (Buerger's disease) is unknown. However, to limit blood vessel destruction in a patient with this disorder, the nurse should instruct the patient to:
    a. limit fluid intake
    b. exercise regularly
    c. elevate extremities
    d. stop smoking

11. A patient with varicose veins is preparing to receive sclerotherapy. The nurse must make sure that the patient:
    a. elevates the feet for two weeks
    b. applies constrictive stockings
    c. avoids ambulating
    d. applies compression bandage for 3 weeks

12. When layers of an artery separate from each other in the presence of an aneurysm, the condition is known as:
    a. fusiform

    b. rupture

    c. dissecting

    d. saccular

13. The danger of arterial embolism exists because:

    a. fluid and electrolyte alterations occur

    b. an infection often develops

    c. arrythmias often result

    d. acute ischemia may result

14. A woman who has had radiation to the axillary lymph nodes may experience:

    a. lymphedema

    b. lymphangitis

    c. infection

    d. fever

ANSWER KEY

Question	Correct answer	Correct answer rationale	Incorrect answer rationales
1.	d	Anemia is not a risk factor.	a, b, and c. Major risk factors include diabetes mellitus, heredity, hypertension, cigarette smoking, elevated serum cholesterol, and obesity.
2.	c	Renal arterial stenosis secondary to cigarette smoking, hypertension, obesity, and high cholesterol can cause chronic renal failure.	a, b, and d. These are incorrect.
3.	a	Secondary hypertension results from preexisting diseases, including glomerulonephritis.	b, c, and d. These are risk factors for primary hypertension.
4.	a	Elevations in blood pressure result directly from increased cardiac output or increased peripheral vascular resistance.	b, c, and d. These conditions would not result in increased blood pressure.
5.	c	Instruct the patient about the importance of complying with medication therapy, the proper techniques for blood pressure measurement, and the need to limit dietary sodium.	a. Fluid restrictions are not a routine part of hypertension management. b. Restricting activity is not correct. d. Infection is not associated with hypertension.
6.	c	Pain, redness, and edema in the calf of a postoperative patient indicate thrombophlebitis resulting from venous stasis.	a, b, and d. The symptoms are not indicative of these disorders.
7.	b	Cardinal signs of pulmonary embolus include sudden onset of chest pain, dyspnea, and cyanosis. A patient with thrombophlebitis is at increased risk for this complication.	a, c, and d. These assessments focus on the extremity, but pulmonary embolism would require cardiovascular and pulmonary assessment.
8.	c	When providing patient teaching, the nurse should tell the patient to elevate the lower extremity above the heart level when lying down.	a, b, and d. These are actions that should be taken in thrombophlebitis.
9.	b	Venous stasis ulcers usually result from chronic venous hypertension.	a, c, and d. These are not causes associated with this disease.

Question	Correct answer	Correct answer rationale	Incorrect answer rationales
10.	d	Thromboangiitis obliterans (Buerger's disease) affects male cigarette smokers between ages 20 and 40. There is no documented evidence that it occurs in nonsmokers.	a, b, and c. These are not associated with the etiology of this disease.
11.	d	Compression bandages must be applied for 3 weeks after sclerotherapy. This encourages circulation.	a. This choice is incorrect because elevating the feet does not encourage healing. b. This choice is incorrect because constriction is always contraindicated in this disorder. This is because the constriction impedes venous return. c. This choice is incorrect because ambulation is encouraged because it facilitates venous drainage.
12.	c	A dissecting aneurysm occurs when layers of the artery separate from each other.	a and d. These choices are incorrect because they are types of aneurysms. b. This choice is incorrect because rupture means that the vessel has opened and the person is bleeding.
13.	d	The danger of arterial embolism is ischemia. This happens as the clot takes up space in the vessel lumen which impairs the flow of blood to the area supplied by the effected artery.	a, b, and c. These choices are incorrect because these situations are not in any way associated with embolism.
14.	a	Secondary lymphedema results from removal of or damage to lymphnodes. This damage may result from radiation which may obliterate lymph tissue.	b. This choice is incorrect because lymphangitis is infection of the lymph nodes. c and d. These choices are not related to this situation.

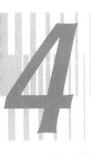

Shock States

I.   Overview of pathophysiologic processes

A.   Description

1.   **Shock is an acute, life-threatening condition in which body tissues are inadequately perfused or unable to utilize oxygen.**

2.   It results in alterations in tissue metabolism and function, from the cellular to the systemic levels.

3.   Shock can be categorized into four major types:

    a.   Hypovolemic

    b.   Cardiogenic

    c.   Obstructive

    d.   Distributive

4.   *Hypovolemic shock* is a state characterized by inadequate amounts of blood volume in the intravascular space.

5.   *Cardiogenic shock* is a condition in which myocardial damage renders the heart unable to pump enough blood to maintain adequate perfusion.

6.   *Obstructive shock* occurs when blood flow is impeded by a mechanical or physical obstruction.

7.   *Distributive shock* refers to conditions involving alterations in the distribution of intravascular volume. It includes three categories:

    a.   Septic

    b.   Neurogenic

    c.   Anaphylactic

B.   Mechanisms of dysfunction

1.   **In all types of shock, inadequate tissue perfusion results in decreased cell oxygenation.**

2.   Decreased cell oxygenation reduces the cell membrane potential and contributes to alterations in cell membrane permeability and the sodium–potassium pump.

3.   As a result, potassium moves out of the cell into the extracellular space, and sodium and water enter the cell.

4.   As sodium accumulates in the cell, the sodium–potassium pump increases its activity, requiring increased amounts of adenosine triphosphate (ATP).

5.   Because of poor oxygenation, production of ATP and cyclic adenosine monophosphate (AMP) declines, causing functions dependent on these substances to cease.

6.   Calcium regulation is affected, which further impairs production of ATP and cyclic AMP.

7.   Because of the sodium flux, cells and major organelles swell, leading to decreased mitochondrial ability and disrupted cellular activity.

8.   Further intracellular membrane changes occur, allowing lysosomes to leak and causing autodigestion of cellular contents.

9.   Eventually, the cell is destroyed and toxic factors such as bradykinin are released, causing additional cellular degradation.

10.   **A shift to anaerobic metabolism causes production of lactate and hydrogen ions to increase, resulting in lactic acidosis.**

11.   Even if perfusion is reestablished, all of the damage cannot be reversed; sec-

ondary cellular injury related to edema and toxic metabolites also can occur.

C. Stages of shock

1. *Compensated or nonprogressive shock:* Vital organs remain adequately perfused because of compensatory mechanisms.

2. *Decompensated or progressive shock:* Vital organs become underperfused and compensatory mechanisms become ineffective, resulting in systemic manifestations.

3. *Irreversible shock:* The extent of shock is so severe that therapeutic interventions become useless; death eventually occurs.

II. Physiologic responses to shock

A. Sympathetic nervous system (SNS) activation

1. **As perfusion decreases, impulses are transmitted to the vasomotor center of the brain, causing SNS activation as a compensatory mechanism.**

2. SNS activation results in vasoconstriction of the arterial bed and increased cardiac inotropic and chronotropic activity.

B. Tachycardia: abnormally rapid heart rate

C. Skin color and temperature changes

1. **In the early stages of shock, blood is shunted to the brain and heart and away from the skin and other organs that tolerate ischemia well.**

2. As a result, the skin appears pale and feels cool.

D. Hypotension: occurs when compensatory mechanisms become inadequate

E. Microcirculatory changes

1. As shock progresses, the venous sphincters are less able to maintain vasoconstriction.

2. Blood flow in the capillary beds becomes sluggish; eventually, microcirculation is blocked.

F. Coagulation abnormalities

1. Metabolic waste products and microaggregates of platelets and clotting factors accumulate in the capillary bed, resulting in clotting.

2. Thrombocytopenia may also occur, particularly in septic shock.

G. Hyperglycemia

1. In response to the release of epinephrine, glycogen is broken down into glucose, which is released into the circulation.

2. Lipolysis results in increased amounts of free fatty acids and increased levels of glucocorticoids, cortisone, and cortisol, contributing to the production of more glucose.

H. Tachypnea: rapid breathing

I. Fluid shifts

1. **To increase fluid retention and improve perfusion, renin is produced by the juxtaglomerular apparatus in the kidneys and antidiuretic hormone (ADH) is produced by the hypothalamus.**

    2.   In addition, activation of the renin-angiotensin system eventually results in further vasoconstriction in an attempt to raise blood pressure.

J. End organ damage, including:

    1.   Impaired removal of waste products secondary to decreased renal function.

    2.   Depression of the reticuloendothelial system resulting in impaired inflammatory and immune response.

    3.   Pulmonary edema and adult respiratory distress syndrome (ARDS).

    4.   Disseminated intravascular coagulation.

    5.   Hepatic dysfunction including fatty infiltrates and decreased clearance.

    6.   Gastrointestinal (GI) problems including ulcerations and enteritis.

    7.   Nutritional deficits secondary to impaired GI function.

    8.   Central nervous system (CNS) damage.

III.   Hypovolemic shock

A. Description: a state characterized by inadequate amounts of blood volume in the intravascular space

B. Etiology

    1.   Hypovolemic shock results from direct or indirect volume losses.

    2.   Direct volume losses include:

        a.   Frank bleeding

        b.   Diarrhea or vomiting

        c.   Diuresis

        d.   Loss of plasma through skin (eg, burns)

    3.   Indirect volume losses include:

        a.   Sequestration of fluid into third spaces (eg, ascites and abdominal obstruction)

        b.   Internal volume losses (eg, hemothorax, hemorrhagic pancreatitis, and splenic rupture)

        c.   Internal fluid shifts (eg, addisonian crisis and hypopituitarism)

C. Pathophysiologic processes and manifestations

    1.   Hypovolemic shock can be categorized as mild, moderate, or severe; symptoms vary according to the severity of the volume deficit.

    2.   Symptoms of mild hypovolemic shock:

        a.   Maximum volume loss is 10%.

        b.   Cardiac output will be decreased, resulting in SNS activation.

        c.   SNS activation is sufficient to maintain normotensive blood pressure and heart rate.

        d.   Skin appears pale, feels cool and clammy because blood is shunted away from it and to vital organs.

        e.   Mucosa is mildly dry.

        f.   Skin turgor is decreased.

        g.   Neurologic manifestations can include anxiety, restlessness, thirst, and weakness.

    3.   Symptoms of moderate hypovolemic shock:

        a.   Volume loss reaches 15% to 40%.

        b.   Cardiac output and blood pressure decrease dramatically.

       c.   Arteriolar vasoconstriction results in decreased perfusion of the kidneys and GI organs.

       d.   Common manifestations include tachycardia, tachypnea, pallor, diaphoresis, hypotension, and CNS activation, including restlessness.

       e.   Other symptoms can include thirst, poor skin turgor, and decreased urine output.

       f.   Although the bone marrow increases production of new blood products, the demand exceeds the ability to replace cells.

  4.   Symptoms of severe hypovolemic shock:

       a.   Volume loss exceeds 45%.

       b.   Compensatory mechanisms are functioning at maximum.

       c.   Vital organs display evidence of impaired perfusion.

       d.   Neurologic manifestations of underperfusion include decreased level of consciousness, confusion, and agitation.

       e.   Metabolic alterations include hyperglycemia and lactic acidosis.

       f.   If shock continues, cell death and severe end organ damage will occur.

D.   Overview of nursing interventions

  1.   **Institute fluid replacement therapy as prescribed. Fluid replacement should be with normal saline because all of the fluid stays in the intravascular space.**

  2.   Administer infusion of blood products, as ordered, for a patient who has experienced frank blood loss.

  3.   Assess for the primary cause of shock in cases of third-space shifting to prevent further volume loss.

  4.   Use military anti-shock trousers (MAST) with a patient who has experienced frank blood loss to cause venocompression and improve venous return.

  5.   Assess hemodynamic status and all major body systems.

  6.   **Monitor the patient's intake and output to ensure adequate fluid replacement.**

IV. Cardiogenic shock

A.   Description: a condition in which myocardial damage renders the heart unable to pump enough blood to maintain adequate perfusion

B.   Etiology

  1.   **Cardiogenic shock is a sequela of myocardial infarction (MI), occurring when 40 to 50% of the myocardium has been destroyed.**

  2.   It also occurs secondary to valvular dysfunction (eg, mitral regurgitation, papillary muscle rupture, ventricular aneurysms, and severe dysrhythmias) or as a result of end-stage cardiomyopathies.

C.   Pathophysiologic processes and manifestations

  1.   Impaired ventricular pumping ability reduces stroke volume and cardiac output.

2. **To compensate for decreased cardiac output, vascular resistance increases to maintain normotension.**

3. Increased resistance increases the workload on the ventricle as blood is forced to pump against increased pressure; this further decreases cardiac output.

4. SNS activation results in the release of catecholamines, further increasing the afterload against which the ventricle must pump.

5. The SNS also increases ventricular contractility, which may further exacerbate ischemia and failure.

6. Left ventricular end diastolic pressure rises and the ventricle distends; this pressure extends to the pulmonary bed and can contribute to pulmonary edema.

7. Hypoxemia and acidosis may occur.

8. Manifestations of compensated shock include:
   a. Alterations in mentation
   b. Restlessness
   c. Weakness
   d. Decreased urine output
   e. Alterations in peripheral perfusion (eg, pallor, cool skin, jugular venous distention, and delayed capillary refill)
   f. Hemodynamic manifestations, such as tachycardia, narrowed pulse pressure, mild hypotension or normal blood pressure, and altered pulmonary function (eg, tachypnea, orthopnea, and crackles)

9. Manifestations of uncompensated shock include:
   a. Increased alterations in mentation
   b. Oliguria
   c. Frank hypotension
   d. Elevated central venous and pulmonary pressures
   e. Pulmonary deterioration (associated with a decrease in tidal volume, increasing pulmonary congestion, and cyanosis)

10. Manifestations of irreversible shock include:
   a. Obtundation
   b. Coma
   c. Anuria or oliguria
   d. Marked tachycardia
   e. Dysrhythmias
   f. Severe hypotension
   g. Deteriorated pulmonary status

D. Overview of nursing interventions

1. Assess hemodynamic and pulmonary systems.
2. Manage invasive monitoring equipment and monitor heart rhythm.
3. Administer vasopressors and diuretics as prescribed.
4. Administer preload and afterload agents as prescribed. (This condition cannot reverse unless appropriate amounts of medications are given.)
5. Prepare patient for insertion of intraaortic balloon pump or ventricular assist device if necessary.
6. Provide supportive care as indicated.

V. Obstructive shock

A. Description: a condition in which blood flow is impeded by a mechanical or physical obstruction

B. Etiology: causes include pulmonary emboli, tension pneumo-thorax, ruptured hemidiaphragm, dissecting aortic aneurysms, pericardial tamponade, and atrial myxoma.

C. Pathophysiologic processes and manifestations

    1. Venous return decreases due to increased pressures around the right atrium or within the chest wall.

    2. Decreased venous return results in less volume available for the ventricles to pump to end organs, causing inadequate perfusion.

    3. Manifestations of obstructive shock resemble those associated with hypovolemic shock (see Section III, C).

D. Overview of nursing interventions

    1. Prepare the patient for chest tube insertion, pericardial tap, or other surgical intervention.

    2. Replace volume with crystalloid or colloids.

    3. Provide supportive therapy as indicated.

    4. Provide swift and accurate care.

VI. Septic shock

A. Description: a type of distributive shock, this condition occurs secondary to septicemia and is characterized by vascular collapse.

B. Etiology

    1. The major cause of septic shock is Gram-negative bacteria.

    2. It also can be caused by Gram-positive bacteria, viruses, fungi, and rickettsiae.

    3. Mortality associated with septic shock is high because it results in multisystem organ failure.

C. Pathophysiologic processes and manifestations

    1. Invading Gram-negative bacteria release toxins called endotoxins.

    2. Endotoxins are lipopolysaccharides that initiate a systemic inflammatory response syndrome (SIRS), activating a number of protein-based systems, including chemical, cellular, and immune or humoral mediators. The chemical mediators include the complement, clotting, kinin, and renin-angiotensin systems.

    3. The complement system increases the production of platelets, leukocytes, and mast cells and the release of anaphylatoxins.

    4. The vasoactive mediators histamine, prostaglandins, brady-kinin, and serotonin also are released, causing massive vasodilation and increased capillary permeability.

    5. The clotting system initiates the production of fibrin clots throughout the body; these clots impair blood flow and decrease perfusion.

6. Activating the renin-angiotensin system results in the release of epinephrine, norepinephrine, and aldosterone, leading to increased sodium and water retention and improved myocardial contractility. In the early stages of septic shock, symptoms include those associated with SNS activation such as tachycardia, tachypnea, and increased cardiac output.

7. Cellular mediators are involved with macrophage, granulocyte, and lymphocytic activity.

8. Immune or humoral mediators such as prostaglandins, tumor necrosis factors, interleukins, and myocardial depressant factors also contribute to cellular destruction and clinical deterioration.

9. In the hyperdynamic phase, symptoms include:
   a. Decreased vascular resistance, while blood pressure is barely maintained
   b. Peripheral vasodilation
   c. Normal to high cardiac output
   d. Hypotension or normotension
   e. Fever
   f. Slight alterations in sensorium (eg, warm flushed peripheral skin and normal capillary refill)
   g. Moderate tachycardia
   h. Tachypnea with adventitious breath sounds
   i. Normal urine output
   j. Hyperthermia

10. In the hypodynamic phase, symptoms include:
    a. Profoundly impaired perfusion
    b. Decreased cardiac output and increased resistance
    c. Mental status changes, such as lethargy and coma
    d. Clammy, pale skin
    e. Hemodynamic manifestations, including tachycardia, dysrhythmias, hypotension, and decreased cardiac output
    f. Pulmonary congestion
    g. Central cyanosis

10. Decreased perfusion results in impaired oxygenation and clotting abnormalities, including disseminated intravascular coagulation (DIC).

11. In the final stage, multiorgan dysfunction occurs.

D. Overview of nursing interventions
   1. Administer appropriate antibiotics or antiviral agents as prescribed.
   2. Administer vasoactive agents as prescribed.
   3. Replace fluid with crystalloid.
   4. Provide supportive care of the pulmonary and cardiac systems as indicated.
   5. Monitor for evidence of end organ damage (associated with a high mortality rate).
   6. After killing the bacteria, manage any sequelae of the infection which are often serious conditions, such as renal failure, life-threatening electrolyte disorders, or cardiac arrhythmias.

    7.   Provide swift and accurate care as every body system is effected by the process.

 VII. **Neurogenic shock**

A. Description

1. **A type of distributive shock, neurogenic shock is characterized by a loss of SNS vasomotor function.**
2. This results in extreme vasodilation throughout the body, creating a maldistribution of blood volume.

B. Etiology
1. Neurogenic shock results from injury to the brain stem or to the spinal cord (high thoracic or low cervical), usually as a result of a traumatic event.
2. It also has been associated with hypoxia, lack of glucose (or excessive insulin), and the depressant action of drugs (particularly anesthetic agents).

C. Pathophysiologic processes and manifestations

1. **CNS system injury disrupts normal regulation of vasomotor tone, causing massive vasodilation throughout the body; this results in pooling of blood in the periphery.**
2. Venous return and cardiac output decrease.
3. The decrease in cardiac output causes inadequate tissue perfusion.

4. Common manifestations include:
    a. **Alterations in mentation, ranging from confusion to coma**
    b. **Alterations in peripheral perfusion, including cool and clammy skin above the lesion and warm, dry skin below (if a spinal cord lesion exists)**
    c. **Normal capillary refill with palpable distal pulses**
    d. **Bradycardia**
    e. **Hypotension**
    f. **Decreased pulse pressure**
    g. **Tachypnea**
    h. **Normal urine output**

D. Overview of nursing interventions
1. Replace fluid with crystalloid or colloids as ordered.
2. Administer vasopressors and antiarrhythmics as prescribed.
3. Administer steroids, as prescribed, depending on the causative injury.
4. Maintain airway and provide pulmonary support.
5. Provide supportive care as indicated for the circulatory system.

 VIII. **Anaphylactic shock**

A. Description

1. **A type of distributive shock, anaphylactic shock is a severe, life-threatening allergic reaction to an antigen or other agent.**

2.   It is characterized by respiratory distress and vascular collapse; onset typically is sudden.

B.   Etiology

1.   **Common causes of anaphylactic shock include:**
     a.   **Reactions to drugs, such as penicillin and hormones**
     b.   **Stings from insects, such as bees and wasps**
     c.   **Ingestion of certain foods, such as peanuts and shellfish**
2.   Anaphylactic shock is considered a Type-I hypersensitivity response that most commonly involves immunoglobulin E.

C.   Pathophysiologic processes and manifestations

1.   After the first exposure to an antigen or foreign agent, antibodies are made.
2.   Infrequently, the first exposure results in symptoms of anaphylaxis; typically, true anaphylactic shock occurs after the second exposure.
3.   In response to the antigen–antibody complex formation, vasoactive mediators such as histamine and leukotrienes are released.
4.   These mediators cause systemic vasodilation and alterations in capillary permeability.
5.   The resultant peripheral pooling of blood and decreased venous return and cardiac output cause cellular hypoperfusion.
6.   Swelling of the airway also can occur due to the inflammatory response, resulting in bronchoconstriction.

7.   **Symptoms of anaphylactic shock include:**
     a.   **Alterations in mentation, including restlessness progressing to coma**
     b.   **Cutaneous manifestations, including urticaria, pruritus, and angioedema**
     c.   **Bronchoconstriction, accompanied by tachypnea, wheezing, and use of accessory muscles**
     d.   **Hemodynamic manifestations, including warm and flushed skin, tachycardia, dysrhythmias, angina, and hypotension**

D.   Overview of nursing interventions

1.   Ensure and maintain a patent airway.
2.   Prepare the patient for endotracheal intubation as indicated.
3.   Administer fluids and vasopressors as prescribed.
4.   Administer antihistamines (Benadryl®) or epinephrine to promote vasoconstriction, as prescribed.
5.   Administer steroids, as prescribed, to reduce the inflammatory response associated with exposure to the allergen.
6.   Provide supportive care as indicated.

Bibliography

Bone, R. C. (1996). Diagnosing sepses: What we need to consider today. *Journal Crit. Illn.*, 11(10): 658–60.

Bone, R. C. (1997). Managing sepsis: What treatments can we use today? *Journal of Crit. Illn.*, 12(1): 15–19, 23–24.

Brar, R. S. et al. (1996). Administering fluid resuscitation effectively for traumatic shock. *Journal Crit Ill.*, 11(10): 672–4, 677–8.

Bullock, B. (1996). *Pathophysiology: Adaptations and alterations in function* (4th ed.). Philadelphia: Lippincott-Raven.

De Jong, M. J. (1997). Clinical snapshot. Cardiogenic shock. *American Journal of Nursing*, 97(6): 40–1.

Ganong, William F. (1997). *Review of medical physiology* (18th ed.). Stanford, CT: Appleton and Lange.

Guyton, Arthur C., & Hall, John E. (1996). *Textbook of medical physiology* (9th ed.). Philadelphia: W. B. Saunders.

Horvath, C. (1994). *Emergency nursing core curriculum* (4th ed.). Chap. 17, Shock emergencies. Philadelphia: W. B. Saunders.

Kinney, M., Packa, D., & Dunbar, S. (1993). *AACN's clinical reference for critical-care nursing* (3rd ed.). St. Louis: C.V. Mosby.

McCance, K. L., & Huether, S. E. (1994). *Pathophysiology: The biologic basis for disease in adults and children* (2nd ed.). St. Louis: Mosby-Year Book.

Porth, C. (1994). *Pathophysiology: Concepts of altered health states* (4th ed.). Philadelphia: Lippincott-Raven.

Sandrock J. (1997). Managing hypovolemia. *Nursing*, Feb. 27 (2), 32aa–bb.

Vincent, J. (1997). Clinical trials in sepses: Where do we stand? Clinical Commentary. *Journal of Critical Care*, March; 12(1): 3–6.

Wardle, E. N. (1996). Experimental and futuristic approaches to treatment of septic shock. Part II. *Care Crit Ill.*, Nov–Dec. 12(6): 21–220.

Wardle, E. N. (1996). Prevention and treatment of septic shock, SIRS, ARDS, and multiorgan failure. *Care Crit. Ill.*, 12(5): 177–80.

STUDY QUESTIONS

1. Inadequate perfusion results in which of the following changes?
   a. decreased cell membrane permeability
   b. reduction in cell membrane potential
   c. movement of sodium out of the cell
   d. increased ADP production

2. The shift to anaerobic metabolism results in:
   a. decreased hydrogen ion production
   b. alkalosis
   c. decreased oxygen utilization
   d. increased lactate production

3. In the early stages of shock, blood is shunted toward the:
   a. brain
   b. skin
   c. muscle
   d. kidneys

4. Activation of the renin–angiotensin system in shock causes:
   a. vasodilation
   b. sodium shifts
   c. fluid retention
   d. glucogenosis

5. In the mild stage of hypovolemic shock, all of the following symptoms are present *except:*
   a. tachycardia
   b. pale skin
   c. decreased cardiac output
   d. normal blood pressure

6. In moderate hypovolemic shock:
   a. lactic acidosis is present
   b. SNS compensation ensures maintenance of blood pressure and cardiac output
   c. bone marrow production of cells decreases dramatically
   d. arteriolar vasoconstriction results in decreased perfusion of the kidneys and GI organs

7. In the compensated stage of cardiogenic shock, anticipate that:

   a. cardiac output is increased
   b. systemic vascular resistance is increased
   c. blood pressure is decreased
   d. systemic vascular resistance is decreased

8. Pulmonary sequelae of cardiogenic shock include:
   a. increased pulmonary congestion
   b. increased tidal volume
   c. tachypnea
   d. decreased pulmonary resistance

9. Distributive shock includes all of the following types of shock except:
   a. anaphylactic shock
   b. septic shock
   c. cardiogenic shock
   d. neurogenic shock

10. The vasoactive mediators released in septic shock contribute to:
    a. increased sodium and water retention
    b. increased capillary permeability
    c. fibrin deposition in the capillary bed
    d. increased production of mast cells

11. A woman brings her husband into the emergency department with urticaria, angioedema, bronchoconstriction, and restlessness. She states they had just finished a fish dinner and this came on suddenly. The nurse should recognize this as:
    a. respiratory distress
    b. allergic reaction
    c. anaphylactic shock
    d. cardiac disorder

12. A nurse caring for a patient with a myocardial infarction discovers the following symptoms in her patient: restlessness, decreased urine output, jugular vein distention, hypotension, crackles, and tachycardia. She knows that these signs are consistent with:
    a. cardiogenic shock
    b. dysrythmia

c. extension of the infarct

d. obstructive shock

13. Which shock state is treated with vaso-pressors and diuretics rather than fluid replacement?

  a. hypovolemic

  b. septic

  c. neurogenic

  d. cardiogenic

14. Loss of SNS motor function resulting in vasodilation, maldistribution of blood volume, and shock occurs in:

  a. septic shock

  b. neurogenic shock

  c. hypovolemic shock

  d. cardiogenic shock

ANSWER KEY

Question	Correct answer	Correct answer rationale	Incorrect answer rationales
1.	b	Inadequate perfusion results in decreased oxygen delivery to the tissue, which reduces the cell membrane potential. This reduction in potential contributes to alterations in membrane permeability and altered sodium–potassium pump processes.	a. Cell membrane permeability actually increases as the cell membrane potential is reduced. c. Sodium moves into the cell and not out of the cell. d. ADP and ATP production are decreased as impaired perfusion occurs.
2.	d	Anaerobic metabolism causes lactic acid to accumulate and contributes to the development of lactic acidosis.	a. Hydrogen ion production increases in anaerobic metabolism. b. Acidosis occurs in anaerobic metabolism, not acidosis. c. Decreased oxygen availability leads to the need for anaerobic metabolism, but the presence of this type of metabolism does not decrease oxygen utilization.
3.	a	In shock, blood is redirected away from "nonvital" organs such as the skin to "vital" organs such as the brain and heart.	b, c, and d. In shock, blood is shunted away from these organs and toward the brain and heart.
4.	c	Activation of the renin–angiotensin system in the kidneys is directed toward increasing the reabsorption of sodium and water and vasoconstriction in order to increase blood pressure.	a. Vasoconstriction, not vasodilation, results from activation of the renin–angiotensin system. b. Sodium is reabsorbed indirectly but is not a major action of the renin–angiotensin system. d. Glucogenesis has nothing to do with the renin–angiotensin system.
5.	a	Tachycardia is not seen in mild stages of hypovolemic shock because the body's compensatory mechanisms are able to maintain normal vital signs and perfusion. Tachycardia does appear with moderate to severe shock.	b, c, and d. All of these symptoms are present with mild hypovolemic shock.
6.	d	In moderate hypovolemic shock, arteriolar vasoconstriction occurs, decreasing perfusion of the kidneys and GI organs.	a. Lactic acidosis does not occur until the severe stage of hypovolemic shock. b. Although the SNS is still functioning in moderate hypovolemic shock, it is not optimally effective because blood pressure and cardiac output cannot be maintained. c. Bone marrow production of cells increases in this stage.

Question	Correct answer	Correct answer rationale	Incorrect answer rationales
7.	b	Systemic vascular resistance increases in cardiogenic shock to compensate for a decreased cardiac output.	a. Cardiac output is decreased. c. Blood pressure is maintained. d. Systemic vascular resistance is increased.
8.	a	As the myocardium fails, left ventricular end diastolic pressure rises. This pressure is transmitted to the pulmonary vasculature resulting in pulmonary edema.	b. Tidal volume is not affected directly. c. Tachypnea may be seen as pulmonary congestion occurs, but it is not a direct sequela of the failure. d. Pulmonary resistance increases as congestion occurs.
9.	c	Distributive shock refers to any condition in which there is abnormal distribution of intravascular volume. This can occur with anaphylactic, neurogenic, and septic shock. In cardiogenic shock, the ventricles are unable to pump efficiently.	a, b, and d. These are incorrect.
10.	b	In septic shock, the vasoactive mediators released function to increase capillary permeability, thereby allowing fluid to move out of the vascular bed and into the interstitial space.	a. Sodium and water are not directly retained in septic shock, but are merely redistributed. c. Fibrin deposition does occur, but this is because of the clotting cascade and not due to vasoactive mediator activity. d. The complement system increases production of mast cells, not vasoactive mediators.
11.	c	These are signs of anaphylactic shock. This type of shock is seen with ingestion of fish, peanuts, penicillin, and hormones. It is also common in bee stings.	a and b. These choices are incorrect because anaphylactic shock is the better choice. A fish allergy will cause anaphylactic shock and respiratory distress is a symptom. e. This choice is incorrect because there is no evidence here of cardiac disorder.
12.	a	Cardiogenic shock occurs when myocardial damage renders the heart unable to pump enough blood to maintain adequate perfusion. Symptoms described in letter a are consistent with cardiogenic shock.	b and c. These choices are incorrect because they may cause cardiogenic shock by reducing the cardiac output, but letter a is the best choice because it supercedes the others. d. This choice is incorrect because it is inconsistent with the scenario and the symptoms described.

Question	Correct answer	Correct answer rationale	Incorrect answer rationales
13.	d	Cardiogenic shock is never treated by infusing fluids. In cardiogenic shock, the heart cannot pump the existing fluid and relief of volume is indicated. Adding volume to a patient in cardiogenic shock can be fatal because the heart cannot pump the volume through out the body.	a, b, and c. These choices are incorrect because these shock states are treated with fluid replacement.
14.	b	Neurogenic shock results in this phenomenon.	a, c, and d. These choices are incorrect because they are not related to loss of SNS motor tone.

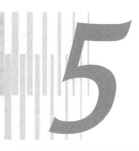

5 Craniocerebral Disorders

I.   Overview of pathophysiologic processes

A. Intracranial pressure and volume disorders

1. **Intracranial pressure (ICP) is the pressure produced by three components within the skull: brain tissue, cerebrospinal fluid (CSF), and blood.**

2. Increased ICP is a disorder that occurs when the volume of any of the three intracranial components rises abnormally.

3. Increased ICP commonly is caused by increases in tissue volume resulting from brain tumors, hematomas, or cerebral edema.

4. Herniation, a shifting of brain contents from a high-pressure compartment (the brain) to one of lower pressure (the spinal canal through the foramen magnum), results from unabated increasing ICP.

5. **Risk factors include any injury or disease to the brain.**

B. Cerebrovascular disorders

1. Cerebrovascular disorders impair blood flow to the brain, either as a result of vessel occlusion or hemorrhaging due to ruptured vessels.

2. **The amount of tissue damage and the resulting type and severity of neurologic deficits depend on the amount of oxygen deprivation and the location and severity of the bleeding.**

3. Cerebrovascular disorders can be ischemic or hemorrhagic.

4. *Ischemic disorders*
   a. Are local, temporary, reversible disruptions of the blood supply resulting from oxygen deprivation
   b. Include transient ischemic attacks (TIA)

5. *Hemorrhagic disorders*
   a. Involve actual bleeding into the brain
   b. Commonly result from ruptured aneurysm or arteriovenous malformation (AVM), a congenital malformation of blood vessels
   c. May also result from the rupture of any cerebral vessel, especially when the vessel is under pressure (as in hypertension)

6. Although categorized as traumatic injuries, hematomas may also be considered cerebrovascular disorders because they result in bleeding into the brain.

7. Common risk factors for CVA and TIA include:
   a. History of hypertension, diabetes, or high cholesterol and triglyceride levels

b. Lifestyle factors such as obesity, cigarette smoking, and lack of physical exercise

8. Other risk factors for CVA and TIA include oral contraceptive use, dehydration, coagulation disorders, sickle cell disease, and hypothyroidism.

C. Head trauma

1. Head trauma refers to any injury to the head that results in injury to the brain.
2. Resulting tissue damage depends on the severity of the injury and the amount of edema present.
3. Types of head trauma include:
   a. Closed head injuries (concussions, contusions, and diffuse axonal injuries)
   b. Hematomas (subdural, epidural, subarachnoid, and intracerebral)

D. Seizure disorders

1. A seizure is a sudden explosive discharge of central nervous system (CNS) neurons; it may be primary or secondary.
2. Epilepsy is a primary disease characterized by seizure activity.
3. Secondary causes of seizures include:
   a. Chemical changes (occurring during drug administration)
   b. Ischemia (occurring during CVA)
   c. Brain injury
4. Risk factors include:
   a. Epilepsy (primary seizures)
   b. Brain diseases or disorders (secondary seizures)

E. Neoplastic disorders

1. Tumors may occur in the brain as primary or metastatic lesions; primary tumors may be extracerebral or intracerebral.
2. *Primary extracerebral tumors* arise from outside the brain tissue such as from the meninges, acoustic nerve, or pituitary and pineal glands.
3. *Primary intracerebral tumors* arise from the brain tissue itself.
4. Brain tumors result in increasing ICP and local tissue destruction, with symptoms such as dizziness, speech and memory defects, and ataxia.
5. There are no specific risk factors for primary tumors; metastatic lesions may result from lung and breast cancer.

II. **Physiologic responses to craniocerebral dysfunction**

A. Decreased level of consciousness

1. **The components of consciousness include content of consciousness and arousal (Display 5-1).**
2. Level of consciousness is directly related to ICP. Abnormal increases in ICP result in decreased level of consciousness, indicating neurologic impairment.
3. Levels of consciousness include:
   a. *Fully oriented and arousable:* The patient arouses spontaneously and is oriented to person, place, and time.
   b. *Confused:* The patient is unable to respond appropriately and clearly;

DISPLAY 5-1
Components of Consciousness

CONTENT OF CONSCIOUSNESS

- Includes moods, awareness of self, awareness of the environment, and cognitive function.
- Is mediated by the cerebral cortex and works in conjunction with the reticular activating system via neuronal pathways that traverse the brain stem.
- Can be altered by any disorder of the central nervous system (eg, CVA, AVM, post-seizure effect [also known as post-ictal], tumor formation, infection, metabolic disorders, head injuries).

AROUSAL

- Involves the state of wakefulness and the ability to respond to external stimuli.
- Is mediated by the reticular activating system.
- Can be altered by the same disorders that affect content of consciousness; typically, these are affected together.
- Level of consciousness is the most sensitive prognostic indicator of brain damage; as damage to the brain progresses, level of consciousness decreases.

disorientation to time occurs first, followed by place and person. Agitation, irritability, and inability to follow commands may also occur.

    c. *Lethargic:* The patient is unable to rouse spontaneously, but requires external stimuli such as voice or touch; confusion also may be evident.

    d. *Obtunded:* The patient sleeps unless aroused by voice or touch; once aroused, the patient displays limited responses to the environment. Verbal responses consist of single-word replies.

    e. *Stupor:* The patient is in a deep sleep or is unresponsive; arousal occurs only with vigorous and continuous stimulation. Spontaneous motor movements are minimal.

    f. *Coma:* The patient displays no response to the external environment, even with noxious stimuli.

B. Abnormal motor responses

    1. Abnormal motor responses typically occur after level of consciousness has become impaired.

    2. Kinds of abnormal motor responses include:

        a. *Abnormal flexion* (decorticate posturing): Upper extremities are flexed and adducted; lower extremities are extended and rotated internally.

        b. *Abnormal extension* (decerebrate posturing): All extremities are extended; upper extremities are hyperpronated.

        c. *Flaccidity:* No motor response is exhibited.

        d. *Purposeful movement:* Patient localizes to pain stimulus (ie, unconsciously attempts to remove source of pain).

        e. *Complete flexion:* In response to pain, patient withdraws or flexes extremities indiscriminately.

3. Focal motor responses most commonly seen in comatose patients include the grasp reflex, sucking reflex, and the Babinski response.

C. **Pupillary changes: ranging from pinpoint fixed to fixed and dilated**

D. **Alterations in oculomotor responses**

1. **In a comatose patient, oculomotor responses indicate an intact brain stem; the absence of responses for more than 48 hours is a strong prognostic indicator of brain death.**

2. Common responses include:

a. *Oculocephalic reflex* (doll's eye response): As the patient's head is turned from side to side, the eyes rotate together to the side opposite the one to which the head is turned. (Abnormal response involves rotation of the eyes together in the same direction as the head.)

b. *Oculovestibular reflex* (also known as cold caloric test or water caloric test): As the patient's ear canal is irrigated with water, the eyes turn toward the side being stimulated. (Abnormal response is absence of eye movement.)

E. **Abnormal breathing patterns**

1. **Alterations in breathing patterns can occur secondary to loss of cerebral, hemispheric, or brain stem control.**

2. Abnormal patterns include:

a. *Cheyne-Stokes respirations:* An alternating pattern of deep and shallow breathing, with periods of apnea; common with diffuse cortical injury or coma resulting from metabolic causes

b. *Central neurogenic ventilation:* A regular hyperpneic pattern, resulting in a low PCO_2 and increased pH; common with increasing ICP and structural damage to the upper brain stem or cerebral cortex

c. *Apneustic ventilation:* A prolonged inspiratory cycle followed by a 2- to 3-second pause, alternating with a prolonged expiratory cycle; found with lesions in the lower pons

d. *Cluster breathing:* Clusters of breaths alternating with irregular periods of apnea; indicates damage to the lower pons or high medulla

e. *Ataxic breathing:* Chaotic respiratory effort; indicates damage to the medullary respiratory control centers

F. **Vital sign changes**

1. In patients with hypothalamic or pituitary injuries or with head trauma, body temperature changes such as hypothermia or hyperthermia may occur.

2. **In patients with increasing ICP, alterations include increasing systolic pressure, decreasing diastolic pressure, and bradycardia. These three symptoms, known as Cushing's triad, commonly occur as pressure on the lower brain stem increases before herniation.**

G. **Agnosia**

1. Agnosia, the inability to recognize an object, may be tactile, visual, or auditory.

2. It involves structural damage in the association centers of the parietal, temporal, and occipital lobes.

H.   Dyspraxia

    1.   Dyspraxia is the inability to execute a planned movement.

    2.   It involves a disruption in the cognitive planning stages of an activity.

I.   Dysphasia

    1.   Dysphasia is the inability to produce or comprehend spoken words.

    2.   It most commonly occurs secondary to vascular events, but may also occur secondary to diffuse cortical injury.

III.   Increased intracranial pressure (ICP)

A.   Description

    1.   ICP is the pressure produced by the brain tissue, CSF, and blood within the skull.

    2.   Normal ICP is 5 to 15 mm Hg or 60 to 180 cm H_2O. (Values depend on the equipment used.)

    3.   Increased ICP exists when the volume of any of the three intracranial components rises, exceeding the brain's inherent compensatory capability (Fig. 5-1).

B.   Etiology

    1.   The most common cause of increased ICP is an increase in tissue volume, typically resulting from a brain tumor, a hematoma, or cerebral edema.

    2.   Increased ICP due to increased CSF volume can result from increased CSF production, impaired reabsorption, or blocked flow.

    3.   Increased ICP caused by increased blood volume results from vasodilation.

C.   Pathophysiologic processes and manifestations

    1.   When ICP increases exceed the brain's compensatory capabilities, compliance decreases and cerebral perfusion pressures deteriorate.

    2.   As cerebral perfusion diminishes, brain tissues experience hypoxia, which results in ischemic damage.

    3. CO_2 accumulates in the tissues, causing acidosis from by-products of anaerobic metabolism.

    4.   The rise in CO_2 causes cerebral vasodilation, which further contributes to a rise in ICP.

    5.   Eventually, if ICP continues to rise unabated, herniation will result (see Section IV).

    6.   Manifestations of increased ICP are generalized, including:

        a.   Decreased level of consciousness

        b.   Abnormal breathing patterns

        c.   Pupillary changes (sluggishly reactive to nonreactive)

        d.   Impaired motor responses

D.   Overview of nursing interventions

    1.   Assess neurologic status frequently to identify rising ICP and determine cerebral perfusion pressure.

    2.   If an ICP catheter has been placed:

        a.   Monitor the wave form.

        b.   Recognize that laying the patient flat, suctioning, and other routine

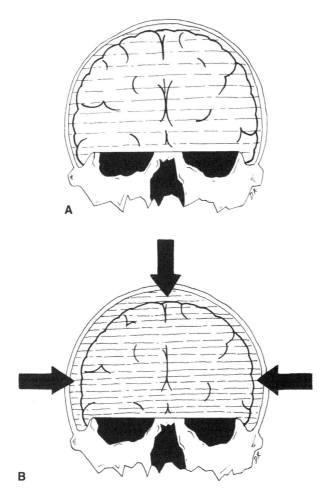

FIGURE 5-1.
(A) A small amount of fluid normally exists in the cranial vault. **(B)** Increasing ICP for any reason compresses brain tissue.

nursing interventions may cause ICP to rise. Note that bearing down, coughing, or Valsalva maneuver may also cause ICP to rise.

3. Maintain the patient's neck, hips, and knees in alignment to improve venous outflow.
4. Maintain the head of the bed at a level to improve cerebral perfusion, with the patient in semi-Fowler's position; this position also allows gravity to drain fluid from the brain.
5. Allow the patient to rest between nursing activities.
6. Administer paralyzing agents (vecuronium), as prescribed, if the patient is moving about so violently as to increase ICP.
7. Hyperventilate the patient to decrease PCO_2 and maintain adequate oxygenation.

8. Administer mannitol or other diuretics and steroids to decrease cerebral edema, as ordered.
9. Restrict fluids to decrease edema.
10. Drain CSF through ICP catheter as appropriate.

IV.   Herniation syndromes

A. Description

1. Herniation is a shifting of brain contents from a compartment of greater pressure to one of lower pressure; typically, contents shift out of the skull and onto the spinal cord through the foramen magnum.
2. Types of herniation include:
    a. *Uncal herniation* (lateral transtentorial): The uncus shifts from the middle fossa through the tentorial notch, compressing the ipsilateral cranial nerve III.
    b. *Central herniation* (transtentorial): The contents shift straight down through the tentorial notch.
    c. *Infratentorial herniation:* This type involves shifting of a cerebellar tonsil through the foramen magnum or upward transtentorial herniation of the brain stem through the tentorial incisura.

B. Etiology

1. Herniation is caused by a rise in ICP beyond the adaptive and compensatory capabilities of the brain.
2. Events that cause increased ICP also contribute to herniation (see Section III,B).

C. Pathophysiologic processes and manifestations

1. As ICP rises, brain contents gravitate toward an area of lower pressure.
2. As tissue movement occurs, cerebral blood flow to the affected area is compromised, contributing to ischemia and hypoxia.
3. Tissue movement also can compress previously unaffected tissue, causing destruction and hemorrhage.
4. A characteristic symptom of all herniation syndromes is increased ICP, which manifests as decreasing level of consciousness, sluggishly reactive to nonreactive pupils, and abnormal motor responses; localized findings also may be present.

5. **Cushing's triad (rising systolic blood pressure, decreasing diastolic pressure, and bradycardia) is considered evidence of impending herniation and occurs as the lower brain stem is compressed.**
6. Common manifestations of *uncal herniation* include:
    a. Ipsilateral ptosis
    b. Dilated pupils
    c. Extraocular muscle paralysis
    d. Contralateral hemiparesis
    e. Bilateral Babinski response
    f. Decreased level of consciousness
7. Typical manifestations of *central herniation* include:
    a. Decreased level of consciousness

      b.   Small reactive pupils, progressing to fixed and dilated pupils

      c.   Contralateral hemiplegia

      d.   Ipsilateral rigidity, progressing into abnormal posturing

8. Symptoms of *infratentorial herniation* include:

      a.   Paresthesia

      b.   Decreased level of consciousness

      c.   Breathing changes

      d.   Ophthalmoplegia and loss of upward gaze

D. **Overview of nursing interventions**

  1. Assess neurologic status for impending herniation.

  2. Undertake the same interventions as for increased ICP (see Section III,D).

V. Hematomas

A. **Description**

  1. A hematoma is a collection of blood in part of the brain (Fig. 5-2).

  2. Typically, a hematoma is located between two layers of the meninges, although it can also occur in the parenchymal tissue.

  3. Types of hematomas include:

      a.   *Subdural hematoma:* Blood collects between the dura mater and the arachnoid mater; this type of hematoma is classified as acute, subacute, or chronic, depending on how quickly blood accumulates.

      b.   *Epidural hematoma:* Blood collects between the dura mater and the skull.

      c.   *Subarachnoid hematoma:* Blood collects between the arachnoid mater and the pia mater.

      d.   *Intracerebral hematoma:* Blood collects within the parenchymal tissue.

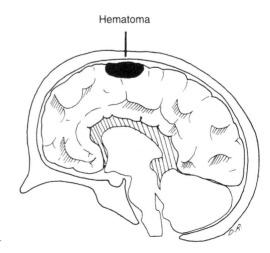

FIGURE 5-2.
Cerebral hematoma.

B. Etiology

1. Subdural hematomas usually are caused by venous bleeding; 50% are associated with skull fractures.
2. Epidural hematomas generally result from arterial bleeding; they also can occur from injury to a meningeal vein or dural sinus.
3. Subarachnoid hematomas usually occur secondary to rupture of intracranial aneurysms and arteriovenous malformations, secondary to head trauma, or from hypertensive bleeding.
4. Intracerebral hematomas may be caused by head trauma or may occur secondary to hypertensive bleeding.
5. **Hematomas also may occur secondary to coagulopathies or in persons on long-term anticoagulant therapy.**

C. Pathophysiologic processes and manifestations

1. Manifestations occur as expanding lesions compress the neural structures and paralyze nerve function.
2. Signs and symptoms vary depending on the location and size of the hematoma.
3. Early signs of hematoma formation include:
   a. Drowsiness
   b. Headache
   c. Restlessness
   d. Impaired cognition
   e. Confusion
4. Classic manifestations of epidural hematomas include a brief period of unconsciousness, followed by a period of lucidity, which then progresses into neurologic deterioration.
5. As the cortex becomes compressed and ICP rises, the emetic centers of the brain may be stimulated, causing vomiting (not associated with nausea).
6. Disorientation becomes more pronounced, and seizures may occur.
7. As the lesion increases in size, manifestations of increased ICP become evident. These include:
   a. Decreased level of consciousness
   b. Pathologic motor responses contralateral to the side of the hematoma
   c. Changes in pupillary response from briskly reactive to sluggishly reactive and, finally, to fixed; pupillary response will be ipsilateral if the hematoma is located on only one side of the brain
8. As damage extends to the cranial nerves, oculomotor responses are lost and a disconjugate gaze is present.

D. Overview of nursing interventions

1. Prepare the patient for surgery, as removal of the hematoma via burr holes is the treatment of choice; provide appropriate postoperative care.
2. Administer mannitol, an osmotic diuretic, to decrease brain edema, as prescribed.
3. Administer steroids, as prescribed, to decrease inflammation.
4. Hyperventilate the patient to decrease PCO_2 (a potent cerebral vasodilator), thereby decreasing ICP.

5. Monitor ICP using an intracranial pressure monitoring device, and institute appropriate interventions (see Section III,D).
6. Identify an expanding hematoma and recognize increased ICP.
7. Identify neurologic deficits and implement a care plan to help the patient compensate.
8. Provide ventilatory and hemodynamic support as indicated.
9. Prevent pulmonary complications with aggressive pulmonary care.
10. Promote skin integrity in a patient with a decreased level of consciousness and impaired mobility.

VI.   **Closed head injuries**

A.   Description

1. Closed head injuries are disorders of the brain in which the skull remains intact and external damage may not be visible.

2. **Damage occurs when pressure from the skull affects the parenchymal tissue or when brain movement within the skull causes shearing and stretching of fibers.**

3. Types of closed head injuries include:
   a. *Concussion:* transient loss of consciousness secondary to blunt trauma to the head
   b. *Contusion:* bruising of the brain
   c. *Diffuse axonal injury:* shearing and stretching of axonal fibers resulting from acceleration-deceleration forces; this is the most severe form of closed head injury

B.   Etiology

1. Closed head injuries are commonly caused by blunt trauma, usually resulting from motor vehicle accidents or falls.
2. Violent shaking can also cause closed head injuries, particularly in children.

C.   Pathophysiologic processes and manifestations

1. Concussion
   a. No structural damage is present on CT or MRI scans.
   b. Symptoms include immediate loss of consciousness lasting less than 5 seconds; loss of reflexes; and transient alterations in respiratory, cardiovascular, and hemodynamic functions (eg, brief apneic period, bradycardia, hypotension)
   c. Within minutes to days, depending on the severity of the injury, a full return to consciousness occurs.
   d. Some manifestations (eg, impaired memory, irritability, forgetfulness, inability to concentrate, headache, fatigue) may last for months.

2. Contusion
   a. Contusions commonly are present under a depressed skull fracture.
   b. CT scan may show evidence of edema or petechial hemorrhages at the site.
   c. In coup/contrecoup injuries, there are two focal areas of bruising injury on opposite sides of the brain.

  d. Manifestations are the same as for concussive injuries, but are generally more severe and longer lasting; a full return to normal may not occur.

 3. Diffuse axonal injury

  a. Manifestations include immediate loss of consciousness and, possibly, abnormal motor reflexes.

  b. Coma may last for up to 3 months; the length of time in a coma is a predictor of eventual outcome.

  c. Patients who do not awaken from a coma within 3 months are considered to be in a permanent vegetative state.

D. **Overview of nursing interventions**

 1. Control edema and subsequent increasing ICP—and prevent possible respiratory failure—by positioning the patient in semi-Fowler's, monitoring pressure, and administering diuretics as ordered.

 2. Maintain skin integrity.

 3. Prevent infection by administering antibiotics.

 4. Provide teaching for the patient and family members regarding potential long-term deficits.

VII. Cerebrovascular disorders

A. Description

 1. **Cerebrovascular disorders include all disorders that disrupt blood flow to the brain, whether due to occluded blood vessels or hemorrhaging resulting from ruptured vessels.**

 2. A hemorrhagic cerebrovascular accident (CVA) occurs when a blood vessel in the brain ruptures for any reason (eg, hypertension, traumatic injury, aneurysm, arteriovenous malformation).

 3. Ischemic CVA is caused by a blood clot in a cerebral vessel which leads to cerebral anoxia, resulting in symptoms of brain dysfunction.

 4. Types of cerebrovascular disorders include:

  a. Ischemic

 1. Transient ischemic attacks (TIA)

 2. Thrombotic/embolic CVA secondary to atherosclerotic disease or embolic events

  b. Hemorrhagic

 1. Hypertensive bleed

 2. Subarachnoid bleed secondary to AVM or aneurysm

B. **Etiology and incidence**

 1. Causes of CVA include thrombotic events (due to atherosclerotic disease) or embolic events (secondary to cardiac valvular disease).

 2. Incidence of thrombotic strokes is higher among males and in persons over age 65; a genetic predisposition appears to exist.

 3. Embolic strokes are caused by emboli that are released from the cardiovascular system and carried to the cerebral circulation, obstructing blood flow to the brain. They are associated with atrial fibrillation, valvular disease, endocarditis, and rheumatic heart disease.

 4. TIA, a signal of impending stroke, is caused by the presence of small thrombi in the cerebral vasculature. The occurrence of TIA precedes a completed stroke in 35% of incidences.

5. Aneurysms are caused by congenital, arteriosclerotic, or traumatic events. Saccular aneurysms, which occur in 2% of the population, typically are found at bifurcations in the circle of Willis; fusiform aneurysms occur most commonly in the basilar arteries or internal carotid arteries.

6. AVMs are congenital, familial, and occur twice as frequently in males than in females; they usually manifest in late adolescence or adulthood. They are a mass of dilated vessels, creating abnormal channels between the arterial and venous systems.

C. **Pathophysiologic processes and manifestations**

1. In ischemic CVAs:
   a. Plaque forms secondary to arteriosclerosis, resulting in a narrowing of the vessel.
   b. Inflammatory disease processes may also damage the vessel wall, contributing to an irregular lumen.
   c. Increased coagulation, decreased blood flow, hypotension, and dehydration can contribute to the formation of thrombi at these narrowed junctures.
   d. Platelet aggregation and fibrin attach to the endothelial lining of the vessel, and clots adhere to the wall.
   e. Over time, the thrombus occludes blood flow, causing ischemic damage to the cerebral tissue fed by the particular artery.
   f. Sometimes, excessive pressure in the cerebral vessels (due to hypertension or trauma) causes rupture of one or more vessels; blood then leaks out into the brain tissue. Damage depends on the extent of the bleeding and subsequent swelling.

2. Manifestations of CVA vary depending on the affected vessel. Symptoms can range from local manifestations to deep coma and include:
   a. Contralateral hemiparesis (internal carotid, anterior cerebral artery, and middle cerebral artery)
   b. Dysphasia (anterior cerebral artery, middle cerebral artery, and internal carotid arteries)
   c. Mental status changes (anterior cerebral circulation, posterior cerebral circulation)
   d. Visual disturbances (posterior cerebral artery, internal carotid arteries, and vertebrobasilar system)

3. **Signs and symptoms of right-sided strokes can include contralateral hemiparesis, spatial-perceptual deficits, impulsive behavior, and left visual field defects.**

4. Common manifestations of left-sided strokes include right-sided hemiparesis; expressive, receptive, or global aphasia; intellectual impairment; slow and cautious behavior; and right visual field defects.

5. In TIA, a temporary disruption of blood flow to the brain causes a transient episode of neurologic dysfunction (eg, brief loss of motor, visual, or sensory function); symptoms usually resolve within 24 hours.

6. Aneurysms and AVMs commonly are asymptomatic before rupture; some focal cranial nerve palsies may occur secondary to compression.

7. In mildly leaking vascular lesions, manifestations include headache, photophobia, and focal neurologic signs.
8. Once rupture occurs, symptoms can include:
   a. Evidence of massive bleeding into the meninges (subarachnoid bleed) or intracerebral bleeding]
   b. Seizures and vomiting
   c. Hemiparesis and ipsilateral pupillary and oculomotor nonreactivity
9. Symptoms of aneurysm and AVM may be related to meningeal irritation (eg, nausea, vomiting, stiff neck, photophobia, blurred vision) or to cerebral edema and increased ICP (eg, seizures, widening pulse pressure, hypertension, and bradycardia).
10. **Two common complications of aneurysms and AVMs are rebleeding and vasospasm.**
    a. **Rebleeding, which occurs within 7 to 10 days after the initial event, is due to degeneration of the fibrin clot. Symptoms are identical to those of the initial hemorrhage.**
    b. **Vasospasm occurs because vasoactive substances in the subarachnoid space shift into the vascular smooth muscle, causing the muscle to contract and become irritable; this decreases the lumen of the vessel and predisposes the patient to further ischemic brain damage. Manifestations of vasospasm include acute deterioration in the preexisting neurologic signs.**

D. **Overview of nursing interventions**
1. *For ischemic disorders*
   a. Administer oxygen to improve oxygen saturation in the blood.
   b. Institute measures to prevent complications (eg, ICP).
   c. Assist the patient with rehabilitation.
   d. Prepare patient for anticoagulant therapy or revascularization procedure.
2. *For hemorrhagic disorders*
   a. Prepare the patient for surgical repair of the aneurysm or AVM if complete rupture has not occurred; provide appropriate postoperative care.
   b. Administer antifibrinolytics, as prescribed, to prolong clot formation and prevent rebleeding.
   c. Recognize vasospasm and administer β-blockers as prescribed.
   d. Monitor blood pressure and control fluid volume.
   e. Assist the patient with rehabilitation.

VIII. **Seizures**

A. **Description**
1. Seizures are sudden electrical discharges from the brain characterized by transient alterations in motor, sensory, cognitive, and brain stem functions.
2. Seizures can be classified as generalized (involving the entire brain) or partial (involving one hemisphere). (See Display 5-2.)
3. Generalized seizures include:
   a. Tonic-clonic (grand mal)

DISPLAY 5-2
Types of Seizures

GENERALIZED

Tonic-clonic
- This type of seizure is characterized by alternating tonic-clonic phases, including muscle contraction with increased tone (tonic) and muscle contraction and relaxation (clonic).
- Constant tonic-clonic seizure activity (status epilepticus) is characterized by no recovery between three episodes of seizures or seizure activity lasting more than 30 minutes.

Absence
- Seizure activity is characterized by abrupt loss of awareness without loss of consciousness; motor activity stops.

PARTIAL

Simple
- Seizure activity is limited to part of the body, and may or may not spread to other areas; consciousness is not impaired.

Complex
- This type of seizure is charactrerized by automatisms (unconsciously controlled behaviors); consciousness is impaired.

---

      b.   Absence (petite mal)
   4.   Partial seizures include:
      a.   Simple (Jacksonian)
      b.   Complex

B. **Etiology**
   1.   Seizures can be caused by:
      a.   Head trauma
      b.   Cerebrovascular disorders
      c.   Congenital malformations
      d.   Perinatal injury
      e.   Infection
      f.   Tumors
      g.   Metabolic disorders
   2.   Seizures can also be idiopathic.

   3.   **Seizures can be precipitated by hypoglycemia, fatigue, stress, illness, drug use, or environmental stimuli.**

C. **Pathophysiologic processes and manifestations**
   1.   Cells in the epileptogenic focus in the brain have a lower seizure threshold, so when stimuli are excessive, they fire with increased amplitude.
   2.   Neighboring cells respond to the increased electrical activity and amplitude, in turn firing uninhibitedly.
   3.   When enough neurons fire, a seizure occurs.

    4. A prodrome or aura (sensory sign indicating a seizure is imminent) commonly occurs before a seizure, whether generalized or partial.

    5. In tonic-clonic seizures, loss of consciousness occurs, accompanied by a brief period of apnea and, possibly, incontinence.

    6. After a generalized seizure, the patient slowly returns to consciousness. During this phase (postictal), the patient may be combative or lethargic.

D. Overview of nursing interventions

    1. During the seizure:

        a. Protect the patient from injury.

        b. Place the patient on the ground in a side-lying position and maintain airway.

        c. Apply oxygen and monitor the patient's responses.

        d. Do not attempt to insert anything in the patient's mouth.

    2. After the seizure:

        a. Administer antiseizure medications as prescribed.

        b. Monitor therapeutic levels of medications.

        c. Educate the patient and family members about factors that precipitate seizure activity.

IX. Brain tumors

A. Description

    1. Brain tumors are intracranial neoplasms; they can be either intracerebral or extracerebral.

    2. Intracerebral tumors arise from the brain itself (ie, neurons, neuroglial cells, blood vessels).

    3. Extracerebral tumors arise from cranial nerves, the pituitary gland, or the meninges.

    4. Intracerebral tumors include:

        a. Glioblastoma multiforme, accounting for 25% of all brain tumors and 55% of all intracerebral masses.

        b. Astrocytoma, accounting for 10% of brain tumors.

        c. Ependymoma, accounting for 5% of all intracranial gliomas in adults and 10% in children.

        d. Medulloblastoma, accounting for 18% of all tumors in children.

    5. Extracerebral tumors include:

        a. Meningioma (15% of all tumors)

        b. Neurilemoma

B. Etiology

    1. The etiology of brain tumors is unknown.

    2. Some tumor growth has been linked to radiation exposure, chemical exposure, and viruses.

C. Pathophysiologic processes and manifestations

    1. Tumors are either encapsulated or nonencapsulated and invasive (Display 5-3).

    2. Nonencapsulated, invasive tumors infiltrate into adjacent tissue and destroy it as they grow.

    3. Encapsulated tumors do not invade neighboring tissue, but rather displace

DISPLAY 5-3
Types of Tumors

ENCAPSULATED

Meningiomas
- Grow slowly
- Originate from the dura and arachnoid mater
- Tend to be benign

Neurilemomas
- Arise from Schwann cells surrounding the axons of the cranial nerves
- Commonly affect cranial nerves V, VIII, and IX

NONENCAPSULATED

Glioblastomas
- Arise from mature astrocytes
- Are highly malignant, vascular, and invasive
- Are associated with the development of necrotic areas with cysts and hemorrhagic sites

Astrocytomas
- Arise from astrocytes
- Grow slowly and are infiltrative
- Commonly occur in the cerebrum and hypothalamus

Ependymomas
- Arise from ependymal cells of ventricular walls
- Tend to grow into the ventricule, particularly the fourth one
- Commonly cause ventricular obstruction

Medulloblastomas
- Arise from embryonic cells
- Grow rapidly
- Typically are found in the fourth ventricle or cerebellum
- Commonly cause ventricular obstruction

---

and compress the tissue as they grow. By doing so, these tumors produce ischemia, edema, and increased ICP.

4. Typical early manifestations of brain tumors can include:
   a. **Headache, papilledema, and vomiting—a triad of symptoms indicating increasing ICP**
   b. **New onset of seizures**
   c. **Alterations in consciousness or cognition**
5. Depending on the tumor's location, focal manifestations may include:
   a. Hemiparesis
   b. Cranial nerve palsies
   c. Dyspraxia

      d. Dysphasia

      e. Personality changes

      f. Gait disturbances

6. Tumors arising from the ventricular wall or compressing on the ventricles will result in a noncommunicating hydrocephalus. This produces dilation of the ventricles proximal to the obstruction, causing atrophy and degeneration of the cerebral cortex and white matter.

7. Manifestations of hydrocephalus are the same as those of rapidly increasing ICP (see Section III, C).

8. Tumors affecting the pituitary and hypothalamic regions will also affect hormonal production.

D.   **Overview of nursing interventions**

1. Prepare the patient for surgery to remove the tumor, if indicated; after surgery, provide appropriate postoperative care.

2. Prepare the patient for chemotherapy and radiation therapy, if indicated.

3. Administer steroids to decrease cerebral edema and anticonvulsant medications to prevent seizures, as prescribed.

4. Monitor for signs of increased ICP, hydrocephalus, and neurologic deterioration.

5. Provide supportive ventilatory, nutritional, and hemodynamic care as indicated.

6. Administer pain medications as ordered.

7. Identify neurologic deficits and implement a care plan to help the patient compensate for these deficits.

8. Provide counseling as needed.

Bibliography

Barker, E. (1994). *Neuroscience nursing.* St. Louis: C. V. Mosby.

Bullock, B. (1996). *Pathophysiology: Adaptations and alterations in function* (4th ed.). Philadelphia: J. B. Lippincott-Raven.

Ganong, William F. (1997). *Review of medical physiology* (18th ed.). Stamford, CT: Appleton and Lange.

Guyton, Arthur C., & Hall John E. (1996). *Textbook of medical physiology* (9th ed.). Philadelphia: W. B. Saunders.

Hickey, J. (1992). *The clinical practice of neurological and neurosurgical nursing* (3rd ed.). Philadelphia: J. B. Lippincott.

Horvath, C. (1994). *Emergency nursing core curriculum* (4th ed.). Chap. 17, Shock emergencies. Philadelphia: W. B. Saunders.

Kinney, M., Packa, D., & Dunbar, S. (1993). *AACN's clinical reference for critical-care nursing* (3rd ed.). St. Louis: C. V. Mosby.

McCance, K. L., & Huether, S. E. (1994). *Pathophysiology: The biologic basis for disease in adults and children* (2nd ed.). St. Louis: Mosby-Year Book.

Porth, C. (1994). *Pathophysiology: Concepts of altered health states* (4th ed.). Philadelphia: Lippincott.

STUDY QUESTIONS

1. Mr. Signa, age 27, has sustained a right-sided frontal/parietal subdural hematoma following a motor vehicle accident. He is generally unresponsive, arouses only with vigorous stimuli, and has minimal spontaneous motor movements. The nurse would categorize his level of consciousness as:
   a. comatose
   b. lethargic
   c. obtunded
   d. stuporous

2. Joey Brown, age 10, was hit in the head with a baseball bat during a game. He experienced a brief period of unconsciousness, but then aroused and was lucid. Two hours later, he began to deteriorate neurologically. The nurse would suspect that he has:
   a. an epidural hematoma
   b. a subdural hematoma
   c. a tonic-clonic seizure
   d. a closed head injury

3. Hyperventilation is recommended if there is any indication of increased ICP. This intervention decreases ICP by:
   a. raising CO_2, which results in vasodilation
   b. lowering O_2, which results in vasoconstriction
   c. raising O_2, which results in vasodilation
   d. lowering CO_2, which results in vasoconstriction

4. An ependymoma commonly results in:
   a. temperature alterations
   b. hydrocephalus
   c. necrotic, cystic areas within the cerebrum
   d. cranial nerve palsies

5. Encapsulated tumors grow by:
   a. displacement and compression of surrounding tissue
   b. infiltration into neighboring tissue
   c. formation of cysts

   d. necrosis and neuronal destruction of surrounding tissue

6. The manifestations of a thrombotic stroke are:
   a. unpredictable
   b. diffuse because of the distribution of thrombi
   c. similar to those of a aneurysm
   d. dependent on the cerebral vessel occluded

7. Ms. Kimmy, age 72, has suffered a right-sided CVA. Her safety is a concern because, based on her diagnosis, the nurse would expect her to exhibit:
   a. impulsive behavior
   b. cautious behavior
   c. right-sided hemiparesis
   d. intellectual impairment

8. Antifibrinolytics are used in the management of hemorrhagic vascular lesions to:
   a. prevent vasospasm
   b. prevent fibrin clot degeneration
   c. decrease meningeal irritation
   d. anticoagulate the patient

9. As ICP rises, compliance:
   a. increases
   b. is not altered
   c. decreases
   d. changes logarithmically

10. Mr. Campbell, age 37, is in the neurologic ICU after aneurysm clipping. His ICP is 17 mm Hg and continues to rise. Which of the following interventions would the nurse *not* want to implement?
    a. maintain the patient's head in alignment
    b. institute muscle paralysis
    c. hyperventilate the patient
    d. maintain the patient's hips and knees in flexion

11. Mr. Smith has been on Coumadin for one year. Which of the following may result:

a. subdural hematoma
b. head injury
c. decreased ICP
d. tumor formation

12. Susan Smith, R.N., is making rounds on the pediatric unit. Joey Jones, 5 years old, drops to the ground having a grand mal seizure. Susan should first:
a. insert a tongue blade into the mouth
b. administer antiseizure medication
c. protect the patient from injury
d. apply oxygen

13. To determine the effectiveness of anti-seizure medications the nurse would:
a. send the patient for a CAT scan
b. draw frequent CBC values
c. monitor postseizure activity
d. determine drug levels

14. There is no structural damage in which condition:
a. tumor
b. contusion
c. CVA
d. concussion

ANSWER KEY

Question	Correct answer	Correct answer rationale	Incorrect answer rationales
1.	d	Patients who are stuporous are unresponsive to anything but vigorous stimuli and have minimal spontaneous motor activity.	a. Comatose patients are unresponsive to any stimuli. b. Lethargic patients are unable to rouse spontaneously, but require external stimuli. c. Obtunded patients sleep unless roused, and have limited responses once they are aroused.
2.	a	The classic presentation of an epidural hematoma is brief unconsciousness, followed by a lucid period, progressing into neurologic deterioration.	b, c, and d. These disorders do not present with these manifestations.
3.	d	CO_2 is a potent vasodilating agent. As cerebral vessels vasodilate, more blood is delivered to the brain, increasing ICP. By blowing off CO_2 and causing vasoconstriction, ICP can be lowered.	a. Increased CO_2 results from hypoventilation, which will result in vasodilation and increase ICP. b. Lowering O_2 will result in hypoxia, which will contribute to cerebral ischemia. c. Raising O_2 will benefit the patient, but does not impact directly on ICP.
4.	b	An ependymoma is a tumor of the ventricle walls. As this lesion increases in size, it may block the ventricles and obstruct CSF outflow, leading to hydrocephalus.	a. Temperature alterations occur with damage to the hypothalamic area only. c. Glioblastoma multiforme causes necrotic cysts. d. Cranial nerve palsies will have no effect on CSF flow.
5.	a	If a tumor is encapsulated in tissue, it grows within the tissue and spreads only by displacement and compression.	b. Unencapsulated tumors grow by direct infiltration. c. This is a by-product of glioblastoma growth, but is not the direct method of tumor growth. d. This may occur as a tumor grows, but is not the best response.
6.	d	Because a thrombotic stroke usually occurs secondary to atherosclerotic plaque formation, the vessels affected can be determined based on the distribution of cerebral blood flow and the areas of the brain supplied by that vessel. Because of this, symptoms vary.	a. Embolic strokes have an unpredictable presentation because there is no way to predict where the emboli will lodge. b. Embolic strokes tend to show diffuse distribution because of the "showering" effect of embolization.

Question	Correct answer	Correct answer rationale	Incorrect answer rationales
			c. Manifestations of aneurysms are in no way similar to those of a thrombotic stroke.
7.	a	Patients with right-sided CVAs tend to demonstrate a lack of judgment and more impulsive behavior than those with left-sided CVAs. This might lead to safety concerns because these individuals tend to make incorrect assessments of their capabilities and are therefore prone to falls.	b. Cautious behavior is seen more commonly in patients with left-sided CVAs. c. A right-sided CVA will have contralateral (ie, left-sided) paralysis. d. Although judgment may be impaired in patients with right-sided CVAs, intellectual impairment is not consistently noted.
8.	b	Antifibrinolytics slow down the breakdown of fibrin, which prolongs clot life. This process stabilizes the clot for a longer time in an attempt to prevent further vascular bleeding.	a. Vasospasm is prevented by the administration of calcium channel blockers. c. Antifibrinolytics will not prevent meningeal irritation, although decreased external stimuli might help. d. Antifibrinolytics do the opposite of anticoagulants.
9.	c	Compliance is a measure of the adaptive capability of the brain to a change in response to external stimuli. As ICP rises, the brain is less able to adapt to this increased pressure and compliance diminishes.	a, b, and d. These responses are incorrect.
10.	d	Flexion of the extremities can impair venous return and therefore cause increased blood flow to the brain; this results in increased ICP. Nursing interventions for a patient with an elevated ICP should be directed toward lowering this pressure.	a, b, and c. All of these interventions decrease ICP.
11.	a	Coagulopathies or persons on long term anticoagulants may develop hematomas.	b, c, and d. These are not sequelae of Coumadin administration.
12.	c	The priority choice is to protect the patient from injury.	a. Never insert anything into the mouth during a seizure. b and d. Medication and oxygen administration are not as important as choice c.

Question	Correct answer	Correct answer rationale	Incorrect answer rationales
13.	d	Determination of therapeutic drug levels and absence of seizures determine effectiveness of therapy.	a and b. A CAT scan and CBC values will not reflect drug efficacy. b. There should be no seizure activity therefore no postseizure activity to monitor.
14.	d	There is no structural damage in concussion.	a, b, and c. Structural damage is noted in these conditions.

6 Neuromuscular Disorders

I. Overview of pathophysiologic processes

A. Upper motor neuron syndromes

1. **Upper motor neuron syndromes are neurologic dysfunctions that result from disruption of the pyramidal motor tracts.**
2. The injury may occur in the motor strip of the cerebrum, the brain stem, the internal capsule, or the spinal cord.

3. **Disruption of the pyramidal tracts will result in flaccidity initially, which is then replaced by spasticity of muscle tone.**
4. Diseases that result in disturbances of upper motor function include central nervous system (CNS) injuries, such as vascular lesions, neoplasms, trauma, inflammatory, and degenerative diseases. (*Note:* See Chapters 5 and 7 for discussions of these types of diseases.)
5. Damage to the spinal cord, by trauma or tumor, is also considered an upper motor neuron injury.
6. There are no particular risk factors for upper motor neuron syndromes.

B. Lower motor neuron syndromes

1. **Lower motor neuron syndromes are those in which the damage occurs in the anterior horn cell of the spinal cord, the axons extending to the muscle, or the myoneural junction (eg, anterior horn cell damage, myoneural junction disorders, and myopathies).**

2. **Dysfunction in the lower motor neuron pathways results in paresis or paralysis and muscle flaccidity.**
3. There is a loss of muscle tone and a reduction in reflexes, which results in hyporeflexia or hypotonia and, eventually, muscle atrophy.
4. Fasciculations and fibrillation of muscle fibers may also occur.
5. Myoneural junction disorders are those in which the anterior horn and fibers are intact, but the defects exist in the synaptic cleft between the terminal axon and the muscle fiber.
6. Insufficient numbers or impaired binding sites, inadequate amounts of neurotransmitting agents, and blockage of binding sites may also result in loss of axonal transmission to the muscle, causing muscle weakness.
7. Multiple sclerosis (MS), amyotrophic lateral sclerosis (ALS), Guillain-Barré syndrome, and myasthenia gravis are lower motor neuron syndromes.
8. Myopathies, such as muscular dystrophy, are diseases in which the muscle itself is damaged.
9. There are no particular risk factors for lower motor neuron syndromes.

II. Physiologic responses to neuromuscular dysfunction

A. Paralysis

1. *Paralysis* is the inability of a muscle group to overcome gravity; it may range from slight paresis or weakness to loss of all muscle ability or paralysis.
2. *Hemiparesis* refers to weakness on one side of the body.
3. *Paraplegia* refers to paralysis of the lower extremities.

4. *Quadriplegia* refers to paralysis of all four extremities.

B. **Flaccidity: a type of hypotonia in which there is lack of muscle movement against resistance; associated with paralysis and atrophy**

C. **Spasticity: a type of hypertonia in which a gradual increase in muscle tone eventually results in excessive resistance to movement**

D. **Atrophy**

  1. Atrophy is a shrinkage in muscle mass that results from lack of use of the muscle and loss of tone.

  2. Because of a lack of neuronal stimulation and, therefore, use, the muscle is eventually replaced by connective tissue and fat. Loss of neuronal inhibition causes a constant condition of muscular contraction, eventually resulting in hypertrophy.

E. **Hypertrophy: enlargement of muscle mass occurring from overuse**

F. **Dystonia: maintenance of an abnormal posture through muscular contractions; occurs when there is sustained and constant muscular contraction without inhibition**

G. **Akinesia**

  1. Akinesias are a decrease in voluntary movements generally seen with damage to the extrapyramidal motor systems.

  2. These may range from *hypokinesia* (decreased movement of expression and locomotion) to *bradykinesia* (slowing of voluntary movements).

H. **Hyperkinesia: excessive movements**

I. **Dyskinesia: abnormal, involuntary movements**

III. Spinal cord injury

A. **Description**

  1. Spinal cord injury refers to any injury in which a segment or the entire cord is damaged.

  2. Such injuries also result in damage to the area of the body supplied by the nerves whose cell bodies within the cord are damaged.

B. **Etiology**

  1. Spinal cord injuries most commonly result from trauma. Acceleration, deceleration, or rotational forces on the vertebrae can:

   a. Disrupt the integrity of the vertebrae and cord

   b. Exert traction on the ligaments

   c. Cause direct damage to the cord within the vertebral canal

  2. Spinal cord tumors cause damage by disrupting blood flow to the cord or by impinging on the nerves.

  3. Syringomyelia, a disease that causes inflammation and degeneration of the cord, destroys fiber tracts beginning in the central cord and moving outward, leading to cavitations within the cord.

  4. Other causes include:

   a. Vascular lesions

   b. Inflammatory disorders

   c. Degenerative diseases

C. **Pathophysiologic processes and manifestations**

1. **Manifestations depend on the location and severity of the spinal cord injury. Table 6-1 describes the functional loss from spinal injury.**
2. In partial cord involvement, only a few neuronal tracts may be affected (eg, in the anterior cord syndrome, only the anterior portion of the cord is affected) with disruption of the pyramidal tracts and loss of pain and temperature sensation below the level of the lesion.
3. In hemisection of the cord, as in Brown-Sequard's syndrome, partial destruction results in ipsilateral paralysis and loss of touch, pressure, vibration, and proprioception below the level of the injury; contralateral loss of pain and temperature sensation also occurs.
4. Complete cord transection results in quadriplegia in lesions above T-1 and paraplegia in lesions below T-1. Loss of all reflexes below the level of injury and loss of sensory input also result.
5. As smooth muscle innervation is lost, manifestations include atony of the bladder and bowel, paralytic ileus formation, loss of genital reflexes, and loss of vasomotor tone.
6. In lesions above T-1, respiratory impairment may result due to paralysis of the intercostals and diaphragm.
7. In acute cord injury, spinal shock may occur and last up to 3 weeks; reappearance of reflex activity indicates the resolution of shock. Initial flaccidity is replaced by spasticity with gradual return of autonomic reflexes.
8. Autonomic hyperreflexia may occur after a spinal cord injury. It results from transection of the autonomic nervous system, which makes autonomic regulation impossible by impeding the balance between the parasympathetic and sympathetic nervous system.
9. Manifestations of increased sympathetic stimulation, not mediated by the parasympathetic nervous system, include hypertension, headache, blurred vision, sweating, flushed skin, and bradycardia. The stimulation may be very simple, occurring in response to sensory stimulation such as a full bowel or bladder or skin stimulation.

D. **Overview of nursing interventions**

1. Assess the patient's level of injury and the sensory and motor responses that still remain.

2. Protect the patient from injury because the ability to respond appropriately to sensory stimuli is impaired.

3. Stabilize the injured segment to prevent extension of the injury.

4. Maintain airway for high cervical lesions and monitor for dysrhythmias.
5. Administer high-dose steroids in acute spinal cord injury and antibiotics, as prescribed.
6. Prepare the patient for vertebral stabilization procedure, tumor debulking or surgical fixation, as indicated.
7. Ensure adequate nutrition, monitoring for return of bowel sounds.
8. Maintain optimal skin integrity.
9. Assist the patient with bowel and bladder function.
10. Educate the patient and staff regarding extent of injury and need for rehabilitation.

TABLE 6-1
Functional Loss from Spinal Cord Injury (Based on Complete Lesions)

LEVEL OF SPINAL INJURY	MOTOR FUNCTION	DEEP TENDON REFLEXES	SENSORY FUNCTION	RESPIRATORY FUNCTION	VOLUNTARY BOWEL AND BLADDER FUNCTION	REHABILITATIVE POTENTIAL
C1-4	• Tetraplegia: loss of all motor function from the neck down		• Loss of all sensory function in the neck and below (C-4 supplies the clavicles.)	• Loss of involuntary (phrenic) and voluntary (intercostals) respiratory function; ventilatory support and a tracheostomy needed	• No bowel or bladder control	• Can be discharged home on a ventilator with home care
C-5	• Tetraplegia: loss of all function below the upper shoulders • **Intact:** sternomastoids, cervical paraspinal muscles, and the trapezius; can control head	C-5, C-6 biceps	• Loss of sensation below the clavicle and most portions of arms, hands, chest, abdomen, and lower extremities • **Intact:** head, shoulders, deltoid, clavicle, portion of forearms (C-5 supplies the lateral aspect of the arm.)	• Phrenic nerve intact, but not intercostal muscles	• No bowel or bladder control	• Use of extremity-powered devices to achieve some upper limb control • Head control facilitates wheelchair balance • Adaptive tools, held in mouth, for typing and writing
C-6	• Tetraplegia: loss of all function below the shoulders and upper arms; lacks elbow, forearm, and hand control • **Intact:** deltoid, biceps, and external rotator muscles of shoulders	C-5, C-6 brachioradials	• Loss of everything listed for a C-5 lesion, but greater arm and thumb sensation • **Intact:** head, shoulders, arms, palms of hands, and thumbs (C-6 supplies the forearm and thumb.)	• Phrenic nerve intact, but not intercostal muscles	• No bowel or bladder control	• Needs assistive devices to use arms (may be able to help feed, groom, and dress self) • Needs a motorized wheelchair • Dependent for all transfers

(continued)

TABLE 6-1
Functional Loss From Spinal Cord Injury (Based on Complete Lesions) (*Continued*)

LEVEL OF SPINAL INJURY	MOTOR FUNCTION	DEEP TENDON REFLEXES	SENSORY FUNCTION	RESPIRATORY FUNCTION	VOLUNTARY BOWEL AND BLADDER FUNCTION	REHABILITATIVE POTENTIAL
C-7	• Tetraplegia: loss of motor control to portions of the arm and hands • **Intact:** voluntary strength in shoulder depressors, shoulder abductors, internal rotators, and radial wrist extensors	C-7, C-8 triceps	• Loss of sensation below the clavicle and portions of arms and hands • **Intact:** head, shoulders, most of arms and hands (C-7 supplies the middle finger.)	• Phrenic nerve intact, but not intercostal muscles	• No bowel or bladder function	• Can perform some activities of daily living (ADLs) • Can use wrist extensor with a special splint to induce finger flexion • Can push a wheelchair with special handgrasps • May be able to drive a specially equipped car
C-8	• Tetraplegia: loss of motor control to portions of arms and hands • **Intact:** some voluntary control of elbow extensors, wrist, finger extension and finger flexors		• Loss of sensation below the chest and in portions of hands • **Intact:** sensation to face, shoulders, arms, hands, and part of chest (C-8 supplies the little finger.)	• Phrenic nerve intact, but not intercostal muscles	• No bowel or bladder function	• Able to do pushups in the wheelchair • Improved sitting tolerance • Can grasp and release hands voluntarily. • Independent in most ADLs • Independent in use of wheelchair • Can use hands for catheterization and rectal stimulation for bowel movements

Level	Motor/Sensory		Respiratory	Bowel/Bladder	Functional Capabilities
T1-6	Paraplegia: loss of everything below the midchest region, including the trunk muscles **Intact:** control of function to the shoulders, upper chest, arms, and hands	Loss of sensation below the midchest area **Intact:** everything to the midchest region, including the arms and hands (T-1 and T-2 supply the inner aspect of the arm; T-4 supplies the nipple area.)	Phrenic nerve functions independently Some impairment of intercostal muscles	No bowel or bladder function	Full control of upper extremities and completely independent in wheelchair Full-time employment possible. Independent in managing urinary drainage and inserting suppositories Able to live in a dwelling without major architectural changes
T6-12	Paraplegia: loss of motor control below the waist **Intact:** shoulders, arms, hands, and long trunk muscles	Loss of everything below the waist **Intact:** shoulders, chest, arms, and hands (T-10 supplies the umbilicus; T-12 supplies the groin area.)	No interference with respiratory function	No bowel or bladder control	In addition to the previously described capabilities, there is complete abdominal and upper back control. Good sitting balance (allows for greater ease of wheelchair operation and athletics)
L1-3	Paraplegia: loss of most control of legs and pelvis **Intact:** shoulders, arms, hands, torso, hip rotation and flexion, and some leg flexion L2-4 (knee jerk)	Loss of sensation to the lower abdomen and legs **Intact:** all of the above plus some sensation to the inner and anterior thigh (L-3 supplies the knee.)	No interference with respiratory function	No bowel or bladder control	Independent for most activities from wheelchair

(continued)

TABLE 6-1
Functional Loss From Spinal Cord Injury (Based on Complete Lesions) (Continued)

LEVEL OF SPINAL INJURY	MOTOR FUNCTION	DEEP TENDON REFLEXES	SENSORY FUNCTION	RESPIRATORY FUNCTION	VOLUNTARY BOWEL AND BLADDER FUNCTION	REHABILITATIVE POTENTIAL
L3-4	• Paraplegia: loss of control of portions of lower legs, ankles, and feet • **Intact:** all of the above, plus increased knee extension		• Loss of sensation to portions of the lower legs, feet, and ankles • **Intact:** all of the above, plus sensation to the upper legs	• No interference with respiratory function	• No bowel or bladder control	• Voluntary control of hip extensors; weak abductors • Walking with braces possible
L-4 to S-5	• Paraplegia: degree varies • Segmental motor control L-4 to S-1: abduction and internal rotation of hip, ankle dorsiflexion, and foot inversion L-5 to S-1: foot eversion L-4 to S-2: knee flexion S1-2: plantar flexion S1-2: (ankle jerk) S2-5: bowel/bladder control	S1-2 (ankle jerk)	• Lumbar sensory nerves innervate the upper legs and portions of the lower legs L-5: medial aspect of foot S-1: lateral aspect of foot S-2: posterior aspect of calf/thigh • Sacral sensory nerves innervate the lower legs, feet, and perineum	• No interference with respiratory function	• Bowel and bladder control possibly impaired • S2-4 segments control urinary continence • S3-5 segments control bowel continence (perianal muscles)	• Can walk with braces or may use wheelchair • Can be relatively independent

Source: Hickey, J. V. (1997). The Clinical Practice of Neurological and Neurosurgical Nursing (4th ed.). Philadelphia: Lippincott-Raven.

IV. Herniated intervertebral disk (Fig. 6-1)

A. Description: a disorder in which the nucleus pulposus protrudes through the annulus fibrosus

B. Etiology

    1. Herniated intervertebral disk occurs secondary to degenerative disk disease or trauma.

        a. Degenerative disk disease occurs because of biochemical alterations in the tissues of the intervertebral disk.

        b. Trauma results from extreme flexion of the trunk, which causes undue stress on the intervertebral disk.

    2. Most herniations occur in the L-4 to S-1 range or in the C-5 to C-7 disks.

C. Pathophysiologic processes and manifestations

    1. Degenerative processes convert the normal intervertebral disk tissue into fibrocartilage tissue. This occurs because of water loss within the disk and fibrosis of tissue.

    2. When herniation occurs, the nucleus pulposus extrudes through the posterior capsule of the disk and compresses the nerve root or the spinal cord.

    3. Compression of the nerve root or cord results in pain and possible loss of sensory or motor function.

    4. Severity of manifestations depend on the level of the disk involved and the severity of the herniation.

    5. Lumbar/sacral involvement is associated with sciatic distribution of pain, which increases with Valsalva maneuvers; limited leg movement and loss of sensory perception may also occur.

    6. Cervical involvement is associated with pain and sensory alterations in the upper arms and hand; other manifestations include neck pain and weakness and atrophy of the biceps or triceps.

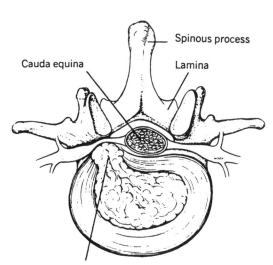

FIGURE 6-1
Ruptured vertebral disk. (From Chaffee, E. E., and I. M. Lytle. 1980. *Basic physiology and anatomy.* Philadelphia: J. B. Lippincott.)

D. Overview of nursing interventions

1. Ensure the patient's comfort during transport to MRI or CAT scan, because movement can cause inflammation.
2. Apply traction as ordered.
3. Maintain bedrest.
4. Administer pain and antiinflammatory agents, as prescribed.
5. Prepare the patient for surgery to stabilize the intervertebral disk or remove it if there is any indication of severe neurologic involvement (eg, decreased deep tendon reflexes or loss of bowel and bladder function); provide appropriate postoperative care.

V.   Multiple sclerosis (MS)

A. Description: a demyelinating disorder of the CNS characterized by periods of exacerbations and remissions

B. Etiology and incidence

1. **MS results from unknown causes; some hypotheses link it to autoimmune pathology.**
2. Genetic predisposition and geographic or environmental factors may contribute to its development.
3. MS commonly occurs in persons ages 20 to 40; it affects more women than men.

C. Pathophysiologic processes and manifestations

1. **Irrespective of the cause, an immune response results in recurrent inflammatory reactions leading to peripheral vasculitis.**
2. This vasculitis causes breakdown of the blood-brain barrier, allowing migration of B lymphocytes into the CNS.
3. Once in the CNS, the B lymphocytes secrete immunoglobulin G antibodies, which increase during exacerbations of the disease process.
4. Macrophages enter the myelin sheath and remove degenerating myelin, forming patchy areas of demyelination. This results in areas of missing myelin called plaques.

5. **Plaques occur predominantly in the white matter, and occasionally in the grey matter; they reduce support of the nerve cells, hindering neuromuscular conduction.**
6. In the acute stages of MS, inflammatory edema around the plaque sites is noted; in the chronic stages, gliosis of the axons occurs, leading to permanent disability.

7. **Manifestations occur intermittently and depend on the area of predominant CNS involvement.**
8. *Corticospinal syndrome* occurs when the corticospinal tracts are affected. Manifestations include symmetric muscular weakness and stiffness, spastic paralysis, and bowel and bladder incontinence.
9. *Brain stem syndrome* occurs when the disease affects the brain stem. Manifestations include dysfunction of cranial nerves III through XII, which re-

sults in ophthalmoplegia, nystagmus, and dysarthria. Facial muscle weakness and paresthesia may also occur.

10. *Cerebellar syndrome* occurs when cells of the cerebellum are affected. Manifestations include spastic gait, ataxia, intention tremors, and hypotonia.

11. *Cerebral syndrome* occurs when cells of the cerebral hemispheres are affected. Manifestations include optic neuritis, impaired vision, and intellectual and emotional deterioration.

D. **Overview of nursing interventions**

1. Educate the patient about the procedures necessary to make the diagnosis (eg, CT scan, MRI, spinal tap).

2. Administer steroids and adrenocorticotropin hormone (ACTH) to control acute exacerbations, as prescribed.

3. Provide symptomatic management of muscular weakness, respiratory difficulty, bowel and bladder atony, and pain.

4. Assist with rehabilitative care to prevent complications of mobility and secondary infectious processes.

5. Refer the patient for physical therapy, which may be useful to assist with muscle strengthening and gait retraining.

6. Teach the patient and family members about the disease process and treatment.

7. Provide counseling as needed.

8. Provide nutrition.

9. Assure safety.

VI. Amyotrophic lateral sclerosis (ALS)

A. **Description:** a fatal disorder marked by degeneration of upper and lower motor neurons; also known as Lou Gehrig's disease

B. **Etiology and incidence**

1. ALS results from unknown causes; studies point to a viral/immune response or metabolic factors as possible causes.

2. ALS commonly begins in the third decade; men are affected more often than women.

C. **Pathophysiologic processes and manifestations**

1. Degeneration of motor neurons occurs without any indication of inflammation.

2. Degeneration reduces the total number of motor neurons in the motor cortex, brain stem, and spinal cord.

3. As degeneration occurs, axonal disintegration, gliosis formation, and scarring of neurons result.

4. Predominant manifestations are:
   a. Generalized muscle weakness
   b. Muscle wasting
   c. Atrophy

5. Paresis begins in one localized muscle group; it extends to include all striated muscle, except the extraocular muscles.

6. Other manifestation may include:

      a. Flaccid and spastic muscle paralysis

      b. Hypotonia

      c. Muscle atrophy and fasciculations

7. Dermatologic manifestations can include loss of skin thickness, nail thickening, decreased hair distribution, and decreased sweat gland activity.

D. Overview of nursing interventions

1. Manage manifestations of the disease, because no cure for ALS exists.
2. Maintain a means of communication as speech dysfunction occurs.
3. Maintain skin integrity and mobility as paralysis becomes progressive.
4. Provide nutritional support and hydration as a priority of care.
5. Monitor and maintain pulmonary status to prevent atelectasis as the diaphragm and accessory muscles weaken.
6. Administer antispasmodics, as prescribed, if spasticity is present.
7. Counsel the patient and family members regarding the terminal progression of the disease.

VII. Guillain-Barré syndrome

A. Description: an inflammatory demyelinating disease characterized by an ascending muscle paralysis that has an acute onset

B. Etiology

1. A cell-mediated immunologic response appears to affect the motor segment of the peripheral nerves.
2. Guillain-Barré syndrome usually is preceded by an upper respiratory or gastrointestinal viral infection.
3. It affects all age groups and sexes equally.

C. Pathophysiologic processes and manifestations

1. In response to the prodromal viral infection, lymphocytes migrate to the nerves and stimulate an autoimmune response.
2. The lymphocytes digest the myelin sheath surrounding the fibers, causing demyelination.
3. The axons are also affected, causing neuronal destruction.
4. Demyelination and axonal degeneration result in decreased innervation of striated muscle and muscle atrophy.
5. Regeneration of the peripheral nerve then occurs, with resultant recovery of neuronal and motor function.
6. In some instances, the cell body has been damaged and regeneration is not possible, leaving residual neuronal deficits.
7. Manifestations occur acutely and progress rapidly.
8. Paralysis and paresthesias begin distally in the legs and progress bilaterally upward until paralysis of the diaphragm occurs, resulting in respiratory distress.
9. Other manifestations include hypotonia and absence of deep tendon reflexes.
10. Autonomic nervous system dysfunction may also be present as indicated by variations in blood pressure, cardiac rhythm abnormalities, and loss of sweating mechanisms.
11. Recovery usually occurs and progresses in reverse order from the onset of symptoms, in a proximal to distal pattern.

D. Overview of nursing interventions
1. Maintain airway and support pulmonary function as highest priorities.
2. Prepare the patient for plasmapheresis during the acute phase, if indicated.
3. Administer steroids, as prescribed, to reduce inflammation.
4. Prevent pulmonary complications.
5. Encourage the patient to move around to prevent complications due to immobility (ie, skin breakdown).
6. Educate the patient and family members regarding the patient's condition, treatment modalities, and the need for rehabilitation after resolution.
7. Provide nutritional support.

VIII. Myasthenia gravis

A. Description: a neuromuscular junction disorder characterized by striated muscle weakness and severe fatigue

B. Etiology and incidence
1. Myasthenia gravis is believed to be an autoimmune disorder; incidence increases in persons who have a preexisting autoimmune disease. It occurs predominantly in women.
2. A thymic tumor has been found in 20% of patients with myasthenia gravis.
3. Receptor-binding antibodies are present in 80% of persons with active myasthenia gravis.

C. Pathophysiologic processes and manifestations
1. The defect in nerve transmission at the neuromuscular junction is caused by defects in the postsynaptic receptor sites.
2. The postsynaptic acetylcholine receptors fail to recognize themselves and an immune response is stimulated, causing release of antibodies to the receptor binding sites.
3. These antibodies attach to the receptor sites and block the binding of acetylcholine released from the terminal axon.
4. Over time, the ongoing autoimmune response destroys the binding sites, decreasing the numbers of available sites.
5. Nerve transmission across the synaptic junction decreases; muscle stimulation also decreases.
6. Onset of symptoms is insidious, beginning with fatigue and mild muscle weakness.
7. Muscles initially affected are those of the eyes, face, and throat, causing diplopia, ptosis, and ocular palsies.
8. Progressive involvement will affect the muscles of mastication, speech, and swallowing. Facial palsies will occur. Manifestations include weight loss secondary to impaired swallowing, drooling, choking, and changes in speech tones secondary to laryngeal involvement.
9. Myasthenic crisis occurs when there is severe and marked increase in muscle weakness, including diaphragmatic paralysis and quadriplegia.
10. Cholinergic crisis occurs when symptoms of myasthenic crisis prompt the patient to ingest increased amounts of anticholinergic medications, causing a toxic reaction.
11. Manifestations of cholinergic crisis include diarrhea, bradycardia, pupillary constriction, increased salivation and sweating, and muscle fasciculations.

D.   Overview of nursing interventions

1.   Teach the patient about electromyography, which assists in diagnosis.
2.   Administer Tensilon®, as prescribed, to cause an immediate improvement in muscle weakness and for purposes of diagnosis.
3.   Administer anticholinergic medications and steroids, as prescribed.
4.   Prepare the patient for plasmapheresis, which may be used as adjunctive therapy.
5.   Provide hemodynamic and pulmonary supportive care as indicated.
6.   Prepare the patient for thymectomy when thymic hyperplasia is present; provide appropriate postoperative care.
7.   Use chemotherapeutic agents, as ordered, for patients with recurrent myasthenic crisis.

IX.   Muscular dystrophy (MD)

A.   Description

1.   The muscular dystrophies are a group of disorders that affect muscle fibers; they are characterized by progressive, symmetric muscle weakness and atrophy, resulting in immobility and deformity.
2.   Types of dystrophies include:
    a.   Duchenne's
    b.   Facioscapulohumeral
    c.   Limb girdle
    d.   Myotonic

B.   Etiology

1.   The dystrophies are genetic disorders that result in biochemical or metabolic alterations.
2.   Duchenne's MD is an X-linked inherited defect thought to occur because of deletion in the DNA chain.
3.   Other theorized causes include:
    a.   An intrinsic defect in muscle fibers causing replacement of muscle with connective tissue
    b.   Abnormalities in enzyme metabolism

C.   Pathophysiologic processes and manifestations

1.   Manifestations present around 3 years of age and are characterized by slowed motor development or progressive weakness and muscle atrophy.
2.   Lack of gross motor control occurs, resulting in frequent falls and difficulty in complex motor tasks.
3.   Hypertrophy of the calf muscles occurs in approximately 80% of cases; toe walking results from weakness of the anterior tibial and peroneal muscles.
4.   Within 5 years, muscle weakness progresses to the trunk and respiratory function is compromised.
5.   Kyphoscoliosis complicates pulmonary status even more; eventually, the child becomes wheelchair-bound.
6.   Other manifestations can include:
    a.   Cardiac manifestations (may occur in as many as 95% of cases)
    b.   Moderate mental retardation
    c.   Smooth muscle dysfunction (manifested by megacolon, volvulus, and malabsorption syndromes)

7. Muscle tissue is replaced by connective tissue and fat, and the number of muscle fibers is decreased. The remaining fibers exhibit necrosis associated with an inflammatory response.

D. **Overview of nursing interventions**

1. Maintain normal function for as long as possible, because no cure for muscular dystrophy exists.
2. Maintain activity with range of motion exercises, use of braces, and prevention of muscle breakdown.
3. Prepare the patient for surgical treatment of contractures, if indicated.
4. Provide pulmonary and hemodynamic support, as indicated.
5. Advise the parents to seek genetic counseling.

Bibliography

Barker, E. (1994). *Neuroscience nursing*. St. Louis: C.V. Mosby.

Bullock, B. (1996). *Pathophysiology: Adaptations and alterations in function* (4th ed.). Philadelphia: Lippincott-Raven.

Cusack T. (1996). Multiple sclerosis: clues to diagnosis and recommended management. *Physician Assistant*, 20(10):24, 27–28, 37–39.

Featherstone, K., Hilton, G., & Jastremski, C. W. (Eds.) (1998). *Society of trauma nurses resource manual for trauma nursing*. Philadelphia: W. B. Saunders.

Ganong, William F. (1997). *Review of medical physiology* (18th ed.). Stamford CT: Appleton and Lange.

Guyton, Arthur C., & Hall John E. (1996). *Textbook of medical physiology* (9th ed.). Philadelphia: W. B. Saunders.

Hickey, J. (1992). *The clinical practice of neurological and neurosurgical nursing* (3rd ed.). Philadelphia: J. B. Lippincott.

Kernnich C. A., & Kaminski H. J. (1995). Myasthenia gravis: pathophysiology, diagnosis and collaborative care. *Journal of Neuroscience Nursing* 27(4):207–18.

Kinney, M., Packa, D., & Dunbar, S. (1993). *AACN's clinical reference for critical-care nursing* (3rd ed.). St. Louis: C.V. Mosby.

McCance, K. L., & Huether, S. E. (1990). *Pathophysiology: A biologic basis for disease in adults and children*. St. Louis: C. V. Mosby.

McCance, K. L., & Huether, S. E. (1994). *Pathophysiology: The biologic basis for disease in adults and children* (2nd ed.). St. Louis: Mosby–Year Book.

O'Donnell L. (1995). Caring for patients with myasthenia gravis . . . find out your role in assessing and managing this debilitating disorder. *Nursing*, 25(3):60–61.

Porth, C. (1994). *Pathophysiology: Concepts of altered health states* (4th ed.). Philadelphia: Lippincott-Raven.

Price, S. A., & Wilson, L. M. (1986). *Pathophysiology: Clinical concepts of disease processes* (3rd ed.). New York: McGraw-Hill.

Tierney, L., McPhee, S., Papadakis, M., & Schroeder, S. eds. (1993). *Current medical diagnosis and treatment*. Norwalk, CT: Appleton & Lange.

Waters R. L. (1996). Functional prognosis of spinal cord injuries, *Journal of Spinal Cord Medicine*, 19(2):89–92.

STUDY QUESTIONS

1. Dysfunction in the lower motor neuron pathways results in:
   a. spasticity
   b. flaccidity
   c. hypertonia
   d. muscle weakness

2. When caring for a patient with a complete spinal cord transection at C-5, the primary nursing concern is:
   a. hemodynamic instability
   b. paralysis
   c. autonomic dysfunction
   d. respiratory distress

3. The manifestations of autonomic hyperreflexia involve:
   a. activation of the sympathetic nervous system
   b. activation of the parasympathetic nervous system
   c. a response to the primary neurologic damage
   d. a normal side effect of spinal shock

4. When intervertebral disk herniation occurs, the manifestations are related to:
   a. extrusion of the posterior capsule
   b. the conversion of the disk tissue into fibrocartilaginous tissue
   c. compression of the nerve root or the spinal cord
   d. degeneration of the vertebral column

5. The need for surgical stabilization of a disk is indicated by the occurrence of:
   a. severe neurologic dysfunction
   b. intractable pain
   c. sensory abnormalities
   d. failure of conservative therapy

6. The pathophysiologic changes that contribute to the occurrence of multiple sclerosis include:
   a. migration of T lymphocytes across the blood-brain barrier
   b. cystic lesions in the myelin
   c. an inflammatory response resulting in secretion of IgG antibodies

   d. degeneration of upper and lower motor neurons

7. Ophthalmoplegia, dysarthria, and facial weakness are indicative of which syndrome in multiple sclerosis?
   a. corticospinal
   b. brain stem
   c. cerebellar
   d. cerebral

8. Amyotrophic lateral sclerosis affects:
   a. upper motor neurons
   b. corticospinal tracts only
   c. lower motor neurons
   d. combined upper and lower motor neurons

9. Recovery from Guillain-Barré occurs:
   a. because of regeneration of the peripheral nerve
   b. because of improved innervation of striated muscle
   c. in rare instances because of cell body destruction
   d. in the distal to proximal direction

10. In myasthenia gravis, the defect in nerve transmission is related to:
    a. the release of norepinephrine instead of acetylcholine in the synaptic junction
    b. an immune response that results in blockage and eventual destruction of receptor sites
    c. a genetic defect in the construction of receptor sites
    d. decreased acetylcholine released into the synaptic cleft

11. Which musculoskeletal disorder is thought to be a genetic disorder?
    a. myasthenia gravis
    b. multiple sclerosis
    c. muscular dystrophy
    d. herniated disk

12. Damage to the anterior horn cells in the spinal cord result in:
    a. muscle flaccidity
    b. muscle spasticity

    c. muscle hypertrophy

    d. increased reflexes

13. Lack of neuronal stimulation to a muscle group resulting in replacement of muscle by connective tissue and fat is called:

    a. spasticity

    b. flaccidity

    c. atrophy

    d. dystonia

14. An important nursing intervention in the care of the patient with ALS is:

    a. maintaining a means of communication

    b. preventing autonomic dysreflexia

    c. managing pain secondary to spinal deformity

    d. Administering anticholinergics

15. Autonomic dysfunction may be noticed in which of the following conditions:

    a. spinal cord injury and intervertebral disc disease

    b. myasthenia gravis and muscular dystrophy

    c. Guillain-Barré and ALS

    d. spinal cord injury and Guillain-Barré

16. Pathophysiologic findings associated with muscular dystrophy may include all of the following except:

    a. cardiac manifestations

    b. increased salivation and lacrimation

    c. mental retardation

    d. megacolor or volvulus

ANSWER KEY

Question	Correct answer	Correct answer rationale	Incorrect answer rationales
1.	b	Lower motor neuron dysfunction occurs in the anterior horn cell of the spinal cord, the myoneural junction, and in the muscles. Disruption in any of these locations results in muscle flaccidity.	a and c. An upper motor neuron lesion results in spasticity and hypertonia. d. Muscle weakness may be noted, but the best response is b.
2.	d	A spinal cord lesion above T-1 completely or partially impairs muscle innervation of the diaphragm and intercostals. This results in poor ventilatory effort and respiratory distress.	a. Hemodynamic instability is a concern, but airway maintenance is of primary importance. b. Paralysis will occur, but pulmonary distress is of primary importance. c. Autonomic dysfunction will be present, but the best response is d.
3.	a	Autonomic hyperreflexia is a condition that occurs in response to sensory stimulation by a resultant activation of the sympathetic nervous system.	b. The manifestations are representative of activation of the sympathetic and not the parasympathetic nervous system. c and d. These are incorrect responses. Autonomic hyperreflexia is neither a normal response to the primary event, nor a normal side effect of spinal shock.
4.	c	As the nucleus pulposus extrudes through the posterior capsule of the disk, the nerve root or the cord is compressed, causing pain and sensory and motor dysfunction.	a. The nucleus pulposus extrudes through the posterior capsule. The capsule does not extrude. b. The disk is fibrocartilaginous, but this does not cause the manifestations. d. Degeneration of the vertebral column may lead to herniation of the disk but is not a direct cause of the manifestations.
5.	a	Significant neurologic involvement, including decreased deep tendon reflexes or loss of bowel or bladder control, is an indicator that surgery is necessary.	b, c, and d. Although all of these might suggest the need for surgical stabilization, the most obvious indicator is neurologic dysfunction.
6.	c	The B lymphocytes in the CNS secrete immunoglobulin G antibodies in response to an unknown agent. The resulting inflammatory response results in movement of macrophages into	a. B lymphocytes and not T lymphocytes have been identified as being active in this process. b. Cysts are not formed, but plaques are.

Question	Correct answer	Correct answer rationale	Incorrect answer rationales
		the myelin sheath and the formation of demyelinated areas.	c. Multiple sclerosis is an upper motor neuron disease and does not affect lower motor neurons.
7.	b	The brain stem syndrome primarily affects cranial nerves III through XII, causing dysfunction of the extraocular muscles and innervation to the muscles of speech. This results in ophthalmoplegia and dysarthria.	a. The corticospinal syndrome is associated with spastic paralysis, bowel and bladder dysfunction, and symmetric muscle weakness. c. The cerebellar syndrome is manifested by spastic gait, ataxia, and intention tremors. d. The cerebral syndrome is associated with impaired vision and intellectual and emotional deterioration.
8.	d	ALS is a combined upper and lower motor neuron disease affecting the motor cortex, brain stem, and spinal cord.	a, b, and c are incorrect.
9.	a	Recovery from Guillain-Barré occurs because of regrowth and repair of the peripheral nerves.	b. Improved innervation of striated muscle does occur with recovery, but this is not the cause of the recovery. c. Recovery does not occur if the cell body is destroyed, but this is a rare occurrence. d. Recovery occurs in the proximal to distal direction.
10.	b	Myasthenia gravis is a neuromuscular junction disorder that is caused by defects in the postsynaptic receptor sites. An immune response releases antibodies to the receptor sites, blocking the binding of acetylcholine and leading to receptor site destruction.	a. Epinephrine is not released into the synaptic junction. c. Myasthenia gravis is not a genetic disease. d. The amount of acetylcholine that is released is not lessened, but there is blockages of the receptor sites.
11.	c	Muscular dystrophy is the only choice that reflects genetic disorders.	a, b, and d. These disorders do not result from genetic defect.
12.	a	Muscle flaccidity results from damage to the anterior horn cells.	b. Muscle spasticity results from damage to the pyramidal tracts. c and d. Muscle atrophy and decreased reflexes will be present.
13.	c	Atrophy is a shrinkage in muscle mass that results from lack of use of the muscle and loss of tone secondary to decreased neuronal stimulation.	a. Spasticity is a type of hypertonia in which there is an increase in muscle tone resulting in excessive resistance to movement. b. Flaccidity is a type of hypotonia

Question	Correct answer	Correct answer rationale	Incorrect answer rationales
			in which there is lack of muscle movement against resistance. d. Dystonia is the maintenance of an abnormal posture through muscular contractions.
14.	a	Speech dysfunction occurs in ALS as motor impairment of muscles needed for language progresses. It is essential to maintain open channels of communication with the patient.	b. Autonomic dysreflexia occurs in spinal cord injuries. c. There is little, if any, pain associated with ALS. d. Anticholinergics are indicated in the treatment of myasthenia gravis, not ALS.
15.	d	Autonomic dysfunction has been documented in both spinal cord injury and Guillain-Barré.	a. Autonomic dysfunction occurs in spinal cord injury, but not in intervertebral disc disease. b. Autonomic dysfunction is associated with neither of these diseases. c. Autonomic dysfunction occurs in Guillain-Barré, but not ALS.
16.	b	Changes in salivation and lacrimation are not associated with muscular dystrophy.	a, c, and d. All of these symptoms may be seen in patients with muscular dystrophy.

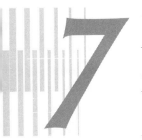

7 Degenerative and Infectious Neurologic Disorders

I. Overview of pathophysiologic processes

A. Degenerative diseases

1. Degenerative diseases occur when cells of the central nervous system (CNS) undergo changes that alter their functioning.
2. The changes usually worsen with age.
3. Symptoms depend on which CNS cells are affected.
4. Alzheimer's disease, Parkinson's disease, and Wernicke' disease are degenerative neurologic diseases.
5. Genetic predisposition may be a risk factor, but generally, no risk factors exist.

B. Infectious diseases

1. Infectious diseases occur when CNS cells are infected with a pathogen.
2. CNS infections follow the same course as infections anywhere else in the body.
3. In the CNS, inflammation is encased in the skull, causing symptoms particular to this phenomenon.
4. Encephalitis, meningitis, and AIDS dementia are infectious neurologic diseases.
5. Risk factors for these diseases vary according to the disease process.

II. Physiologic responses to degenerative and infectious neurologic dysfunction

A. Alterations in content of consciousness
1. Changes in content of consciousness may be acute or chronic.
2. Acute changes include organic brain syndromes, delirium, and clouding of consciousness. Chronic changes include dementia and vegetative states (Display 7-1).

B. Memory impairment: Recent or remote recall may be affected.

C. Disorientation: inability to correctly identify time, person, and place

D. Hallucinations: subjective sensory misperceptions that occur in the absence of relevant external stimuli; may be visual, auditory, tactile, or involve the senses of smell or taste

E. Illusions: misinterpretations of sensory stimuli

F. Delusions: false beliefs based on a misinterpretation of sensory stimuli

G. Hypersomnia: excessive drowsiness and sleep from which arousal occurs easily

H. Language comprehension deficits: decreased ability to comprehend spoken language or to name objects; typically seen with amnesiac dementias associated with temporal lobe damage

I. Distractibility: loss of concentration contributing to an inability to carry out complex or sequential intellectual tasks

J. Dyspraxia: inability to execute a planned activity; may result from an inability to sequence the individual components of the activity and plan for its execution

DISPLAY 7-1
Alterations in Content of Consciousness

TYPE

Acute alterations:
- Organic brain syndromes: disorders of perception and interpretation of external stimuli.
- Delirium: a state characterized by disorientation, delusions, and hyperactivity of the autonomic nervous system
- Clouding of consciousness: a state of limited awareness, sometimes accompanied by lethargy or irritability

Causes
- Direct injury to nervous tissue
- Overactivity of a previously inactive brain center
- Exposure to exogenous agents (e.g., chemicals or bacteria)

Manifestations
- Impaired short-term memory
- Distractibility
- Disorientation
- Alterations in perception (illusions, delusions)
- Impaired intellectual functioning and judgment
- Alterations in activity levels (hyperactive, hypoactive, lethargic)
- Alterations in autonomic junction (tachycardia, diaphoresis, dilated pupils)

TYPE

Chronic alterations:
- Dementia: a condition chaacterized by alterations in content of consciousness, but not normal
- Vegetative state: a condition in which no cerebral function exists, but sleep–wake cycles are present and autonomic junction is intact

Causes
- Tissue destruction
- Inflammation
- Biochemical imbalances
- Slow-growing viruses
- Genetic predisposition

Manifestations
- Inability to acquire new information or knowledge
- Impaired short-term memory
- Impaired ability to learn

K. Alterations in behavior: includes personality changes and inappropriate affect; commonly seen with frontal lobe injuries

L. Alterations in visual-spatial relationships: inability to recognize visual-spatial relationships; commonly seen with dementias altering the cerebral cortex

III. Alzheimer's disease

A. Description

    1. Alzheimer's disease is a chronic, irreversible, organic mental disorder.

    2. It starts with memory losses and eventually progresses to severe neurologic manifestations.

B. Etiology and incidence

    1. The cause of Alzheimer's disease is unknown.

    2. Several theories about its cause exist.

        a. One theory holds that degenerative neuronal changes are due to chemical and enzymatic disparities, such as the loss of the enzyme choline acetyltransferase, which results in decreased acetylcholine.

        b. Another theory, the latent virus theory, is based on the isolation of prions (submicroscopic proteinaceous infectious particles) in the tissues of patients with the disease.

        c. Because a genetic predisposition to the disease appears to exist, an additional theory holds that Alzheimer's disease may involve an autosomal dominant gene.

        d. Other theories include the involvement of antibrain antibodies, autoimmune responses, and an extra gene on chromosome 21.

    3. Alzheimer's disease typically affects persons over age 65. When onset occurs before age 50, it is considered presenile dementia of the Alzheimer's type; after age 65, it is considered senile dementia.

    4. Incidence of Alzheimer's disease increases with age.

C. Pathophysiologic processes and manifestations

    1. Alzheimer's disease is characterized by the presence of neurofibrillary tangles (distorted and twisted protein fibers within the neuron) and the degeneration of large numbers of terminal axons.

    2. These changes, commonly found in the cortex, result in a fibrous core and contribute to senile plaque formation.

    3. The severity of the disease appears to be associated with the number of fibrous plaques.

    4. Onset is insidious; early symptoms include memory loss, forgetfulness, and mood swings.

    5. Memory loss progresses until confusion and disorientation occur.

    6. Higher intellectual functions (eg, ability to make judgments, think abstractly, and recognize visual-spatial relationships) begin to deteriorate.

    7. As the ability to concentrate and analyze diminishes, dyspraxia may become apparent.

    8. Personality changes (eg, hostility, depression, and emotional lability) occur.

9. Motor changes, such as flexion posturing, may also occur.

D. Overview of nursing interventions

1. Assess neurologic deficits and evaluate the patient's ability to compensate for them.

2. **Help the patient compensate for neurologic deficits with the use of memory aids.**

3. Help the patient maintain existing cognitive functions.

4. Ensure adequate nutritional status.

5. Assist with personal hygiene.

6. **Maintain a safe environment and monitor patient as Alzheimer's patients have been known to wander from their homes.**

7. **Provide counseling for the patient and family members. Because of the potential genetic relationship, counseling is essential.**

IV. Parkinson's disease

A. Description

1. Parkinson's disease is a chronic disorder of the basal ganglia.

2. Types include primary and secondary Parkinson's disease.

B. Etiology

1. The cause of Parkinson's disease is unknown.

2. Primary Parkinson's disease occurs after age 40 and peaks at age 60; it affects men and women equally.

3. Secondary Parkinson's disease occurs secondary to other disorders (eg, infection, drug toxicity, and neoplasm); it usually is reversible.

C. Pathophysiologic processes and manifestations

1. In Parkinson's disease, the dopaminergic pathways (neural pathways that respond to the inhibitory neurotransmitter dopamine) sustain degenerative changes. The amount of cyclase-linked dopamine receptors in the basal ganglia also decreases.

2. Depletion of these dopamine-linked fibers results in a deficiency of dopamine, which is required for extrapyramidal function.

3. A relative increase in some excitatory neurotransmitters also occurs, resulting in a biochemical imbalance between inhibitory and excitatory neuronal transmission.

4. This imbalance disrupts normal motor function, causing constant excitatory muscle stimulation.

5. Symptoms occur bilaterally but asymmetrically, and are insidious at onset.

6. Characteristic manifestations include:

   a. **Tremors (asymmetric, rhythmic, and low-amplitude): These commonly occur at rest and lessen with voluntary movement; as the disease progresses, tremors become more pronounced and symmetric.**

   b. **Muscle rigidity (involuntary contraction of striated muscle inhibiting voluntary movement): These usually are accompa-**

nied by brief, jerking motor contractions called "cogwheel" activity.

    c. Akinesia (decreased or absent voluntary movements): associated with severe fatigue

    d. Bradykinesia (slowness of voluntary movements): characterized by difficulty in initiating or continuing movements

    e. Hypokinesia (decreased frequency of movements)

    f. Dysphagia (difficulty swallowing) as esophageal muscles are affected

7. Posture also is affected and is characterized by alterations in postural fixation, equilibrium, and righting.

    a. Alterations in postural fixation result in neck and head flexion, rendering the patient unable to maintain a straight position when upright.

    b. **Alterations in equilibrium or righting ability result in a festinating gait; the patient takes short, accelerating steps in an attempt to maintain an upright position while walking.**

8. Autonomic manifestations include diaphoresis, orthostatic hypotension, constipation, and urinary retention.

9. Secondary manifestations include:

    a. Disturbance in fine motor control resulting in impaired handwriting and clumsiness with activities of daily living

    b. Blurred vision and fixed upward and lateral rotation of the eyes

    c. Masklike face and decreased blinking

    d. Generalized weakness and fatigue

10. In the late stages of the disease, dementia occurs.

D. **Overview of nursing interventions**

1. Administer dopamine precursors (Levodopa®), dopamine decarboxylase inhibitors (Sinemet®), and anticholinergic agents as prescribed.

2. Assess neurologic deficits and determine the patient's ability for self-care.

 3. **Assess nutritional status (because of dysphagia and constipation).**

4. Ensure a safe environment.

 5. **Encourage the patient to wear elastic stockings and change positions slowly to compensate for orthostatic hypotension.**

6. Assist with rehabilitation.

V.   Wernicke's disease (also known as Wernicke-Korsakoff syndrome)

A. **Description: a degenerative disease associated with nutritional deficits and characterized by gait disturbances, confusion, and cranial nerve palsies**

B. **Etiology and incidence**

1. Wernicke's disease is caused by a deficiency of thiamine.

 2. **Groups at high-risk include:**

    a. **Chronic alcoholics who generally maintain poor nutritional intake**

    b. **Persons with malabsorption syndromes**

    c. **Malnourished persons**

3. Age of onset ranges from 30 to 70; incidence is higher among men.

C. **Pathophysiologic processes and manifestations**

1. Thiamine (vitamin B_1) is essential for neuronal metabolism; if metabolism is altered, energy cannot be produced and vital neuronal activities cease.

2. Degeneration of neurons is commonly found in the thalamus, hypothalamus, the fourth ventricle, the cerebellum, and the vestibular division of cranial nerve VIII.

3. Symptoms can include:
   a. Alterations in consciousness
   b. Oculomotor dysfunction (including ophthalmoplegia, nystagmus, and conjugate gaze palsy)
   c. Ataxia (impaired muscular coordination)
   d. Anterograde amnesia (inability to retain new information)
   e. Retrograde amnesia (inability to retrieve information from memory)

 4. **Korsakoff psychosis, which is characterized by amnesia and confabulation (invention of experiences to compensate for memory gaps), may also occur.**

5. Rarely, severe neurologic deterioration can lead to coma.

D. **Overview of nursing interventions**

1. Administer thiamine as prescribed.
2. Assess neurologic status and evaluate deficits.
3. Provide a safe environment.
4. Assist the patient with rehabilitation.

 5. **For a patient with a history of alcoholism, consider the need for adequate nutrition.**

VI. Encephalitis

A. **Description: an acute infection of the nervous system resulting in the rapid onset of altered states of consciousness**

B. **Etiology**

1. Encephalitis is caused by a virus.
   a. The most common causative agents are herpes simplex type I and arthropod-borne viruses (eg, Eastern equine encephalitis or St. Louis encephalitis).
   b. Arthropod-borne agents are associated with seasonal incidence; all other viral agents occur year round.

2. Encephalitis also may result from a secondary complication of systemic viral diseases (eg, poliomyelitis and mononucleosis) or from a viral illness such as rubella.

3. Rarely, encephalitis results from vaccination with a live attenuate virus vaccine (eg, measles, mumps, and rubella).

4. Exposure to toxins such as carbon monoxide may also lead to symptoms of encephalitis.

C. **Pathophysiologic processes and manifestations**

1. The pathophysiologic processes of neuronal damage vary according to the agent involved.

a. Herpes simplex type I is found most commonly in the temporal and frontal lobes and results in hemorrhagic necrosis.
b. Arthropod-borne viruses cause diffuse neuronal degeneration, with a secondary inflammatory process producing edema and necrosis of tissue.

2. As neuronal destruction, edema, and hemorrhage occur, intracranial hypertension increases; herniation may occur eventually.

3. Manifestations are of acute onset and include:
   a. Changes in mentation, including confusion and delirium
   b. Fever (always present)
   c. Seizures and coma (may occur as disease progresses)
   d. Increased intracranial pressure

4. Other symptoms can include:
   a. Cranial nerve palsies
   b. Paresthesia and paresis
   c. Abnormal reflex activity

D. Overview of nursing interventions

1. Assess neurologic status and document progression of neuronal deterioration.
2. Administer antiviral agents intravenously as prescribed.

3. Recognize and manage increased intracranial pressure.
4. Provide supportive ventilatory and hemodynamic care as indicated.
5. Assist the patient with rehabilitation.

VII. Meningitis

A. Description

1. Meningitis is an infection of the meninges including the spinal cord or brain; a secondary inflammatory process affecting neuronal tissue and the cerebral vasculature also may occur.

2. Types include:
   a. Bacterial meningitis
   b. Aseptic meningitis
   c. Fungal meningitis

B. Etiology and incidence

1. Bacterial meningitis primarily affects the pia mater and arachnoid. It results from infection with *Neisseria meningitidis, Streptococcus pneumoniae,* and *Haemophilus influenzae.*
   a. These agents occur worldwide and affect mainly children and adolescents.
   b. Pneumococcal meningitis mainly affects persons over age 40 and in epidemic distributions.
   c. Typically, these agents gain access to the meninges through the bloodstream or by direct extension from an infected area such as the sinuses.

2. Aseptic meningitis results from coxsackie virus, poliomyelitis, herpes simplex type I, and adenoviruses. It occurs only in the meninges.
3. Fungal meningitis results from cryptococcosis, coccidioidomycosis, candidiasis, and aspergillosis. It typically affects persons with preexisting immunosuppression.

C. **Pathophysiologic processes and manifestations**
   1. In *bacterial meningitis:*
     a. Bacteria from the bloodstream invades the meninges, initiating an inflammatory response.
     b. This inflammatory response leads to vascular edema and increased permeability of vessel walls.
     c. Meningeal vessels are hyperemic, and the inflammatory response delivers neutrophils to the subarachnoid space.
     d. A purulent exudate forms and is distributed to the cranial and spinal nerves and into the perivascular spaces of the cortex.
     e. Within the cortex, the number of microglia and astrocytes increases.
   2. In *aseptic meningitis,* inflammation of the meninges results either from a virus or from other causes (eg, encephalitis, subarachnoid bleeding, or cerebral abcess).
   3. In *fungal meningitis:*
     a. A granulomatous reaction contributes to the development of granulomas at the base of the brain.
     b. Fungi may also extend into the tissues, causing arteritis, thrombosis, and infarction.
     c. Meningeal fibrosis may develop, leading to permanent cranial nerve dysfunction.
   4. Manifestations of meningitis vary depending on the causative agent.
   5. Symptoms of bacterial meningitis include:
     a. Meningeal irritation, including stiff neck, headache, Brudzinski's sign, and Kernig's sign
     b. Photophobia
     c. Nuchal rigidity
     d. Fever
     e. Elevated white cell count
     f. Alterations in consciousness
   6. Symptoms of aseptic meningitis include:
     a. Mild throbbing headache
     b. Photophobia
     c. Mild nuchal rigidity
     d. Fever
     e. Malaise
   7. Characteristic manifestations of fungal meningitis include a slowly occurring dementia and the absence of fever.

   8. **In meningococcal meningitis, a petechial rash may be present.**

D. **Overview of nursing interventions**
   1. Administer the appropriate antibiotic, antiviral, or antifungal agents as prescribed.

2. Ensure patient safety, particularly those who exhibit altered levels of consciousness.

3. **Decrease stimuli to alleviate pain, photophobia, and neuronal irritability.**
4. Provide supportive care as indicated.
5. Keep the patient comfortable.

VIII.   AIDS dementia

A. **Description: progressive cognitive dementia associated with the presence of the human immunodeficiency virus (HIV).**

B. Etiology
   1. AIDS dementia occurs concomitantly with other systemic manifestations of HIV disease and as a single entity.
   2. It occurs in all age groups, affecting both men and women.
   3. Transmission of HIV occurs via blood and body secretions and has a higher incidence among persons engaging in unsafe sexual practices and using intravenous drugs.

C. Pathophysiologic processes and manifestations
   1. Manifestations are progressive and can include:
      a. Impaired cognition (eg, diminished intellectual capacity, decreased insight and judgment, and general loss of all higher intellectual functions)
      b. Behavioral changes (eg, apathy, social withdrawal, emotional lability, and irritability)
      c. Alterations in motor function (eg, progressive extremity weakness, deterioration in handwriting, impaired coordination)
   2. In the later stages of the disease, hallucinations, severe dementia, psychomotor retardation, ataxia, paresis, and seizures may occur.

   3. **AIDS dementia, unlike the systemic manifestations of AIDS, is believed to result from direct infiltration of HIV into the nervous tissue and not from a immunosuppression. In a few instances, HIV DNA has been isolated in neuronal tissue.**
   4. Cortical atrophy has been detected on microscopic examination; diffuse pallor of white matter also has been found.

D. Overview of nursing interventions
   1. Assess neurologic deficits and identify existing capabilities.
   2. Evaluate the patient's ability for self-care.
   3. Administer Retrovir®, DDI, other antireplicative agents or protease inhibitors as prescribed.
   4. Administer antibiotics to fight systemic infection as prescribed.

   5. **Ensure the patient's safety, because judgment is impaired and motor dysfunction may occur.**
   6. Institute seizure precautions.

Bibliography

Barker, E. (1994). *Neuroscience nursing.* St. Louis: C. V. Mosby.

Bedos, J., Chastang, C., Lucet, J., Kalo, T., Gachot, B., & Wolff, M. (1995). Early predictors of outcome for HIV patients with neurological failure. *Journal of the American Medical Association,* 274:35–40.

Bullock, B. (1996). *Pathophysiology: Adaptations and alterations in function* (4th ed.). Philadelphia: Lippincott-Raven.

Ganong, William F. (1997). *Review of medical physiology* (18th ed.). Stamford, CT: Appleton and Lange.

Guyton, Arthur C., & Hall John E. (1996). *Textbook of medical physiology* (9th ed.). Philadelphia: W. B. Saunders.

Jenkyn L. R., Coffey D. J., & Reeves A. G. (1996). Parkinsons and Alzheimers: New tools, new attitudes in patient care. *Geriatrics, 51*(1):65–72.

Kinney, M., Packa, D., & Dunbar, S. (1993). *AACN's clinical reference for critical-care nursing* (3rd ed.). St. Louis: C.V. Mosby.

McCance, K. L., & Huether, S. E. (1994). *Pathophysiology: The biologic basis for disease in adults and children* (2nd ed.). St. Louis: Mosby–Year Book.

McKeogh M. (1995). Dementia in HIV disease—a challenge for palliative care? *Journal of Palliative Care, 11*(2):30–3.

Porth, C. (1994). *Pathophysiology: Concepts of altered health states.* (4th ed.). Philadelphia: Lippincott-Raven.

Rosenberg D. M., McLaulin B., Bennett M., & Mathisen K. (1996). Diagnosing HIV dementia: a retrospective analysis. *Journal of the Association of Nursing in AIDS Care,* 7(6):57–66.

Salzman E. W. (1996). Living with parkinson's disease. *New England Journal of Medicine,* 3343:114–16.

Tapper, V. J. (1997). Pathophysiology, assessment and treatment of Parkinson's disease. *Nurse Practitioner: American Journal of Primary Health Care, 22*(7):76–80.

Tierney, L., McPhee, S., Papadakis, M., & Schroeder, S. (eds.). (1993). *Current medical diagnosis and treatment.* Norwalk, CT: Appleton & Lange.

STUDY QUESTIONS

1. A state of disorientation characterized by delusions and hyperactivity is called:
   a. dementia
   b. organic brain syndrome
   c. delirium
   d. clouding of consciousness

2. A vegetative state is manifested by all of the following symptoms *except:*
   a. presence of delusions
   b. absent intellectual activity
   c. intact sleep–wake cycles
   d. intact autonomic function

3. Which of the following terms described a false, fixed misbelief based on misinterpretation of sensory stimuli?
   a. illusion
   b. delusion
   c. hallucination
   d. hypersomnia

4. Neurofibrillary tangles are degenerative changes noted in Alzheimer's disease that contribute to:
   a. decreased amounts of acetylcholine
   b. proteinaceous infectious particles
   c. senile plaque formation
   d. autoimmune responses

5. Early manifestations of Alzheimer's disease include:
   a. alterations in judgment
   b. dyspraxia
   c. paratonia
   d. memory loss and forgetfulness

6. The manifestations of Parkinson's disease are due to:
   a. imbalance between excitatory and inhibitory neurotransmitter activity
   b. increased activity of the dopaminergic pathway
   c. damage in the caudate and putamen
   d. damage at the level of the striated muscle

7. Postural alterations in Parkinson's disease are characterized by all of the following *except:*
   a. difficulty with righting
   b. orthostatic hypotension
   c. festinating gait
   d. short, accelerated steps

8. It is believed that AIDS dementia is due to:
   a. an immunosuppressive effect
   b. degeneration in axonal conduction
   c. direct HIV infiltration in neuronal tissue
   d. macrophage activity

9. Herpes simplex encephalitis results in:
   a. diffuse neuronal degeneration
   b. inflammation
   c. cerebral edema
   d. hemorrhagic necrosis

10. Bacterial meningitis results in the formation of a:
    a. slowly occurring dementia
    b. purulent exudate
    c. granuloma
    d. thrombosis

11. An acute alteration in consciousness is most likely due to:
    a. biochemical imbalance
    b. slow growing viruses
    c. direct injury to nervous tissue
    d. genetic predisposition

12. Dyspraxia is a manifestation most commonly associated with:
    a. Alzheimer's disease
    b. Parkinson's disease
    c. encephalitis
    d. meningitis

13. Fungal meningitis is characterized by:
    a. fever
    b. increase in numbers of microglia and astrocytes
    c. necrosis of tissue
    d. a granulomatous reaction

14. Acute onset of confusion and delirium can be anticipated with which disease process?
    a. AIDS dementia
    b. encephalitis
    c. Parkinson's disease
    d. Wernicke's disease

ANSWER KEY

Question	Correct answer	Correct answer rationale	Incorrect answer rationales
1.	c	Delirium is a state of disorientation that is characterized by hyperactivity, aggressive behavior, delusions, and possibly hallucinations.	a. Dementia is a state of diminished judgment and cognitive capability, but without any alterations in arousal. b. Organic brain syndrome is a disorder of perception and interpretation of external stimuli. d. Clouding of consciousness refers to a condition of limited awareness that may be combined with lethargy or irritability.
2.	a	A vegetative state is one in which all cerebral function is gone, yet sleep–wake cycles are still present. Autonomic function is also intact, but higher integrative/intellectual activity is absent. Delusions are not present in a vegetative state.	b, c, and d. These are characteristics of a vegetative state.
3.	b	The definition of a delusion is a false, fixed misbelief based on misinterpretation of sensory stimuli.	a. An illusion is a misinterpretation of sensory stimuli. c. A hallucination is a subjective sensory misperception in the absence of relevant external stimuli. d. Hypersomnia is excessive drowsiness and sleep.
4.	c	Neurofibrillary tangles are distorted and twisted protein fibers within the neuron. Degeneration of numerous bundles of these fibers results in a fibrous core that contributes to plaque formation.	a. There may be decreased amounts of acetylcholine in patients with Alzheimer's disease, but this does not occur secondary to neurofibrillary tangles. b. The presence of proteinaceous particles lends credence to the belief that Alzheimer's disease is due to latent virus activity. d. Although an autoimmune process has been hypothesized, no evidence exists that neurofibrillary tangles lead to this process.
5.	d	Memory loss, forgetfulness, and mood swings are consistent with the early development of Alzheimer's disease.	a, b, and c. These are considered late manifestations of Alzheimer's disease.

Question	Correct answer	Correct answer rationale	Incorrect answer rationales
6.	a	Parkinson's disease results from degeneration of the basal ganglia, decreasing the production of dopamine, an inhibitory neurotransmitter. Because of this decrease, there is an imbalance in the relationship between excitatory and inhibitory neurotransmitter activity.	b. There is decreased activity of the dopaminergic pathway in Parkinson's disease. c. The primary damage is in the basal ganglia, not the caudate and putamen. d. The damage does not occur at the level of the muscle, but rather at innervation of that muscle.
7.	b	Posture is affected in Parkinson's disease, and this contributes to difficulty with righting, postural fixation, and equilibrium. Orthostatic hypotension is not considered a postural abnormality.	a, c, and d. These are associated with postural alterations.
8.	c	HIV DNA has been isolated in the neurons of some patients with AIDS dementia, leading to the belief that AIDS dementia is due to direct HIV infiltration, instead of a condition related to immunocompetence.	a, b, and d. These are incorrect responses.
9.	d	Herpes simplex encephalitis results in hemorrhagic necrosis, particularly in the frontal and temporal lobes.	a. Encephalitis is an infectious, not a degenerative process. b. Inflammation is present but is a secondary characteristic of the infectious process. c. Cerebral edema does occur, but it is a secondary characteristic.characteristic.
10.	b	Bacterial meningitis is associated with the production of a purulent exudate.	a. Bacterial meningitis may result in acute dementia but not a slowly progressive one. c. Fungal meningitis results in granulomas. d. Fungal meningitis also has been known to result in the formation of thrombi.
11.	c	The causes of acute alterations include direct injury to nervous tissue, overactivity of a previously inactive brain center and exposure to exogenous agents.	a, b, and d. All of these are causes of chronic alterations. Other causes include tissue destruction, and inflammation.
12.	A	Dyspraxia is the inability to execute a planned activity secondary to an inability to sequence the individual components of the activity and plan for its execution. This is most notable in Alzheimer's disease.	b, c, and d. Dyspraxia is not of particular importance in any of these diseases.

Question	Correct answer	Correct answer rationale	Incorrect answer rationales
13.	d	Granulomas develop at the base of the brain in fungal meningitis. Arteritis, thrombosis and infarction can also occur.	a. Fever is generally associated with bacterial meningitis. b. An increase in the number of microglia and astrocytes are associated with bacterial meningitis. c. Meningeal fibrosis, rather than necrosis, is associated with fungal meningitis.
14.	b	Encephalitis is associated with the acute onset of mental status changes.	a, c, and d. All of these can lead to confusion and delirium, but the changes occur slowly, not acutely.

8 Musculoskeletal Disorders

I.   Overview of pathophysiologic processes

A. Soft tissue disorders

   1. Soft tissue disorders affect the tissue surrounding the skeletal system, including ligaments, tendons, muscles, and joints.

   2. Injuries to these structures will limit mobility and cause pain.

   3. Sprains and strains and dislocations are soft tissue disorders.

   4. Persons at risk for soft tissue injuries include:
      a. Elderly people
      b. Patients with conditions that limit physical mobility
      c. People who engage in athletic sports

B. Skeletal disorders

   1. Skeletal disorders are diseases of the bone.

   2. Fractures, tumors, and some metabolic conditions, such as osteoporosis and bone cancers, are skeletal disorders.

   3. Risk factors for skeletal disorders include:
      a. History or potential for trauma or falls
      b. History of poor nutrition
      c. Postmenopausal status
      d. Diagnosis of cancer with bone lesions

C. Inflammatory disorders

   1. Conditions that result from metabolic disorders affecting the bone are considered inflammatory disorders.

   2. Inflammatory disorders include osteomyelitis, osteoarthritis, and gouty arthritis.

   3. Risk factors include:
      a. Genetic predisposition to arthritis
      b. Inborn error of purine metabolism
      c. Deep-tissue infection
      d. Diabetes
      e. Chronic immunosuppression

II.   Physiologic responses to musculoskeletal dysfunction

A. Pain (localized)

B. Immobility

C. Inflammation (redness, heat, and tenderness)

III. Sprains and strains

A. Description

1. A sprain is a rip or tear in the ligaments surrounding a joint; in a severe sprain, the ligaments may completely tear or rupture.
2. A strain is a stretching injury to a muscle or its supporting tendons.

B. Etiology

1. Sprains and strains commonly occur in conjunction with skeletal trauma, even without injury to the bone.
2. Sprains result from overuse, misuse, or excessive twisting or rotation on joint movement. Any joint may be sprained, but the most common sites are the ankle and knee.
3. Strains result from mechanical overloading, excessive forcible stretching, or unusual muscle contractions. Common sites for strains are the cervical spine, the lower back, and the feet.

C. Pathophysiologic processes and manifestations

1. Tendons and ligaments are composed of dense connective tissue with a limited blood supply. This tissue is primarily made up of intercellular bundles of collagen fibers aligned for directional pull.
2. A pull or twist in the opposite direction results in trauma to the soft tissue; this causes inflammation, pain, and, possibly, loss of mobility (which may occur hours after the injury).
3. Ecchymosis may be present as small blood vessels rupture.
4. After the injury, capillaries permeate the injured area, supplying the fibroblasts with the substances needed to produce great amounts of collagen.
5. Gradual healing of the long collagen bundles restores strength; healing occurs over weeks, varying with the degree of injury.
6. Figure 8-1 illustrates degrees of sprain on the knee joint.

D. Overview of nursing interventions

1. Elevate the affected area to reduce edema.
2. Apply ice at the time of injury to limit inflammation and tissue destruction, to decrease pain, and to reduce muscle spasm.
3. Use compression wraps to limit edema and reduce pain from movement, making sure the wrap is not so tight as to impair blood flow.
4. Have the patient rest the injured tissue to minimize hemorrhaging within the joint or muscle and to reduce swelling.
5. Manage pain (an important part of treatment).
6. Maintain adequate nutrition and fluid intake.

IV. Dislocations

A. Description

1. A dislocation refers to the displacement of a bone from its correct articulating position within a joint.
2. A subluxation is a partial dislocation in which the ends of the bone are in partial contact with the joint.

B. Etiology

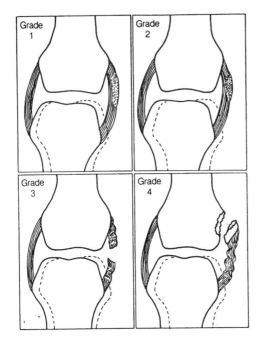

FIGURE 8-1.
Degrees of sprain on the medial side of the right knee: grade 1, mild sprain of the medial collateral ligament; grade 2, moderate sprain with hematoma formation; grade 3, severe sprain with total disruption of the ligament; and grade 4, severe sprain with avulsion of the medial femoral condyle at the insertion of the medial collateral ligament. (Adapted from Spickler, L. L. [1983]. Knee injuries of the athlete. *Orthopedic Nursing,* 2(5), 12–13; Porth, C. M. (1994). *Pathophysiology: Concepts of Altered Health States* (4th ed.) Philadelphia: Lippincott, p. 1205.)

1. Dislocations may be congenital, or they may result from injuries (traumatic) or disease (pathologic).
2. Traumatic dislocations commonly are caused by rotational injuries, which are typically seen in athletes.
3. Pathologic dislocations commonly are caused by arthritis, rheumatoid arthritis, or osteoarthritis.
4. Other causes of dislocations include paralysis, neuromuscular diseases, and use of neuromuscular drugs.
5. Common sites for dislocations include the hip (congenital, pathologic), knee, and shoulder (traumatic).

C. Pathophysiologic processes and manifestations
1. A sensation of "popping" or "giving out" at the affected site typically occurs after dislocation. Patients who experience recurrent dislocations may sense an impending dislocation.
2. Common manifestations include pain in the affected area, limited joint movement, and observable deformity.
3. An outwardly rotated leg is a common sign of hip dislocation.

D. Overview of nursing interventions
1. Assess all infants for congenital hip displacement.
2. Assist the physician in reducing the dislocation, as necessary.
3. Immobilize the joint, as ordered, to promote healing.
4. For a patient with a knee dislocation:
   a. Teach the patient appropriate exercises for strengthing the quadriceps to prevent recurrences.
   b. Instruct the patient on using a knee brace for activity.

5. Provide patient teaching covering:
    a. Causes of the dislocation and the potential for recurrences
    b. Need for follow-up care
    c. Importance of exercises
    d. Application of brace (if indicated)
6. Prepare the patient for surgery if necessary.

V. Fractures

A. Description
1. A fracture is a break or loss of continuity in a bone.
2. It results from the placement of more force or stress on the bone than it can absorb.

B. Etiology
1. Fractures may be caused by sudden traumatic injury, fatigue or stress from overuse or repeated wear (stress fracture), or weakening from disease or tumor (pathologic).
2. Fractures are classified according to type and location (Fig. 8-2 and 8-3).

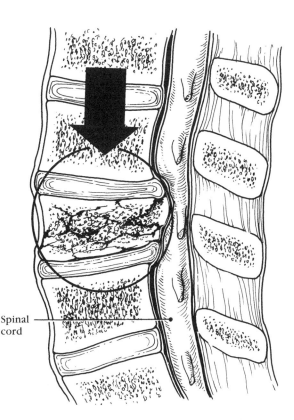

FIGURE 8-2.
Compression fracture in the lumbar vertebrae. (from Bullock, B. L. [1996] *Pathophysiology: Adaptations and Alterations in Function* (4th ed.). Philadelphia: Lippincott-Raven, p. 859)

Spinal cord

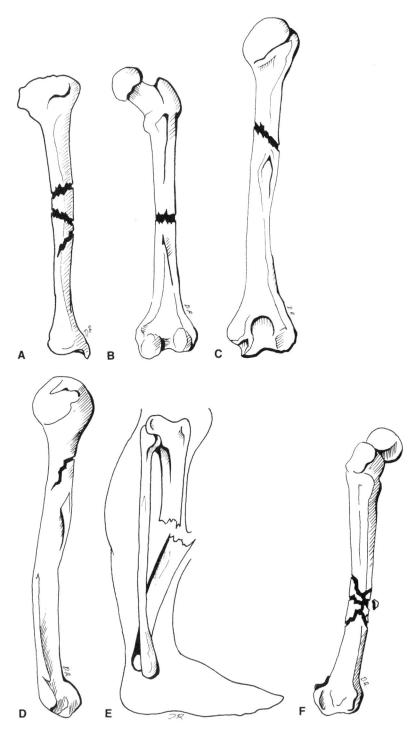

FIGURE 8-3.
Types of fractures. **(A)** Spiral fracture of a long bone. **(B)** Transverse fracture of the femur. **(C)** Lateral fracture of a long bone. **(D)** Oblique fracture. **(E)** Compound fracture of the tibia. **(F)** Bone fragments present in compound fracture.

C. **Pathophysiologic processes and manifestations**
1. When the fracture occurs, local numbness and muscle flaccidity occur due to temporary loss of nerve function; this may last only a few minutes.
2. Subsequent muscle spasms in the area of the fracture cause pain, swelling, and tenderness at the site.
3. A disruption in the periosteum and the blood vessels serving the bone marrow, cortex, and surrounding tissues occurs; the damaged ends of the interrupted bone and surrounding soft tissue bleed, contributing to swelling.

4. **Bone tissue necrosis adjacent to the fracture results in inflammation; the inflammatory response causes vasodilation, exudation of plasma and leukocytes, and infiltration by mast cells.**
5. If nerves, muscles, ligaments, and tendons are damaged from the trauma, loss of function in the affected area occurs.

6. **Deformity may be present; the type of deformity varies depending on the affected bone and type of force applied.**
   a. Bending forces and unequal muscle pulls cause angulation in long bones.
   b. Rotational forces and unequal pulls of attached muscles can twist the longitudinal axis of the bone out of position.
7. Shortening of the extremity occurs when muscles pull on the long axis of the extremity, causing fractured fragments to override each other.
8. Crepitus, a grating sound created by bone fragments rubbing against each other, may be heard or palpated.
9. In compound fractures, visible bleeding may occur; pelvic or femur fractures may cause hypovolemic shock because blood loss here can be significant.

10. **The process of bone healing begins with the formation of a hematoma (clot) between the fractured bone ends within the medullary canal and under the periosteum. The length of this process varies depending on the degree and site of injury, the patient's age and condition, and the underlying pathology. Fig. 8-4 illustrates the healing process of a fracture.**
11. Complications of fractures include nonunion, fat embolism, and compartment syndrome (see Section VI for a discussion of compartment syndrome).
12. Nonunion refers to a failure of the bone to grow together and close the gap between the broken ends. In this condition, the gap fills with dense fibrous and cartilaginous tissue rather than with new bone.
13. Occasionally, a fluid-filled space within the fibrous tissue resembles a joint. This condition is called pseudoarthrosis ("false joint").

14. **Fat embolism refers to a condition in which fat globules originating in the bone marrow at the injury site are thought to enter the circulation; this condition is potentially lethal, particularly when it occurs in the long bones. Major symptoms of fat embolism are respiratory insufficiency, cerebral involvement, and petechial rash.**

D. **Overview of nursing interventions**
1. Use a splint to immobilize the fracture and prevent further injury.

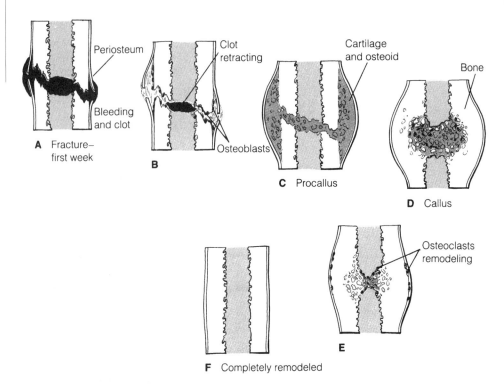

FIGURE 8-4.
Healing of a fracture. **A.** Immediately after fracture, blood seeps into the area and a hematoma forms. **B.** After 1 week, osteoblasts begin to form as clot retracts. **C.** After about 3 weeks, a procallus begins to form and stabilizes the fracture. **D.** From 6 to 12 weeks, a callus forms with bone cells. **E.** In 3 to 4 months, osteoclasts begin to remodel the fracture site. **F.** With normal apposition, the bone will be completely remodeled in 12 months. (Bullock, B. L. [1996]]. *Pathophysiology: Adaptations and Alterations in Function* (4th ed.). Philadelphia: Lippincott-Raven.)

2. Assist the physician with closed reduction if necessary; afterward, immobilize the affected body part using a splint, cast, or traction.
3. Prepare the patient for surgery if closed reduction is impossible.
4. Monitor the patient for complications related to the fracture as well as for problems associated with periods of immobility.
5. Medicate the patient appropriately, as fractures are very painful.
6. Instruct the patient on how to care for himself or herself.
7. Arrange for home care and physical therapy as needed.

VI. **Compartment syndrome**

A. Description: an abnormal increase in pressure within a confined anatomic space, resulting in impaired circulation, nerve injury, and loss of muscle function
B. Etiology and incidence

1. Compartment syndrome can result from a decrease in compartment size or an increase in compartment volume.

 2. **Decrease in compartment size can result from constrictive dressings or casts.**

3. Increase in compartment volume can result from swelling or bleeding.

4. Patients at risk for compartment syndrome include those with fractures or crushing injuries of the limbs; the legs and forearms are the most common sites.

C. **Pathophysiologic processes and manifestations**

1. Normal intracompartment pressure is about 6 mm Hg; pressures above 30 mm Hg are considered high enough to impair capillary perfusion.

2. If pressure increase is sufficiently high and remains unrelieved for several hours, permanent damage to nerve and muscle cells, with resulting loss of function and limb contractures, may occur.

3. Severe pain, caused by the stretching of the skin and soft tissue, occurs. Patients may describe it as deep, throbbing, and nonstop.

4. Paresthesia occurs as nerves are compressed. Patients often describe it as a burning or tingling sensation, or as a loss of feeling.

5. Limited muscle movement or diminished reflexes occur with muscle ischemia.

 6. **Distal pulses may be present and normal; this occurs because the major arteries palpated in pulse-taking lie outside the muscle compartment.**

7. Muscle trauma releases myoglobin, an intracellular muscle protein, into the urine causing a dark, red-brown pigmentation.

D. **Overview of nursing interventions**

1. Assess at-risk patients frequently.

2. Instruct the patient in the use of a pain-rating scale; interpret the degree and type of pain according to the patient's evaluation.

3. Assist the physician with invasive pressure measurement using a wick catheter or needle placed directly into the muscle compartment.

4. Remove any constricting material to reduce pressure.

5. Avoid elevation of the extremity because it decreases arterial pressure, thus reducing the amount of tissue pressure needed to stop circulation.

6. Prepare the patient for fasciotomy, if indicated, to allow blood flow.

VII. **Osteoporosis**

A. **Description**

 1. **Osteoporosis is a condition in which an abnormal increase in bone resorption (reabsorption) causes a decrease in bone density.**

2. Although the rate of bone formation may remain normal, demineralization (with loss of calcium and phosphate salts) causes the bone to become brittle and porous; resulting structural weakness leads to pathologic fractures.

B. **Etiology and incidence**

1. Osteoporosis may be primary or secondary to other disorders.

2. Primary osteoporosis occurs between age 51 and 70 and is six times more common in women (postmenopausal osteoporosis) than in men. A possible causative factor is a hormonal deficiency (estrogen in women, androgen in men).

3. Senile osteoporosis occurs after age 79 and is twice as common in women as in men; onset is more gradual than the postmenopausal type. Causation may be related to a reduction in vitamin D synthesis due to aging.

4. Risk factors include:
    a. Early menopause
    b. Family history
    c. Malnutrition
    d. Sedentary lifestyle
    e. Nulliparity

5. Incidence of primary osteoporosis is greater among whites and Asians than in African Americans; this may occur because white and Asian women have less original bone mass than African-American women.

6. Secondary osteoporosis accounts for fewer than 10% of cases; associated causes include malabsorption syndromes, corticosteroid excess, prolonged heparin therapy, diabetes mellitus, osteogenesis imperfecta, malignancy, chronic renal failure, and immobility.

C.   Pathophysiologic processes and manifestations

1. X-ray reveals decreased radiodensity and the presence of vertebral fractures.

2. Serum calcium, phosphorus, and PTH (parathyroid hormone) are normal.

3. Alkaline phosphatase may be normal or slightly elevated.

4. Imaging reveals areas of demineralization, particularly marked in the spine, pelvis, and femoral neck and head; vertebral compression is common.

5. Affected people often remain asymptomatic for years.

6. **Height loss and the discovery of unsuspected fractures on x-ray may be the first diagnostic clues.**

7. Significant fractures of the hip, ribs, clavicle, or other bones may occur with minimal or no precipitating trauma.

8. Vertebral collapse causes kyphosis or hunchback, resulting in considerable loss of height.

D.   Overview of nursing interventions

1. Assess the patient to determine the underlying cause.

2. Increase intake of calcium and vitamin D with supplements, as prescribed.

3. Administer estrogen to reduce rate of bone resorption, as prescribed.

4. Administer calcitonin, as prescribed, to inhibit osteoclast activity and to reduce the rate of calcium release from the bone.

5. Administer etidronate to suppress osteoclast-induced bone resorption, as prescribed.

6. Measure the patient's height periodically to assess stabilization or progression of the disease.

7. Prepare high-risk patients for screening using computed tomography (CT) or magnetic resonance imaging (MRI) scan.

8. Provide patient teaching covering:

    a. Recognition of risk factors
    b. Adequate dietary intake of calcium and other minerals, protein, and vitamin D
    c. Importance of mild exercise and activity
    d. Prevention of further injuries
    e. Management of present condition

VIII. Osteomyelitis

A. Description

1. Osteomyelitis is an infection of the bone resulting in a breakdown of the bone structure, decalcification, and tissue necrosis.
2. It can be acute or chronic.
3. This disease also can spread throughout the bone, including the marrow, cortex, and periosteum.

B. Etiology

1. The most common causative organism is *Staphylococcus aureus.*
2. Other causative organisms include streptococci, *Haemophilus influenzae, Pseudomonas, Escherichia coli,* and various fungi.

3. **Organisms can invade the bone by way of direct trauma (compound fracture, orthopedic surgery, penetrating wound) or by way of skin abscesses, urinary tract infections, dental caries, or otitis media.**
4. Bloodborne osteomyelitis (hematogenous osteomyelitis) commonly occurs in children and adolescents.
5. Chronic osteomyelitis (infection persisting for more than 8 weeks) may result from inadequately treated acute bone infections and can persist for years.

C. Pathophysiologic processes and manifestations

1. Infection begins in the soft, medullary tissue, usually in the long bones of the legs. Granulocytic leukocytes then infiltrate the area.
2. Leukocyte destruction by the bacteria causes release of a proteolytic enzyme, which contributes to tissue necrosis.
3. Inflammation at the site provokes blood vessels to thrombus, which results in pain, heat, and swelling in the extremity and causes devascularization, bone ischemia, and eventual necrosis.
4. In chronic osteomyelitis, the necrotic bone separates from the viable bone, forming a fragment called a sequestrum. As new bone is laid down, the periosteum of the new bone forms an encasement called an involucrum around the sequestrum.
5. Sinuses in the involucrum allow pus to escape from inside; some pockets of infection are walled off allowing organisms to remain dormant for long periods.
6. New granulation may close sinuses, but infection within will build pressure that causes reopening or formation of new channels.

7. **Full healing is accomplished only when all necrosed bone has been discharged or excised.**
8. Xray will show evidence of periosteal elevation and sequestrum; bone scan will show these changes earlier than x-ray.

    9.   Pathologic fractures caused by weakened bone shaft may occur.

D.   **Overview of nursing interventions**

    1.   **Prevent infection by maintaining meticulous asepsis for patients who have undergone orthopedic surgery.**

    2.   Provide prompt care for all skin wounds.

    3.   Administer antibiotics, as prescribed, after identifying causative organism through wound culture.

    4.   Prepare the patient for surgery to remove sequestra, if indicated.

    5.   Leave wounds open for drainage; continuous wound irrigation systems may be left in place after surgery.

IX. Osteoarthritis

A.   **Description: a chronic disorder characterized by degeneration of joint cartilage and hypertrophy of the bone at the articular margins (Fig. 8-5)**

B.   **Etiology and incidence**

    1.   Mechanical and hereditary influences contribute to the occurrence of osteoarthritis.

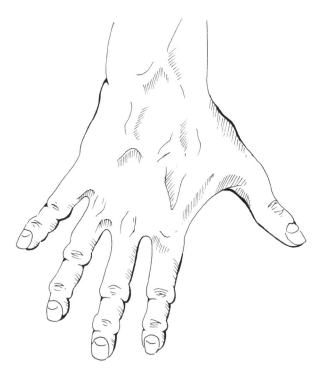

FIGURE 8-5.
Osteoarthritis. Joint inflammation.

2. It may also occur secondary to another articular disease, such as a traumatic or sports injury.

3. Osteoarthritis, which commonly affects the hips and knees, is the most widely occurring form of joint disease.

4. X-rays typically reveal some feature of the disease in the weight-bearing joints of up to 90% of the population over age 40, particularly in overweight persons.

C. **Pathophysiologic processes and manifestations**

1. Early morning stiffness is a classic sign.

2. Joint pain, the most common symptom, is associated with exercise and weight bearing and is generally relieved by rest.

3. Articular inflammation may be present at times, but is minimal.

4. Severity of symptoms increases with age. There are no systemic symptoms, which helps rule out inflammatory disorders, such as rheumatoid arthritis, which are associated with similar symptoms of joint discomfort.

5. Weather changes are associated with aching in the joints.

6. Motion can produce a "grating" sound in the joint.

7. Limitation of movement occurs over time.

8. Heberden's and Bouchard's nodes may occur when the interphalangeal joints are involved; painless at first, these may later become red, swollen, and tender. Numbness, loss of dexterity, and swelling also occur.

D. **Overview of nursing interventions**

1. **Administer aspirin and nonsteroidal anti-inflammatory medications, as prescribed, to relieve joint pain and inflammation.**

2. Administer intra-articular injections of corticosteroids to provide transient relief of symptoms, as ordered.

3. Reduce joint stress by using supportive devices (eg, crutches, braces, walker, cane, cervical collar) and by encouraging rest after activity, use of moist heat, paraffin dip for hands, and massage.

4. Encourage the patient to engage in as much activity as tolerable.

5. Provide patient teaching covering

    a. Need for weight loss

    b. Avoidance of overexertion

    c. Use of medications and assistive devices

    d. Importance of exercise

    e. Maintenance of safe environment

X. **Gout (gouty arthritis)**

A. **Description**

1. Gout is a metabolic disorder of uric acid formation and excretion causing excess levels of uric acid in the blood and other body fluids, including the synovial fluid.

2. It can be primary or secondary.

3. **Gouty arthritis occurs when uric acid reaches a high concentration, leading to crystallization in the synovial fluid, which then causes joint pain and inflammation. This type of arthritis, which is extremely painful, may be acute or chronic.**

B.   Etiology and incidence

1.   Primary gout is a familial disease that results from a disorder in purine metabolism.

2.   Secondary gout is associated with acquired causes of hyperuricemia, such as renal disease, multiple myeloma, diuretic therapy, advanced carcinoma, and psoriasis.

3.   Gout also is associated with a sluggish rate of kidney filtration, possibly from deposits of urate crystals in the renal tubules.

4.   Gouty arthritis occurs in some, but not all, persons with hyperuricemia; males over age 30 account for 90% of all cases.

5.   The most commonly affected joint is the great toe; other common sites include the knees, ankles, and feet. More than one joint may be affected during a single attack.

C.   Pathophysiologic processes and manifestations

1.   Normally, purines are synthesized to purine nucleotides, which are used in the synthesis of essential nucleic acids; uric acid is a breakdown product of purine nucleotides.

2.   An accelerated rate of purine synthesis or purine breakdown results in overproduction of uric acid; this raises serum uric acid levels, causing symptoms of gout.

3.   Intense pain, the primary manifestation of an acute attack, results from deposition of monosodium urate crystals in and around the joint.

4.   The joint is strikingly tender, warm, and dark red.

5.   Fever commonly is present.

6.   Tophi, small subcutaneous nodules composed of urate crystal aggregates, commonly occur along the pinna of the ear and on the hands and feet; aspirate of a tophus will reveal crystals of sodium urate.

7.   Renal calculi, due to sodium urate crystallization and deposition in the renal interstitium, occur in up to 20% of patients.

8.   After the initial attack, asymptomatic periods up to several years can occur; repeated attacks may become more frequent over time. Functional loss and disability occur with chronic gouty arthritis.

9.   Serum uric acid levels are elevated (>7.5 mg/dL) unless the patient is on uric-acid-lowering drug therapy.

D.   Overview of nursing interventions

1.   For an acute attack:

a.   **Have the patient rest with no weight bearing until the attack has subsided.**

b.   **Administer pain medications as prescribed; assist with hydrocortisone injections directly into the joint, if ordered.**

c.   **Administer anti-inflammatory medications (colchicine, indomethacin, phenylbutazone), as prescribed.**

2.   For long-term management:

a.   Encourage a high fluid intake (>3 L/day) to reduce risk of renal calculi.

b.   Administer antihyperuricemic medications (allopurinol, colchicine) to reduce serum urate concentrations, as prescribed.

c.   Recommend a low-purine diet.

    d.   Provide patient teaching on appropriate activity levels, proper use of medications, care during exacerbations, and continuing health care.

XI.   **Bone tumors**

A.   **Description**

    1.   Bone tumors are those found in the skeletal framework; they can be primary or secondary.

    2.   Bone tumors are classified as benign or malignant.

B.   **Etiology and incidence**

    1.   The cause of bone tumors is unclear.

    2.   Primary bone tumors may arise from bone cells or osteoblasts, cartilage, fibrous tissue, or marrow; these kinds of tumors are uncommon, affecting only about 1% of the population. Adolescents have the highest rate of incidence, mainly of osteogenic sarcoma and Ewing's sarcoma.

    3.   Secondary bone tumors related to malignant metastatic lesions are more common; incidence is higher in persons over age 60. As cancer treatments prolonging life continue, the incidence of these tumors is rising.

C.   **Pathophysiologic processes and manifestations**

    1.   A common manifestation of a bone tumor is a palpable mass or hard lump; tumors near the surface (eg, anterior tibia) are more likely to be felt.

    2.   Pain may or may not be present; generally, skeletal pain that is unrelieved by rest, feels worse at night, and lasts, continuously or intermittently, over several days is suggestive of malignancy. In patients with diagnosed cancer, pain in the bones is a significant indicator of metastases.

    3.   Pressure from the tumor on a peripheral nerve may cause neurologic signs such as decreased sensation, numbness, and limited movement.

     4.   Pathologic fractures can occur with benign or malignant tumors. These fractures are secondary to bone destruction, a primary pathologic feature of bone tumors.

    5.   Benign tumors cause the least amount of bone damage because of their symmetric, controlled growth pattern. They may, however, compress or displace surrounding bone tissue and blood supply, weakening the bone structure and may lead to pathologic fractures.

    6.   As a malignant tumor erodes the bone cortex, new bone formation between the bone surface and the periosteum occurs. Bone layers are also added to the exterior bone surface to additionally strengthen the cortex.

    7.   Bone contour visibly changes. Continued penetration of the cortex elevates the periosteum, stimulating unusual patterns of bone formation, which can be visualized on x-ray or scan.

    8.   Increased serum alkaline phosphatase levels may be present because bone lysis releases alkaline phosphatase.

    9.   Hypercalcemia may be present because bone destruction releases calcium, a major cation of bone structure.

D.   **Overview of nursing interventions**

    1.   Promote early detection by carefully assessing reports of skeletal pain, swelling, or "bumps."

2. Note increased serum alkaline phosphatase levels and presence of hypercalcemia.
3. Use x-ray, CT scans, and MRI to visualize and locally stage tumors, as ordered.
4. Determine tumor type through bone biopsy, as ordered.
5. Prepare the patient for selected treatment modalities (eg, chemotherapy, surgery, radiation therapy, immunotherapy, hormonal therapy).
6. Provide effective, individualized pain relief, as ordered, because pain can be severe, unrelenting, and debilitating.
7. Prevent pathologic fractures.
8. Educate the patient and family members about treatment modalities and the patient's condition.
9. Provide emotional support for the patient and family members.

Biliography

Bullock, B. (1996). *Pathophysiology: Adaptations and alterations in function* (4th ed.). Philadelphia: Lippincott-Raven.

Ganong, William F. (1997). *Review of medical physiology* (18th ed.). Stamford, CT: Appleton and Lange.

Guyton, Arthur C., & Hall, John E. (1996). *Textbook of medical physiology* (9th ed.). Philadelphia: W. B. Saunders.

Kinney, M., Packa, D., & Dunbar, S. (1993). *AACN's clinical reference for critical-care nursing* (3rd ed.). St. Louis: C. V. Mosby.

McCance, K. L., & Huether, S. E. (1994). *Pathophysiology: The biologic basis for disease in adults and children* (2nd ed.). St. Louis: Mosby-Year Book.

Porth, C. (1994). *Pathophysiology: Concepts of altered health states* (4th ed.). Philadelphia: Lippincott-Raven.

Radioactive relief for cancer bone pain. *Am J Nurs.,* 94(2): 58, February 1994.

Roth, S. H. Pharmacologic approaches to musculoskeletal disorders. *Clinics of Geriatric Medicine,* May 4 (2):441–61.

Silver, J. J., Einhorn, T.A. (1995). Osteoporosis and aging. *Clinical Orthopedics,* July(316):10–20.

Tierney, L., McPhee, S., Papadakis, M., & Schroeder, S. (eds.). (1993). *Current medical diagnosis and treatment.* Norwalk, CT: Appleton & Lange.

STUDY QUESTIONS

1. Ms. Chambers, age 82, will be discharged from the hospital 4 days after closed reduction of a fractured femur. Her right leg is in a long leg cast. Which of the following assessment findings should be of greatest concern to the nurse?
   a. temperature 97°
   b. respiratory rate of 16
   c. ecchymosis of several toes
   d. discrete, small, red spots on the skin

2. After having an x-ray, Mr. Gray, age 32, learns that his ankle is sprained. Mr. Gray asks the nurse, "What is a sprain?" Which of the following replies is most appropriate?
   a. "A sprain is an overstretching of the joint muscles."
   b. "A sprain is an injury to soft tissue and is minor compared to a fracture."
   c. "A sprain is an injury to the tendons and muscles caused by rotational pull."
   d. "A sprain is an injury to the ligaments of the joint caused by overuse or twisting motion."

3. Which of the following patient statements would alert the nurse to the presence of osteoarthritis?
   a. "All the joints in my body are aching constantly."
   b. "When my hips ache, moderate exercise really seems to reduce the pain."
   c. "When I woke up this morning, I felt so stiff it was hard to get out of bed."
   d. "I'm feeling tired most of the time and sometimes have a fever at night."

4. The nurse is reviewing the patient history for Ms. Hampton, age 64, checking for risk factors for osteoporosis. Use of which of the following medications would increase Ms. Hampton's risk for the disease?
   a. colchicine
   b. prednisone
   c. furosemide
   d. vitamin D

5. A patient in the emergency room is told he has a comminuted fracture of the right radius. The nurse should explain to him that this means there is:
   a. splintering on one side of the bone
   b. a palpable bone protrusion under the skin
   c. a break of the bone in two parts under intact skin
   d. fragmentation of the bone under the intact skin

6. Mr. Jeffers, age 62, is admitted with an acute attack of gout. The nurse should focus assessment on:
   a. degree of swelling in affected joint
   b. patient's description of the pain
   c. ability to maintain activities of daily living (ADL)
   d. range of motion in the affected joint

7. Mr. Potts, age 23, is being prepared for discharge. He has been treated with antibiotics for extensive osteomyelitis of the right femur. The nurse should base patient teaching primarily on the knowledge that:
   a. Group sports are less important for young men of this age than for teenagers.
   b. Stress to the bone must be minimized to reduce the risk of pathologic fracture.
   c. Osteomyelitis will be likely to recur if the patient continues contact sports activities.
   d. Young men of this age are not likely to accept any limitations to activity.

8. Ms. Moss, age 28, has multiple trauma. She is out of bed in a chair 8 days after

fracture of the femur. She is in a long leg cast. When assessing Ms. Moss, the nurse suspects fat embolism. Which of the following actions should the nurse undertake initially?

a. administer oxygen
b. call the physician immediately
c. bivalve the cast to release pressure
d. return the patient to bed with the assistance of ancillary personnel

9. After receiving his usual analgesic, a patient hospitalized with a fracture of the humerus complains his pain is greater than ever. Assessment of the limb reveals palpable distal pulses, no impingement of the digits by the cast, and rapid capillary refill. The patient complains of pain when his fingers are extended. At this time, the most appropriate analysis by the nurse is:

a. The patient may be becoming habituated to his usual analgesic.
b. The patient may need his analgesic more frequently in smaller doses.
c. Some increase in pain can be anticipated due to the rush of blood to the affected part during the healing process.

d. Progressive pain may be indicative of a serious complication.

10. Which laboratory studies are altered in bone cancer?

a. calcium and alkaline phosphatase
b. potassium and alkaline phosphatase
c. magnesium and calcium
d. creatinine and blood urea nitrogen (BUN)

11. The danger of compartment syndrome is:

a. loss of distal pulses
b. increased muscle movement
c. a cold tingling sensation in the extremity
d. muscle ischemia

12. A nurse is caring for a patient with compartment syndrome. She is planning to get the patient out of bed and is sure to avoid:

a. assessing the patient's pain
b. elevating the extremity
c. removing constricting garments
d. assessing circulation

ANSWER KEY

Question	Correct answer	Correct answer rationale	Incorrect answer rationales
1.	d	Petechial rash is a classic sign of fat embolism; biopsy of petechiae has revealed the presence of lipid particles.	a. Temperature is within normal limits. b. Respiratory rate is within normal limits. c. Ecchymosis would be consistent with trauma. The age of the bruise would be determined by inspection of color. Assessment of circulation and sensorineural status of foot should be done.
2.	d	This statement best describes a sprain.	a. This statement describes a strain. b. Sprains can be serious, taking weeks to recover. Severely torn ligaments may require surgery. c. This statement is more descriptive of a strain.
3.	c	Stiffness occurs after periods of rest.	a. Systemic symptoms are uncommon, although multiple joints may be involved. b. Pain is provoked by activity in osteoarthritis. d. Systemic symptoms are not usual in osteoarthritis.
4.	b	Steroids increase the risk of osteoporosis, possibly through their effect on the excretion rate of calcium and phosphorus.	a, c, and d. These medications are not known to increase the risk of osteoporosis.
5.	d	This statement best describes a comminuted fracture.	a. This statement describes a greenstick fracture. b. This statement describes a bone fracture out of alignment. c. This statement describes a complete fracture.
6.	b	Pain is a cardinal symptom; it is always subjective.	a. Swelling is anticipated and will resolve with treatment. c. This is not a priority at this time. d. Range of motion will be limited during the acute attack.
7.	b	Knowing that stress to the bone must be minimized will guide the nurse in helping the patient plan activities.	a. This may be somewhat true if the patient is not still emotionally adolescent, but it is neither specific to the patient nor a priority. c. Contact sports may increase the risk for injury or pathologic frac-

Question	Correct answer	Correct answer rationale	Incorrect answer rationales
			ture but will not cause osteomyelitis. d. This is an absolute statement, not appropriate to any specific patient.
8.	a	Oxygen is given for the respiratory distress that occurs with fat embolism. It will reduce hypoxia as well as reduce the surface tension of fat globules that settle in the lung.	b. The physician should be called as soon as possible, but this is not the initial action. c. This action is incorrect. It would have no effect on a fat embolism. d. This action is appropriate, but it is not the initial action.
9.	d	Although most of the assessment was normal, the symptoms of progressive pain and pain on passive extension of the fingers are early indications of compartment syndrome and require immediate medical intervention.	a. There is no basis for this observation. b. This administration method may be more desirable, but increasing pain in a patient previously relieved with analgesic is not normal. c. This is not necessarily a true statement in this situation.
10.	a	Serum calcium and alkaline phosphatase are often elevated in bone cancer.	b, c, and d. Elevations in potassium and magnesium are not necessarily associated with bone cancer. Creatinine and blood urea nitrogen are associated with renal function.
11.	d	The danger of compartment syndrome is compression of blood vessels and nerves leading to muscle ischemia.	a. Distal pulses may be present because the major arteries that are palpated when pulse taking lie outside of the compartment. b. Muscle movement is usually decreased. c. A burning tingling sensation is usually present.
12.	b	In compartment syndrome, avoid elevating the extremity because it decreases arterial pressure, thus reducing the amount of tissue pressure needed to stop circulation.	a and d. A patients pain and circulation should always be assessed. c. Constricting clothing must be removed to reduce pressure.

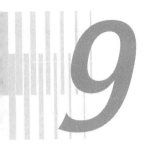

9 Skin Disorders

I. Overview of pathophysiologic processes

A. Infectious and inflammatory disorders

1. Infectious and inflammatory skin disorders either cause the immune system to react to the presence of an antigen, causing a hypersensitivity reaction, or cause the body to react to infection.

2. These disorders may result from exposure to an allergen or from a bacterial, viral, or fungal infection.

3. Dermatitis (of any etiology), eczema, acne, lichen planus, psoriasis, pityriasis rosea, warts, herpes, and bacterial and fungal infections are classified as infectious and inflammatory skin disorders.

4. Risk factors include exposure to a substance that would cause an infection or an inflammatory response.

B. **Parasitic diseases**
  1. Parasitic diseases are invasions of the skin by parasites.
  2. These diseases can occur in any person at any time, because the parasites leap or jump from one person to the next.
  3. As the parasites lay eggs, infestation rapidly becomes extensive.
  4. The sole risk factor for acquiring parasitic diseases is having close contact with a person who has parasites.

C. **Trauma**

  1. **Trauma (an opening to the skin) is significant because it breaks the body's first line of defense.**
  2. Skin trauma results from cuts, scrapes, stab wounds, or other injuries.
  3. Burns are the most severe type of skin trauma.
  4. There are no specific risk factors for burns.

D. **Skin cancer**

  1. **The incidence of skin cancers has been rising for several years; it is attributed to exposure to ultraviolet rays.**
  2. Types of skin cancers associated with prolonged, unprotected exposure to ultraviolet rays include basal cell, squamous cell, and melanoma; most are easily treatable.

  3. **Kaposi's sarcoma is a type of skin cancer associated with immunosuppressed patients, particularly those with human immunodeficiency virus (HIV).**

II. **Physiologic responses to skin dysfunction (Figure 9–1)**

A. **Lesions**
  1. Lesions are any identifiable changes in skin structure.
  2. Vascular lesions include:
      a. *Petechiae:* small (less than 1 cm) deposits of blood in the skin
      b. *Purpura:* large (greater than 1 cm) deposits of blood in the skin
      c. *Telangiectasia:* tiny, dilated, superficial blood vessels
      d. *Hemangioma:* two common types include bright-red strawberry and port-wine stain; strawberry lesions commonly disappear in early childhood, but port-wine stains do not.
  3. Other lesions include:
      a. *Macule:* small (up to 1 cm), flat, nonpalpable area of changed color (eg, freckle or petechiae)
      b. *Papule:* small, palpable, elevated lesion that may vary in color (eg, nevus)
      c. *Nodule:* large (greater than 1 cm), raised, solid, lesion that is often deeper and firmer than a papule (eg, swollen lymph node)
      d. *Plaque:* large (greater than 1 cm) solid elevated lesion on the skin surface
      e. *Wheal:* transitory, usually irregularly shaped area of localized redness and edema that occurs as a normal response to skin trauma
      f. *Vesicle* (blister): small (less than 1 cm) skin elevation that contains serous fluid (eg, herpes blister)

Primary Lesions

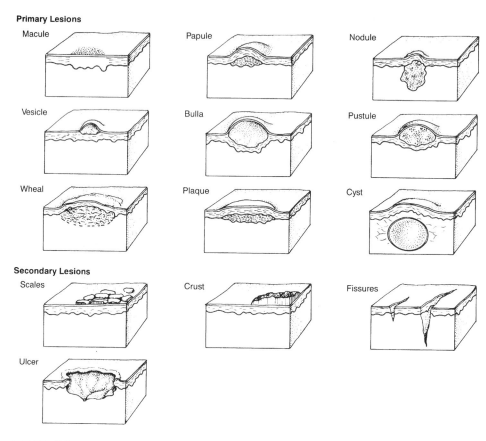

Secondary Lesions

FIGURE 9-1.
Type of skin lesions. (*Source:* Smeltzer, S. C. and Bare, B. G. (1992). *Brunner and Suddarth's Textbook of Medical-Surgical Nursing* [7th ed.]. Philadelphia: J.B. Lippincott.)

g. *Bulla:* large (greater than 1 cm) vesicle filled with fluid
h. *Pustule:* vesicle filled with purulent fluid
i. *Cyst:* tumor containing liquid or semisolid material

B. Excoriation: epidermal loss due to abrasion

C. Ulcer: irregularly shaped skin cavity with epidermal destruction

D. Scar: deposition of connective tissue resulting from dermal destruction

E. Skin tags: soft, brown or flesh-colored appendages of horny skin outgrowth

F. Fissures: crack in epidermis that extends to the dermis

G. Scales: debris on skin surface

H. Crust: dried exudate

I. Senile lentigines: brown age marks or liver spots; usually seen on sun-exposed areas

J. Vitiligo: patchy areas of depigmentation with smooth, definite borders; seen in dark-skinned people

K. Keloids: disfiguring, ropelike hypertrophic scars that develop after skin injury; more prevalent in black-skinned people

L. Alopecia: hair loss generally involving the scalp, eyebrows, and eyelashes

M. Inflammation: nonspecific, local response to injury characterized by redness, heat, swelling, pain, and impaired function

N. Pruritus: itching sensation described as prickling or burning; associated with circulating allergens or the local release of proteins in the skin

III. Seborrheic dermatitis

A. Description

1. Seborrheic dermatitis is a chronic, inflammatory, scaling eruption; lesions occur chiefly on the scalp, face, upper trunk, and skinfolds.
2. It is characterized by periodic remissions and exacerbations.
3. In infants, it is called cradle cap; in adults, it is called dandruff (if it occurs on the scalp).

B. Etiology and incidence

1. Seborrheic dermatitis is associated with a genetic predisposition that is exacerbated by physical or emotional stress.
2. Incidence is higher in middle-aged or older adults.

C. Pathophysiologic processes and manifestations

1. Seborrheic dermatitis involves vasodilation and inflammatory cell discharge in the epidermal layer of the skin.
2. Lesions appear as patches of sallow or greasy skin, with or without scaling and redness.
3. When scaling occurs (due to increased cell mitosis), it can be dry, moist, or greasy.
4. Manifestations include pruritus and irritation.

D. Overview of nursing interventions

1. For mild cases:
   a. Provide shampoos or soaps containing sulfur.
   b. Use castor or mineral oils to moisturize the skin.
2. For extreme cases:
   a. Administer topical corticosteroids, as prescribed.
   b. Administer topical antibiotics to manage secondary infection, as prescribed.
3. Provide patient teaching on managing and preventing secondary infection.
4. Instruct patient to use sunscreen.
5. Teach patient how to administer medications, if prescribed.

IV. Contact dermatitis

A. Description and etiology

1. Contact dermatitis is a skin inflammation caused by exposure to either an allergenic substance or an irritant; duration of exposure may be short or prolonged.

    2. With successive recurrences, the disorder becomes chronic.

B. **Pathophysiologic processes and manifestations**

    1. After the irritant or allergen initially contacts the skin, a reaction occurs. Usual manifestations include erythema, exudate, scaling, and pruritus.

    2. In *allergic contact dermatitis*

        a. A cell-mediated response or a delayed hypersensitivity response occurs.

        b. The allergen binds with a protein to form an antigenic molecule.

        c. Sensitization occurs on first exposure, and manifestations occur after reexposure to the allergen.

        d. Activation of the antigenic complex in the cutaneous tissue initiates an inflammatory response; symptoms include swelling and vesicle formation.

    3. In *irritant contact dermatitis*

        a. The stratum corneum is damaged, allowing the irritant to be absorbed into the skin.

        b. Manifestations are the same as for allergic dermatitis.

C. **Overview of nursing interventions**

    1. **Assist with identification of the allergic substance or irritant; instruct the patient to avoid it in the future.**

    2. Administer topical or oral antihistamines, as prescribed, to inhibit inflammatory response and ease pruritus and discomfort.

    3. Administer topical corticosteroids, as prescribed, in severe cases.

    4. Assess for evidence of secondary infection; if present, administer antibiotics as prescribed.

    5. Instruct the patient on prevention of secondary infection and pharmacologic management.

V. Eczema

A. **Description**

    1. Eczema is a common form of chronic dermatitis.

    2. It can be classified into two types:

        a. Atopic (also called atopic dermatitis)

        b. Nummular

B. **Etiology and incidence**

    1. Eczema is associated with a family history of asthma or allergic responses.

    2. It most commonly occurs in childhood, but it also occurs in adults; nummular eczema commonly develops in elderly men.

C. **Pathophysiologic processes and manifestations**

    1. In *infantile atopic eczema*

        a. Lesions begin in the cheeks and progress to the extremities and trunk, usually leaving the diaper area clear.

        b. Lesions start as vesicles, which can result in oozing and crusting of excoriated areas.

    2. In *adult atopic eczema*

        a. Markedly dry skin that is extremely itchy develops.

    b.   Scratching results in excoriation, lichenification (thickening), and even scarring; as a result, leathery areas of hypo- or hyperpigmented color are left in the antecubital and popliteal parts of the body.

  3. In *nummular eczema*

    a.   Lesions develop as coin-shaped papulovesicular patches on the arms and legs.

    b.   Excoriation and subsequent bacterial infections can lead to lichenification.

    c.   The skin develops an inflammatory response to noxious stimuli; common manifestations include vasodilation, swelling of the upper dermal layer, and damage to the epidermal layer.

D. **Overview of nursing interventions**

  1. Administer antipruritic medications, antihistamines, and topical corticosteroids as prescribed.

  2. Assess for secondary bacterial infection; if present, administer antibiotics as prescribed.

  3. Apply open wet dressings to resolve pruritus.

  4. Assess skin integrity.

  5. Counsel the patient regarding altered body image.

  6. Teach patient how to administer medication effectively.

VI. Acne

A. **Description**

  1. Acne is a localized inflammatory skin disorder characterized by papules, comedones (whiteheads and blackheads), and pustules.

  2. Types include:

    a.   *Acne vulgaris:* commonly seen in adolescents, with lesions on the face, neck, and upper body

    b.   *Acne conglobata:* chronic form resulting in scarring

    c.   *Acne rosacea:* chronic form occurring in older adults and resulting in reddening of the nose and cheeks; nose can also develop hyperplasia

B. **Etiology**

  1. The cause of acne is unknown; however, it is theorized that it may result from the oversecretion of sebum from the sebaceous glands and hormonal dysfunction.

  2. **Precipitating factors may include use of certain cosmetics, ingestion of certain drugs, exposure to oils or grease, contact with clothing, and emotional stress.**

C. **Pathophysiologic processes and manifestations**

  1. The sebaceous glands hypertrophy and produce more sebum.

  2. Keratinization of the hair follicle also occurs, obstructing the gland and causing sebum retention.

  3. Comedones form and enlarge; they may rupture, discharging their contents into the dermis or to the surface.

  4. If discharge into the dermis occurs, a papular nodule or cyst may develop.

  5. Permanent scarring results eventually.

D. Overview of nursing interventions
1. Administer topical medications such as systemic antibiotics or retinoic acid, as prescribed.
2. Assess for the presence of a secondary bacterial infection; if present, manage appropriately.
3. Teach the patient about facial hygiene and management of pustules.
4. Identify concerns regarding body image and encourage the patient to develop a positive self-image.
5. Teach the patient about precipitating factors.
6. Teach the patient how to maintain a normal, well-balanced diet.
7. Instruct patient to avoid fatty and greasy foods.

VII. Lichen planus

A. Description: chronic papulosquamous disorder of the skin and mucous membranes
B. Etiology and incidence
1. The cause of lichen planus is unknown; however, exacerbation is associated with certain drugs and chemicals.
2. Lichen planus affects adults and usually has a duration of 15 to 24 months.
C. Pathophysiologic processes and manifestations
1. Within the dermis, an inflammatory response is initiated.
2. Lymphocytic infiltration and hyperkeratosis occur, resulting in vacuolation and cell degeneration.
3. Lesions (which are found in the buccal mucosa about half the time) are pruritic papules with a reddish purple coloration.
4. Whitish grey lines, called Wickham's striae, may also be present.
5. Larger scaly plaques may eventually develop.
D. Overview of nursing interventions
1. Administer topical steroids and antipruritic agents, as prescribed.
2. Assess for secondary bacterial infections; if present, manage appropriately.
3. Teach the patient to avoid skin trauma and ensure good mouth care.

VIII. Psoriasis

A. Description: chronic inflammatory papulosquamous condition resulting in silvery, scaly patches due to epidermal overgrowth
B. Etiology
1. The cause of psoriasis is unknown; however, it is theorized that genetic or biochemical alterations may be involved; there is a familial predisposition.
2. Onset occurs between the ages of 10 and 40.
C. Pathophysiologic processes and manifestations
1. When keratinocytes mature, they move up and out from the inner layer to replace the skin surface. As they move, they flatten, dehydrate, and become keratinized.
2. In psoriasis, this process is speeded up so that, instead of epidermal replacement occurring every 21 days, it occurs every 5 days.

3. Vasodilation of dermal vessels and leukocyte accumulation into the dermis result in erythema.
4. Because of the increased mitotic rate, keratinization does not occur and the skin's protective mechanism is impaired.
5. Lesions most commonly occur on the elbows, knees, and scalp and are clearly demarcated.

D. **Overview of nursing interventions**
1. For mild cases:
    a. Use emollients to soften skin.
    b. Administer steroids, as prescribed.
2. For severe cases:
    a. Administer antimetabolites and topical steroids, as ordered.
    b. Use ultraviolet light and tar preparations, as indicated.
3. Administer antibacterial agents, as prescribed.
4. Administer keratolytics, as prescribed, to soften or remove the horny or dead outer skin layer.
5. Assess skin integrity.
6. Institute measures to prevent secondary injury.

IX. **Pityriasis rosea**

A. **Description: inflammatory skin disease characterized by clusters of macules and papules surrounded by erythematous areas**
B. **Etiology and incidence**
1. The cause of pityriasis rosea is not known.
2. Lesions occur most commonly in the spring and fall; young adults are primarily affected.
3. Pityriasis rosea is not contagious and is self-limiting, lasting about 6 weeks.
C. **Pathophysiologic processes and manifestations**
1. The initial lesion is usually solitary (herald patch) and is associated with scaling.
2. Lesions commonly occur on the trunk and upper extremities; they occur less often on the face.
3. Initial lesions, which may be macular and papular, enlarge and begin to fade as successive crops of new lesions appear.
4. Pruritus is common; fatigue and headache may also be present.
D. **Overview of nursing interventions**
1. Administer antipruritics, antihistamines, and topical steroids, as prescribed.
2. Assess skin integrity; administer emollients to resolve dryness and scaling.
3. Encourage the patient to discuss changes in body image.

X. **Verrucae (warts)**

A. **Description**
1. Verrucae are a family of common benign skin tumors composed of exaggerated or irregularly thickened normal skin that is raised above the skin surface.

> 2. Types include:
>   a. *Verrucae vulgaris* (common dry warts)
>   b. *Verrucae plantaris* (plantar warts)
>   c. *Condyloma acuminata* (genital or moist warts)

B. **Etiology: caused by the human papilloma virus (HPV)**

C. **Pathophysiologic processes and manifestations**

1. *Verrucae vulgaris* vary in size from a small, pinhead-size growth to large patches (mosaic); these are commonly seen on the hands, especially in children.
2. *Verrucae plantaris* occur on the soles of the feet, extending deep into the thick skin; pressure from walking causes pain.
3. *Condyloma acuminata* are found in the anogenital area in adults and are typically sexually transmitted. (When these are found in the anal area in children, sexual abuse may be suspected.)

D. **Overview of nursing interventions**

1. **Teach the patient that the warts are contagious and emphasize the importance of having them removed to avoid contaminating others.**
2. Prepare the patient for cryosurgery or sharp dissection of certain warts, if indicated.
3. Administer caustic agents, if indicated.
4. Educate the patient and sexual partner about the transmission of genital warts and prevention of recurrence.

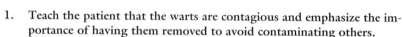

XI.   Herpes

A. **Description**

1. Herpes lesions appear as painful vesicles that progress to ulcers.
2. Lesions can occur at any site on the body but are found most commonly on the lips, mouth, face, and genitals.
3. Herpes zoster is an acute viral infection in which lesions manifest along a unilateral nerve root segment or dermatome.

B. **Etiology**

1. Herpes is caused by two types of herpes simplex virus (HSV) infections.
   a. HSV type I (common fever blisters)
   b. HSV type II (genital herpes); HSV type II is considered a sexually transmitted disease. (See Chapter 18, Sexually Transmitted Diseases, for more information.)
2. Transmission occurs by way of direct contact with a lesion.
3. Infections can be primary or secondary (recurrent).
4. Precipitating events include weather extremes, sunlight, hormonal changes, and local trauma.
5. Herpes zoster is caused by reactivation of the varicella virus; it most commonly occurs in adults over age 50.

C. **Pathophysiologic processes and manifestations**

1. Primary infection with HSV results in vesicles and pain; within a few days, vesicles open and dry up.
2. The first manifestation of herpes zoster is pain localized over a particular

nerve distribution area; erythema and vesicles then occur, lasting about 3 weeks. Fever, malaise, and paresthesia may also be present.

D.   **Overview of nursing interventions**

1.   Administer antiviral agents and systemic steroids, as prescribed.
2.   Administer analgesics to manage pain, as prescribed.
3.   Assess for postherpetic neuralgia; if present, manage appropriately.
4.   Assess disease severity.
6.   Assess for evidence of secondary bacterial infection; if present, manage appropriately.
7.   Instruct patient on the disease process, what factors bring on an occurrence, and how to avoid contaminating others.

XII.   Bacterial infections (pyodermas)

A.   **Description and etiology**

1.   Bacterial infections include a variety of acquired skin lesions characterized by erythema and pustules; most common causative organisms are Gram-positive staphylococci and beta-hemolytic streptococci.
2.   Types include:
     a.   *Folliculitis:* staphylococcal infection in one or more hair follicles
     b.   *Furuncle* (boil): acute inflammation of a hair follicle that has spread to the surrounding tissue
     c.   *Carbuncle:* extension of a furuncle into several follicles
     d.   *Stye* (hordeolum): folliculitis of one of the stiff hairs of the eyelid
     e.   *Impetigo:* superficial staphylococcal or streptococcal skin infection; it is communicable in the young and is especially common in children living in an unclean environment

B.   **Pathophysiologic processes and manifestations**

1.   Normally the skin's surface is acidic and contains resident bacteria that do not harm the host.
2.   Skin infection occurs when an imbalance exists, such as with a superimposed systemic illness or the administration of certain medications that allow the resident bacteria to invade the skin and cause damage.
3.   *Folliculitis* results in pustule formation; inflammation occurs, resulting in erythema.
4.   A *furuncle* manifests as a deep, coin-sized erythematous pustule. The lesion is painful and usually develops a cellulitis with a white center on the skin surface.
5.   A *carbuncle* is a group of infected hair follicles. This subcutaneous infection develops into a red, painful mass, which can spread causing septicemia; it occurs most commonly on the back and upper neck.
6.   A *stye* manifests as a pink, swollen area on the eyelid.
7.   In *impetigo,* pruritic red macules develop into vesicles and bullae, which form a honey-yellow-colored crust; leaking fluid from the pustules causes the lesions to spread. Secondary bacterial infections can lead to ulcer formation and impaired wound healing.

C.   **Overview of nursing interventions**

1.   Administer antibacterial agents, as prescribed.

2. Prepare patient for surgical incision and drainage of pustule, if indicated.
3. Apply warm soaks to ease discomfort and encourage drainage.
4. Apply normal saline wet to dry dressings or apply antibiotic soaks to ulcerated areas, as indicated.
5. Teach the patient about the cause of the lesions.
6. Educate the patient about preventing impetigo.

XIII. Fungal infections

A. Description
1. Fungal infections are commonly superficial skin infections occurring in areas of the body where keratin is abundant (eg, stratum corneum, nails, and hair).
2. Types include:
    a. Tinea pedis (athlete's foot): affects the foot
    b. Tinea capitis: affects the scalp
    c. Tinea corporis (ringworm): affects the torso, neck, chest, and legs
    d. Tinea ungulum: affects the nails
    e. Candidiasis: affects the skin, nails, mouth, vagina, or gastrointestinal or respiratory tracts

B. Etiology and incidence
1. Fungi are organisms that are transmitted by direct physical contact.
2. Tinea infections occur on the integumentary system from a fungus and are classified according to their location on the body.
3. Candidal infections are caused by *Candida albicans,* which thrives in a warm, moist environment.

C. Pathophysiologic processes and manifestations
1. *Tinea pedis* appears as scaling lesions between the toes and on the soles of the feet; eventually, these lesions can fissure.
2. *Tinea capitis* is manifested by pruritus and scaling and often leads to hair loss.
3. *Tinea corporis* presents as a circular red patch with an elevated border that may be erythematous and scaly.
4. The initial lesions of *tinea ungulum* give an opaque quality to the nail tissue, which thickens, cracks, and finally becomes distorted in shape.
5. *Candidal infections* present as a rash with red macules that have well-defined borders; these borders erode and result in scaling. Cutaneous candidal infections occur in the inter-triginous areas of obese or diabetic persons.
6. Thrush is produced by *C. albicans;* it presents as creamy white areas on the inflamed mucous membranes of the mouth.

D. Overview of nursing interventions
1. Administer antifungal agents (topical or oral), as prescribed.
2. Administer keratolytic agents for noninflammatory scaling, as prescribed.
3. Assess for evidence of secondary infection; if present, manage appropriately.
4. Provide patient teaching covering:
    a. Need for good hygiene

      b.   Avoidance of scratching

      c.   Modes of transmission

XIV. Scabies

A. Description

   1.   Scabies is an acquired parasitic skin disorder.

   2.   It is characterized by the formation of burrows in the skin, found most commonly between the fingers, inside the wrists and elbows, and along the belt line.

B. Etiology

   1.   Scabies is caused by the *Sarcoptes scabiei* mite.

   2.   It is spread by direct skin contact and *not* by contact with clothing, bedding, or other objects.

C. Pathophysiologic processes and manifestations

   1.   The female mite burrows into the skin and lays eggs.

   2.   When the eggs hatch into larvae, they move to the skin surface, burrowing as they search for food or protection.

   3.   Scratching causes the mites to burrow deeper, which further exacerbates the itching sensation.

   4.   Pruritus, the chief manifestation, is generally more severe at night.

   5.   Other manifestations include:

      a.   Papules

      b.   Secondary excoriations

      c.   Crusting and lichenification (may occur with chronic infestation)

D. Overview of nursing interventions

   1.   Administer topical lindane 1% or permethrin cream 5%, as prescribed.

   2.   Administer crotamiton 10% cream for children or pregnant or lactating females, as prescribed.

   3.   Assess for secondary infection and manage symptoms, if present.

   4.   Educate the patient and family members regarding transmission, prevention, and personal hygiene.

XV. Pediculosis

A. Description

   1.   Pediculosis (lice infestation) is an acquired parasitic skin disease characterized by small red macules and papules.

   2.   Classifications include:

      a.   Pediculosis capitis (head lice)

      b.   Pediculosis corporis (body lice)

      c.   Pediculosis pubis (pubic lice)

B. Etiology

   1.   Pediculosis is caused by a louse.

   2.   It is transmitted by way of direct skin contact or by contact with contaminated objects, bedding, and clothing.

C. Pathophysiologic processes and manifestations

1. Lice live on the skin surface but inject their digestive juices and excreta into the skin, causing a sensitivity reaction.
2. The eggs, called nits, are deposited along hair shafts.
3. The primary manifestation is severe pruritus with secondary excoriation.
4. In pediculosis corporis, papules may also be present.

D. Overview of nursing interventions

1. Administer lindane or pyrethrine (RID) lotion or shampoo, as prescribed.
2. Remove nits with a comb.
3. Educate the patient and family members regarding transmission, management, and prevention of reinfestation.
4. Administer accurate doses of the solution, because some medications used to kill nits also damage the central nervous system.

XVI. Burns

A. Description and etiology: traumatic skin injuries resulting from heat, electrical current, chemicals, friction, shearing forces, or excessive sunlight exposure

B. Classification

1. Burns are classified according to depth and extent of injury.
2. Classifications of the depth of burns include:
   a. First-degree (partial thickness)
   b. Second-degree (superficial or deep partial thickness)
   c. Third-degree (full thickness)
3. A *first-degree burn* involves destruction of the epidermis resulting in localized pain and redness. Healing is complete and occurs within 5 to 10 days.
4. A *superficial second-degree burn* involves destruction of the epidermis and the upper third of the dermis; it is characterized by pain and blister formation. Healing is complete but requires extended time to occur.
5. A *deep second-degree burn* involves destruction of the epidermis and dermis, leaving only the epidermal skin appendages within the hair follicles. The skin may be waxy white in appearance and require grafting or prolonged periods for recovery.
6. A *third-degree burn* involves destruction of the entire epidermis and dermis and typically involves fat and muscle; the skin may be white, charred, or leathery in appearance. This burn requires skin grafting and prolonged periods for recovery.
7. The extent of injury is calculated according to the rule of nines for adults and the pediatric rule of nines for children. A more detailed estimation is possible using the Lund and Browder chart (Fig. 9-2).

C. Pathophysiologic processes and manifestations

1. Pathophysiologic processes of burn injuries can be grouped into two phases:

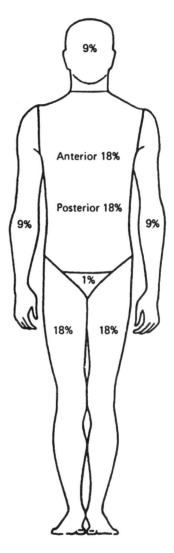

FIGURE 9-2.
The Rule of Nines used for estimating the percentage of body burns in the adult.

      a. Resuscitative phase
      b. Postresuscitative phase
  2. *Resuscitative phase*
      a. **Immediately after a burn injury, fluid shifts occur secondary to the direct damage to the microcirculation; as a result, changes in membrane permeability occur and vasoactive substances are released.**
      b. **Rapid leakage of fluid from the vascular space to the interstitium occurs, resulting in loss of circulating blood volume and massive edema.**
      c. **This loss is most obvious in the first 6 to 8 hours after injury.**

Capillary integrity is generally restored by 24 to 36 hours after injury, and fluid loss diminishes.

    d. The loss of circulating volume is termed *burn shock* and is potentially lethal.

    e. Cardiac output decreases, resulting in hypotension.

    f. A disruption in the transmembrane potential on a cellular level results in sodium–potassium pump impairment, causing intracellular swelling.

    g. Catecholamines are released into the circulation, resulting in tachycardia, peripheral vasoconstriction, and increased systemic vascular resistance.

    h. Edema around the face and neck can result in airway obstruction; circumferential burns of the extremities can cause decreased perfusion to the distal extremities and limb loss.

    i. The metabolic rate increases, resulting in a hypermetabolic state associated with increased oxygen consumption.

    j. Hyperglycemia and hypothermia may also occur.

    k. Pulmonary complications include bronchoconstriction, increased alveolar edema, and hypoxia.

    l. Immunoglobulins decrease in number, and defects in the structure of white cells have been noted, resulting in a suppressed immune response.

    m. Anemia and coagulopathies also occur.

3. *Postresuscitative phase*

    a. Mucosal irritation persists, leading to increased mucus production and decreased pulmonary clearance capacity.

    b. Obstruction of smaller airways occurs, leading to atelectasis and pneumonia.

    c. Hypermetabolism continues with resultant increased temperature and protein catabolism; this continues until burn covering is done by the formation of new skin.

    d. Wound infection is a dangerous complication because the body has lost its primary defense against invasion and the immune response is suppressed.

D.   **Overview of nursing interventions**

1. Ensure volume replacement to prevent hypovolemic shock and shock-induced organ failure.

    a. Administer isotonic crystalloid for fluid resuscitation, calculating quantities based on the Parkland formula (4 mL × kg body weight × % burn surface area = total fluid requirement for 24 hours).

    b. Replace 50% of this total in the first 8 hours after injury, 25% in the second 8 hours, and 25% in the last 8 hours.

    c. Taper fluid replacement in the second 24 hours after injury to the particular needs of the patient.

2. Evaluate the effectiveness of fluid resuscitation by monitoring urine output, cardiovascular responses, and acid–base balance.

3. Assess cardiovascular status and monitor for tachycardia and hypo-

volemia; note that cardiac monitoring is particularly important in electrical burns because of the incidence of dysrhythmias.

4. Ensure pulmonary support (eg, institute intubation and mechanical ventilation for patients with facial and neck burns or those with inhalation injuries, as indicated).

5. Monitor oxygenation status by way of arterial blood gases.

6. Monitor for the presence of carboxyhemoglobin when inhalation injury is suspected.

7. Maintain pulmonary hygiene to prevent secondary pneumonia and acute respiratory distress syndrome (ARDS).

8. Administer bronchodilators to offset bronchospasm and obstruction, as prescribed.

9. Monitor metabolic needs and ensure adequate nutrition (eg, total parenteral nutrition or enteral feedings).

10. Prepare the patient for debridement and escharotomy (surgical removal of eschar or dead tissue to relieve underlying pressure caused by edema).

11. Provide wound management (eg, bathing the patient in a hydrotherapy tank followed by debridement and scrubbing the wound bed); afterward, apply topical agents such as silver sulfadiazine, sulfamylon, or silver nitrate to the burns, as prescribed.

12. Prepare the patient for grafting procedures and ensure adequate pain management.

13. Ensure aseptic technique in all procedures because burn patients are particularly prone to sepsis.

14. Provide for physical therapy to prevent contractures and loss of function.

15. Educate the patient and family members regarding degree and severity of injury, procedures, and progress.

16. Provide emotional support and prepare the patient for rehabilitation.

 XVII. Skin cancer

A. Description: primary skin lesions that develop into cancer; classifications include basal cell, squamous cell, melanoma, and Kaposi's sarcoma (see Section XVIII for a discussion of Kaposi's sarcoma)

B. Etiology and incidence

1. The cause of skin cancer is unknown, although most dermatologic carcinomas are associated with increased lifetime exposure to the sun (specifically ultraviolet radiation) or with a history of previous radiologic therapy.

2. Basal cell carcinoma occurs most commonly in light-skinned people.

3. Incidence of malignant melanoma is increasing and is thought to be due to the thinning ozone layer.

C. Pathophysiologic processes and manifestations

1. *Basal cell carcinoma* presents as a single firm, skin-colored nodule with a raised perimeter; small telangiectatic vessels are common. Invasion of vessels, lymph nodes, and bone may occur.

2. *Squamous cell carcinoma* is classified as intraepidermal or invasive; it

presents as scaly, slightly elevated lesions that develop into ulcers with irregular borders.

3. *Malignant melanoma* is a rare tumor of the melanocytes; it arises from nevi or as new moles, presenting as a slightly elevated black or brown lesion with an irregular border and uneven surface that tends to ulcerate and bleed.

D. **Overview of nursing interventions**

1. Prepare the patient for chemosurgery, cryosurgery, or sharp dissection, if indicated.
2. Administer antineoplastic agents or radiotherapy, as prescribed.
3. Provide supportive therapy for the patient undergoing chemotherapy or radiation therapy.
4. Educate the patient and family members regarding the importance of limiting sunlight exposure.
5. Educate the patient regarding the selection and use of sunscreens.

XVIII. Kaposi's sarcoma

A. **Description and etiology**

1. Kaposi's sarcoma is a type of skin cancer commonly associated with immunosuppression.

2. **Although it occurs most often in acquired immunodeficiency syndrome (AIDS) patients, it also can occur in patients who are immunosuppressed for any reason (eg, patients receiving chemotherapy and organ-transplantation patients).**

B. **Pathophysiologic processes and manifestations**

1. Immunosuppression reduces the body's defenses against other cells, including cancer cells, allowing these cells to grow.
2. Kaposi's sarcoma appears as a purple lesion, which at first is macular.
3. As the disease progresses, the purple macular lesion may become more nodular.
4. The lesions may remain in one area, such as the legs.
5. In the rapidly progressive form of the disease, lesions spread symmetrically over the entire body.
6. Lesions may itch or hurt.
7. Biopsies are needed to make the diagnosis.
8. Occasionally, the lesions may extend under the skin to the lymph nodes.

C. **Overview of nursing interventions**

1. Administer chemotherapy, if prescribed.
2. Provide comfort and care for the patient with AIDS (see Chapter 20, Immunologic Disorders).
3. Be sure to follow appropriate protocol, as there are many drugs being developed for treatment.

Bibliography

Bullock, B. (1996). *Pathophysiology: Adaptations and alterations in function* (4th ed.). Philadelphia: Lippincott-Raven.

Brody, M. B. et al. (1997). Varicella-zoster virus infection: The complex prevention-treatment picture. *Postgraduate Medicine 102*(1): 187–90, 92–4, 227–8.

Ganong, William F. (1997). *Review of medical physiology* (18th ed.). Stamford, CT: Appleton and Lange.

Germonpre, P. et al. (1996). Hyperbaricoxygen therapy and piracetam decrease the early extension of partial thickness burns. *Burns 22*(6):468–73.

Guyton, Arthur C., & Hall, John E. (1996). *Textbook of medical physiology* (9th ed.). Philadelphia: W. B. Saunders.

Harkins, L. (1997). Protocols for contact dermatitis. *Lippincott's Primary Care Practitioner. 1*(1):97–99.

Kinney, M., Packa, D., & Dunbar, S. (1993). *AACN's clinical reference for critical-care nursing* (3rd ed.). St. Louis: C. V. Mosby.

Krenek, G. et al. (1996). Eczema: nuts and bolts of management. *Consultant 36*(3):486–488, 491, 493.

McCance, K. L., & Huether, S. E. (1994). *Pathophysiology: The biologic basis for disease in adults and children* (2nd ed.). St. Louis: Mosby-Year Book.

Porth, C. (1994). *Pathophysiology: Concepts of altered health states* (4th ed.). Philadelphia: Lippincott-Raven.

Pyner, T. (1997). Know how guide to eczema/dermatitis. *Nursing Times, 93*(13):30–1.

STUDY QUESTIONS

1. A 32-year-old male firefighter received second-degree burns on the anterior and posterior trunk and on both arms. Using the rule of nines, which of the following estimates best approximates the percentage of burn surface area?
   a. 36%
   b. 44%
   c. 54%
   d. 63%

2. Characteristics of second-degree deep partial-thickness burns include:
   a. formation of wet, thin-walled blisters immediately after surgery
   b. tissue destruction involving possibly the entire dermis
   c. tissue destruction involving the epidermis, dermis, and subcutaneous tissue
   d. superficial tissue destruction

3. Recommended fluid replacement for the initial 24 hours after injury is:
   a. 4 mL × kg body weight × % burn surface area
   b. 6 mL × kg body weight × % burn surface area
   c. 8 mL × kg body weight × % burn surface area
   d. 10 mL × kg body weight × % burn surface area

4. The nurse would describe the procedure of escharotomy to the patient as:
   a. draining excess fluid
   b. grafting new skin
   c. cutting through dead tissue
   d. application of sulfamylon

5. Intracellular swelling after severe burns is related to:
   a. increased cardiac output
   b. disruption in the transmembrane potential
   c. a hypermetabolic state
   d. decreased immunoglobulin

6. The initial manifestations of which one of the following disorders include erythema, exudate, scaling, and pruritus?

a. seborrheic dermatitis
b. allergic dermatitis
c. contact dermatitis
d. scabies

7. Lichenification refers to:
   a. skin excoriation
   b. skin hyperpigmentation
   c. pruritus and itchiness
   d. skin thickening

8. Psoriasis may be caused by all of the following *except:*
   a. contact with an infected person
   b. biochemical alteration
   c. genetic predisposition
   d. familial predisposition

9. When assessing a patient for skin cancer, the nurse should note that an ulcerated nodule with an indurated base describes:
   a. basal cell carcinoma
   b. Kaposi's sarcoma
   c. melanoma
   d. squamous cell carcinoma

10. When providing patient teaching on the typical course of treatment for basal cell carcinoma, the nurse should instruct the patient on:
    a. usual sites of metastasis
    b. methods of photoprotection
    c. expected radiation therapy
    d. growth process of this type of cancer

11. A patient who presents with Kaposi's sarcoma has which coexisting problem?
    a. immunosuppression
    b. tuberculosis
    c. herpes
    d. HIV

12. A nurse performing an assessment notices inflamed mucous membranes in the mouth and creamy white areas. The nurse recognizes this as:
    a. *Tinea capitis*
    b. *Candida albicans*
    c. leukoplakia
    d. sarcoptes scabiei

13. Pain over a nerve distribution area, followed by erythema and vesicles, fever and malaise describes which viral skin disorder:
    a. herpes simplex
    b. carbuncle
    c. impetigo
    d. herpes zoster

14. Which of the following conditions can occur when resident bacteria invades the skin and causes damage?
    a. herpes zoster
    b. herpes simplex
    c. sarcoptes scabiei
    d. folliculitis

ANSWER KEY

Question	Correct answer	Correct answer rationale	Incorrect answer rationales
1.	c	9% per arm, 1% anterior, and 18% posterior trunk.	a, b, and d. These estimates are incorrect. Using Lund and Browder's chart, the total would be 40%.
2.	b	a. indicates superficial second-degree burns.	c. indicates third-degree burns. d. indicates first-degree burns.
3.	a	Replace 50% of this total in the first 8 hours after injury; replace 25% of this total in each of the second and third 8-hour periods after injury. Thereafter, fluid re-replacement is tailored to the patient's individual needs.	b, c, and d. These are incorrect.
4.	c	Escharotomy refers to cutting through dead tissue (eschar) to relieve pressure caused by edema.	a. Draining excess fluid is not done for burns. b. Grafting may be done for deep second- and third-degree burns, but cannot be done over dead tissue. d. Sulfamylon is used as a medication on dressings.
5.	b	A disruption in the transmembrane potential on a cellular level results in sodium–potassium pump impairment, causing intracellular swelling.	a. In burns, there is a decreased cardiac output. c. A hypermetabolic state leads to increased O_2 consumption. d. Decreased immunoglobulin leads to suppressed immune function.
6.	c	Contact dermatitis is a skin inflammation caused by contact with an allergen, thus stimulating the immune system to react accordingly.	a. Seborrheic dermatitis appears as patches of sallow, greasy skin with or without scaling and redness. b. Allergic dermatitis involves hives. d. Scabies manifests as papules with crusting.
7.	d	Lichenification, seen in adult atopic dermatitis and scabies, refers to skin thickening.	a, b, and c. These are incorrect responses.
8.	a	Psoriasis is not a contagious disease and is not spread by contact with lesions.	b, c, and d. All of these are potential causes.

Question	Correct answer	Correct answer rationale	Incorrect answer rationales
9.	d	Squamous cell carcinoma appears as an ulcerated nodule with an indurated base.	a. Basal cell carcinoma appears as waxy, grayish-yellow nonindurated lesions. b. Kaposi's sarcoma appears as multiple purplish-reddish plaques. c. Melanoma typically is a darkly pigmented lesion with irregular borders.
10.	b	The patient needs to understand the importance of limiting sun exposure and methods to achieve this.	a. Basal cell carcinoma typically does not metastasize. c. Radiation is not a recommended treatment. d. Basal cell carcinoma does not have a rapid growth.
11.	a	Kaposi's sarcoma is a type of skin cancer associated with immuno-suppression. Immunosuppression can result from many etiologies.	b, c, and d. These choices are incorrect. Herpes and tuberculosis are not associated with Kaposi's sarcoma. Immunosuppression (which occurs with HIV) infection leads to the development of Kaposi's sarcoma. HIV is one possible cause of immunosuppression.
12.	b	*Candida albicans* is described in the stem. This is a fungal infection that thrives in a warm, moist environment.	a. This choice is incorrect because *tinea capitis* is pruritis and scaling that occurs on the scalp. c. This choice is incorrect because leukoplakia is the presence of white patches on the mucous membrane. a. This choice is incorrect because sarcoptes scabiei is the parasite that causes scabies.
13.	d	The symptoms described are those of herpes zoster which is a reactivation of the varicella virus.	a. This choice is wrong. Herpes simplex occurs on the mucous membranes and is caused by the herpes simplex virus. b and c. These choices are incorrect because both carbuncle and impetigo are bacterial infections, and their symptoms are different than those described in the stem.
14.	d.	Folliculitis is a staphylococcal infection in one or more hair follicle. It is the only choice that describes a bacterial infection.	a, b, and c. These choices are incorrect because both herpes conditions are caused by a virus, and Sarcoptes scabiei is a parasite.

10

Eye, Ear, Nose, and Throat Disorders

I.   Overview of pathophysiologic processes

A.   Structural disorders
1.   These disorders affect or alter an organ's structure; structural deformities may or may not affect function.
2.   Structural disorders of eye, ear, nose, and throat include retinal detachment, cataracts, nasal fractures, and tumors.
3.   Risk factors vary with the specific disorders.

B.   Functional disorders
1.   These disorders affect or alter the function of an organ or organs; infections commonly affect function.
2.   Functional disorders of the eye, ear, nose, and throat include glaucoma, otitis externa and media, hearing loss (conductive, neurosensory, and Meniere's disease), sinusitis, epistaxis, and inflammation of pharyngeal structures.
3.   There are no particular risk factors.

II.   Physiologic responses to eye, ear, nose, and throat disorders

A.   Responses to eye disorders
1.   Alterations in vision: may be produced by structural changes and may range from decreased vision to blindness; blurred or halo vision may occur and portions of the visual field may be lost.
2.   Pain: results from structural disorders.

B.   Responses to ear disorders
1.   Hearing loss: can result from structural or functional disorders.

2. Drainage: occurs in the presence of infection.

3. **Vertigo: sensation in which the person feels himself or his surroundings moving in space; results from disturbances in equilibrium (eg, middle ear disorders).**

4. Erythema: redness due to infection or inflammation.

C. **Responses to nose disorders**

1. Mucopurulent nasal drainage: produced by the nasal mucosa as a result of an infection, typically viral or bacterial.

2. Nasal obstruction: reduction in the passageway through the nasal cavity caused by edema of the nasal mucosa.

3. Mucosal erythema: increased redness of the nasal mucosa due to irritation.

D. **Responses to throat disorders**

1. Pain: produced by inflammation and infection within the three divisions of the throat

2. Airway or esophageal obstruction: reduction in the airway or esophagus produced by inflammation, infection, neoplasm, or disruption of bony structures or soft tissue within the throat.

3. Dysphagia: inability to swallow food (fluids are usually tolerated)

4. Voice changes: due to alterations in air movement.

5. Sore throat: caused by inflamed or infected tissue.

III. **Retinal detachment**

A. **Description: separation of the retina from the posterior part of the eye; threatens visual function**

B. **Etiology**

1. **The most common cause of retinal detachment is trauma, such as blunt injury.**

2. Age-related degenerative changes also may cause detachment.

3. Other causes include vascular or metabolic diseases.

C. **Pathophysiologic processes and manifestations**

1. The part of the retina containing the rods and cones separates from the layer of the eye that nourishes them.

2. The most common detachments are those that result from tears.

3. The vitreous humor is normally jellylike; however, with age, its acid concentration changes and liquefies the part of the eye that maintains the eye's shape and holds its structures together. As this process continues, the posterior structures in the eye can move forward, tearing the retina.

4. **The patient may complain of flashing lights or "floaters" early in the process; these symptoms occur as blood and other cells are reflected by the rods and cones.**

D. **Overview of nursing interventions**

1. Prepare patient for surgery to reattach the retina; afterward, provide appropriate postoperative care.

2. Provide a safe environment.

IV. Cataracts

A. Description: alteration in the lens from normally clear to opaque; opacity leads to vision loss

B. Etiology

1. The most common cause of cataracts is aging, which typically causes the nucleus of the lens to become brown-yellow.

2. **Overuse of steroids or Cushing's disease can also cause cataracts.**

3. Physical changes of the lens also may result in a loss of transparency.

C. Pathophysiologic processes and manifestations

1. Changes in tiny fibers that extend from the ciliary body to the outer portion of the lens distort the visual image.

2. Coagulation may result from a protein that will decrease the amount of light entering the retina, resulting in cloudy vision.

3. As the lens becomes opaque, symptoms include glare, poor night vision, and blurred vision.

4. Pupillary color may change to yellow, grey, or white.

D. Overview of nursing interventions

1. Instruct the patient to avoid bright sunlight or light by wearing dark sunglasses or a hat.

2. Tell the patient to avoid driving at night.

3. Prepare patient for surgery, if indicated; afterward, provide appropriate postoperative care.

4. Instruct the patient that surgery should be done only when absolutely necessary.

V. Glaucoma

A. Description

1. Glaucoma is a condition marked by increased intraocular pressure (IOP); if left untreated, damage to the optic nerve may result.

2. Normal IOP is 13 to 22 mm Hg; in glaucoma, these pressures rise.

3. Glaucoma may be open-angle or closed-angle, depending on the aqueous humor's ability to drain out of the eye's anterior chamber.

4. Glaucoma also may be primary or secondary.

5. Primary open-angle glaucoma is usually a bilateral disease in which there is increased IOP and a normal drainage angle.

B. Etiology

1. Glaucoma may be congenital or acquired.

2. Primary congenital glaucoma results from maldevelopment of the trabeculum and the iridotrabecular junction.

3. Primary closed-angle glaucoma results from the obstructed outflow angle of the peripheral iris.

4. Secondary open-angle glaucoma results from long-term steroid use, uveitis, blockage of the trabecular system, trauma, or tumors.

C. Pathophysiologic processes and manifestations

1. When the aqueous humor is unable to drain out of the eye, pressure builds up and is referred to the eye's posterior chamber.
2. As a result, the iris flattens out and may obstruct the outflow of aqueous humor from the anterior chamber through the trabecular system, the Schlemm canal, and the venous plexus.
3. Open-angle glaucoma is usually asymptomatic, which makes it difficult to diagnose; by the time visual field changes occur, there is significant optic nerve damage.
4. Symptoms of glaucoma include:
   a. Blurred vision
   b. Halo vision
   c. Pain in the eye (due to the rapid rise in IOP)
   d. Changes in the eye's appearance (eg, redness)
5. Pupillary block closed-angle glaucoma is a medical emergency. If left untreated, blindness can result.

D. Overview of nursing interventions
1. Administer medications (eg, pilocarpine eye drops) to decrease IOP, as prescribed.
2. Instruct the patient on the proper methods of administering eye drops and ointments.
3. Administer pain medications, as needed.

VI. Otitis externa

A. Description: inflammation and infection of the outer auditory canal
B. Etiology
1. Otitis externa is caused by bacterial invasion.
2. It is associated with swimming or swimming in contaminated water (swimmer's ear).
3. When the cerumen (protective earwax) dissolves, an increased risk for developing otitis externa exists.

C. Pathophysiologic processes and manifestations
1. Fluid builds up in the ear, causing pain and a sense of fullness; hearing loss may also result.
2. Other symptoms may include discharge and itchiness.

D. Overview of nursing interventions
1. Administer analgesics for pain, as prescribed.
2. Assess the discharge and administer antibiotic ear drops, as prescribed.
3. Irrigate the ear canal to clear it.
4. Instruct the patient to avoid contact with water for approximately 2 weeks.

VII. Otitis media

A. Description: inflammation and infection of the middle ear; most commonly seen in infants and young children
B. Etiology

1. Otitis media is caused by blockage of the eustachian tubes due to mucosal edema and hypertrophied lymph tissue, and impaired mucociliary function.

   2. Common causative agents are *Streptococcus pneumoniae, Streptococcus pyogenes,* and *Haemophilus influenzae.*

   3. In the pediatric population, otitis media occurs due to the position of the eustachian tube, which is shorter and straighter than in adults.

   4. Supine positioning increases the risk of infection spread because the organisms will move with gravity.

   5. Aerotitis is a form of otitis media that results from barotrauma (injury caused by pressure changes encountered with flying and deep-sea diving).

C. Pathophysiologic processes and manifestations

   1. Commonly, an attack of otitis media follows a cold or respiratory infection.

   2. As with any infection, fever is typically present.

   3. Inflammation of the inner ear structures is rated after otoscopic examination, with exudate noted behind the eardrum as swollen, red, or yellow; this exudate may become so large that the tympanic membrane ruptures.

   4. Lymph glands behind the ears or on the neck may be swollen.

   5. The child may complain of pain or may pull at the ear.

   6. As eustachian obstruction progresses from mucosal swelling, microbes multiply.

D. Overview of nursing interventions

   1. Administer analgesics for pain, as indicated.

   2. Administer antibiotics, as prescribed.

   3. Provide hydration.

   4. Administer antipyretics, as prescribed.

   5. Prepare the child for myringotomy (incision of the tympanic membrane) with tube insertion, if indicated; afterward, provide appropriate postoperative care.

VIII.   Conductive hearing loss

A. Description: inability of sound to reach the inner ear as a result of obstruction (eg, fluid, pus, wax); onset may be sudden or progressive

B. Etiology

   1. Sudden conductive hearing loss usually results from infection or trauma to the ear (otitis media, ruptured tympanic membrane).

   2. Progressive conductive hearing loss results from
       a. Otosclerosis (a disorder occurring at the point where the stapes attaches to the otic capsule)
       b. Cerumen impaction

C. Pathophysiologic processes and manifestations

   1. Changes in hearing may be sudden or progressive.

   2. The patient frequently asks for statements to be repeated or may give inappropriate responses to questions.

3. Signs and symptoms may be related to the cause of the hearing loss, such as fever and leukocytosis in the presence of infection.
4. If otitis media is the cause, symptoms may include:
    a. Itching
    b. Discharge
    c. Fluid
    d. Throbbing and pressure in the ear
    e. Fever
    f. Red, bulging, or retracted tympanic membrane

5. **If otosclerosis is the cause, tinnitus may be present and reduced air conduction on the Rhinne test is noted.**
6. If cerumen is excessive, it will be visible on otoscopic examination.

D. **Overview of nursing interventions**
1. Determine the cause of the hearing loss and initiate interventions, as indicated.
2. Inform the patient that once the causative agent has been treated or repaired, hearing should return to normal.
3. Provide alternative methods of communication if required.
4. Assist with procedures such as ear irrigation, if indicated.
5. Administer pain medications and antibiotics, as prescribed.

IX.   Neurosensory hearing loss

A. Description: hearing loss resulting from cochlear or neural damage (also known as perceptive hearing loss); onset may be sudden or progressive

B. Etiology

1. **Sudden neurosensory hearing loss can result from trauma to the eighth cranial nerve, the cochlea, or from ototoxicity (the aminoglycoside antibiotics, including gentamicin and tobramycin, are highly ototoxic).**
2. Progressive neurosensory hearing loss can result from aging, noise, acoustic tumors, and Meniere's disease (see Section X for a discussion of Meniere's disease).

C. **Pathophysiologic processes and manifestations**
1. Hearing loss may be unilateral or bilateral.
2. Symptoms may include tinnitus, dizziness, and pain.
3. Testing with a tuning fork will demonstrate this type of hearing loss.

D. **Overview of nursing interventions**
1. Provide alternative methods for communication (eg, use sign language or speak slowly enough for the patient to read lips).
2. Administer analgesics for pain relief, as prescribed.
3. For a patient who is dizzy, provide a safe environment and encourage the patient to seek assistance when ambulating.
4. Use hearing aids when possible.
5. The patient with hearing loss is deprived of necessary stimulation; the nurse must communicate at all times, using special means as necessary.

X. Meniere's disease

A. Description: inner ear disorder involving a triad of symptoms of vertigo, tinnitus, and hearing loss

B. Etiology

   1. Meniere's disease is idiopathic, but it may be associated with middle ear infection.
   2. It affects men more than women.
   3. It may result from a head trauma.

C. Pathophysiologic processes and manifestations

   1. Circulatory disturbances in the vessels supplying the inner ear may occur.
   2. The membranous portion of the labyrinth may be dilated.
   3. In addition to the triad of vertigo, tinnitus, and hearing loss, symptoms may include nausea and vomiting, which are present primarily during acute attacks.
   4. Symptoms affect balance (vestibular) as well as hearing.
   5. Meniere's disease may be treated and may recur.

D. Overview of nursing interventions

   1. Administer diuretics, as prescribed.
   2. Administer vasodilators, as prescribed.
   3. Provide a safe environment.
   4. Provide nutrition and hydration.
   5. Be prepared to send the patient for hearing assist devices if deafness occurs.

XI. Nasal fractures

A. Description: any break in the nasal bony structure that may result in a deformity or obstruction

   1. Trauma may result from falls, blows, vehicular accidents.

B. Etiology: usually due to blunt trauma from falls, blows, or motor vehicle accidents

C. Pathophysiologic processes and manifestations

   1. As with any traumatic injury, pain, swelling, and ecchymosis occur.
   2. Bleeding may occur.
   3. Depending on the nature of the fracture, the nose may appear to be deformed.
   4. Blood or bone may obstruct air passage.
   5. Hematomas may occur inside or outside of the nose.

D. Overview of nursing interventions

   1. Administer analgesics for pain management, as prescribed.
   2. Assess for bleeding and monitor amount.
   3. Assess respiratory rate, character, and quality for possible obstruction.

   4. Assess drainage for presence of cerebrospinal fluid.

XII. Sinusitis

A. Description: inflammation and infection of the sinuses; may be acute or chronic

B. Etiology

1. Acute sinusitis
    a. Usually results from a viral or bacterial upper respiratory infection; once the infection has spread into the sinuses, increasing mucosal edema blocks the sinus ostium, rendering the sinuses unable to drain the purulent matter
    b. Is commonly caused by *Streptococcus pneumoniae, Haemophilus influenzae,* and *Staphylococcus aureus*
    c. Typically lasts less than 3 weeks
2. Chronic sinusitis
    a. Results from chronic blockage of the sinus ostium; it is often related to allergies and hypersensitivity reactions
    b. Lasts longer than 3 months

C. Pathophysiologic processes and manifestations

1. Microbe invasion of the sinuses causes inflammation, edema, and congestion with fluid; as the organisms multiply, these processes eventually occlude drainage areas.
2. Sinus pressure and pain increase, and drainage becomes purulent.
3. If a condition that obstructs drainage already exists (eg, deviated septum or polyps), sinusitis does not resolve easily and often recurs.

D. Overview of nursing interventions

1. Administer antibiotics, as prescribed.
2. Institute treatment measures based on the patient's symptoms.
3. Administer pseudoephedrine and ephedrine spray (with caution), as prescribed.
4. Provide pain relief with analgesics, as prescribed.

XIII. Epistaxis

A. Definition: nosebleed due to hypertensive or nonhypertensive causes; may originate in the anterior or posterior nose

B. Etiology

1. Anterior epistaxis is caused by drying, ulceration, crusting of the septal mucosa, trauma, or cocaine use.
2. Posterior epistaxis is due to hypertension; structural, neoplastic, or metabolic causes (e.g., septal perforation, hemophilia, hereditary hemorrhagic telangiectasia, thrombocytopenia, coagulopathies, cancer); trauma; or cocaine use.

C. Pathophysiologic processes and manifestations

1. Nasal bleeding can be profuse.
2. A group of vessels in the anterior septum commonly ruptures from direct trauma.

3. Bleeding that occurs from the larger posterior vessels is usually from a systemic disease or disorder.
4. Bleeding from the posterior nose usually results in blood trickling down the throat.

D. Overview of nursing interventions

1. Instruct the patient to sit upright with the head tilted forward.
2. Spray the nose with 0.25% phenylephrine hydrochloride, as prescribed, to cause vasoconstriction.
3. Instruct the patient to avoid using tissues or cotton gauze in the nares because these are difficult to remove and may further irritate the mucosa.
4. Assess breathing and oxygen saturation.
5. Assess nasal packing for color, odor (if any), and amount of drainage (if any).
6. Monitor the position of a Foley catheter placed for posterior epistaxis.

XIV. Inflammation of pharyngeal structures

A. Description and etiology

1. Inflammation of the pharyngeal structures includes:
    a. Pharyngitis (inflammation of the pharynx)
    b. Tonsillitis (inflammation of the tonsils)
    c. Adenoiditis (inflammation of the adenoids)
    d. Laryngitis (inflammation of the larynx)
2. These disorders can be caused by bacteria (streptococcus), viruses (rhinovirus, Epstein-Barr, adenovirus), or a spirochete (syphilis).
3. Acute pharyngitis is most commonly known as strep throat.
4. Chronic pharyngitis is the constant inflammation of the pharynx typically seen in persons who smoke, use their voice excessively, or work in dusty areas.
5. Peritonsillar abscess is an infection in the space above the tonsils; it usually follows acute tonsillitis.
6. Laryngitis is usually caused by increased use of the voice, dust, smoke, chemicals, or an upper respiratory infection.

B. Pathophysiologic processes and manifestations

1. Infectious organisms cause excessive mucus secretion.
2. Bacteria accumulate, multiply, and remain in the back of the throat, leaving exudates in the throat.
3. The mucosa becomes red, inflamed, and may be dotted with pustules.
4. Symptoms may include:
    a. Irritation and fullness in the throat
    b. Fever
    c. Hoarseness
    d. Difficulty swallowing
    e. Snoring
    f. Mouth breathing
    g. Cough
5. If the person has tonsils, the tonsils and adenoids will be involved, with pustules appearing on the tonsils.

6. If left untreated, the infection may extend into the palate and abscess.
7. In laryngitis, the inflammation cannot be visualized.

C. **Overview of nursing interventions**
1. Administer antibiotics, as prescribed.
2. Provide relief from throat pain with gargles or analgesics, as ordered.
3. Instruct patient to avoid irritants that may precipitate inflammation.
4. Instruct the patient to avoid talking whenever possible.

XV.   Throat cancer

A. **Definition: malignant neoplasms in the throat; most common type is squamous cell carcinoma**

B. **Etiology: predisposing factors include cigarette smoking and chronic hoarseness**

C. **Pathophysiologic processes and manifestations**
1. Cancer of the throat may occur in the esophagus, pharynx, or larynx.
2. Cancers in the throat may metastasize quickly when the throat muscle is involved by spreading to the lymph glands.
3. Cancers of the larynx and vocal cords are removed surgically with fairly good prognosis if contained.
4. The course, treatment, and prognosis of head and neck cancers varies with the tissue type of cancer which may originate in the tongue, palate, jaw, lip, cheek, pharynx, larynx, lymph nodes, and salivary glands.
5. Manifestations can include
    a. Persistent cough
    b. Pain and burning in the throat when drinking hot liquids or citrus juices
    c. Dysphagia
    d. Dyspnea
    e. Weight loss
    f. Foul-smelling breath
    g. Pain radiating to the ear

D. **Overview of nursing interventions**
1. Provide supplemental nutrition for the patient with dysphagia.
2. Monitor and assess breath sounds, arterial blood gases, and oxygen saturation for hypoxia.
3. Assess the patient for respiratory distress.
4. Provide mouth care to eliminate foul-smelling breath.
5. Administer analgesics for pain, as prescribed.
6. Prepare the patient for chemotherapy, radiation therapy, or surgery, as indicated.

Bibliography

Bullock, B. (1996). *Pathophysiology: Adaptations and alterations in function* (4th ed.). Philadelphia: Lippincott-Raven.

Ganong, William F. (1997). *Review of medical physiology* (18th ed.). Stamford, CT: Appleton and Lange.

Guyton, Arthur C., & Hall, John E. (1996). *Textbook of medical physiology* (9th ed.). Philadelphia: W. B. Saunders.

Kinney, M., Packa, D., & Dunbar, S. (1993). *AACN's clinical reference for critical-care nursing* (3rd ed.). St. Louis: C.V. Mosby.

McCance, K. L., & Huether, S. E. (1994). *Pathophysiology: The biologic basis for disease in adults and children* (2nd ed.). St. Louis: Mosby-Year Book.

Porth, C. (1994). *Pathophysiology: Concepts of altered health states* (4th ed.). Philadelphia: Lippincott-Raven.

Price, S. A., & Wilson, L. M. (1992). *Pathophysiology: Clinical concepts of disease processes* (4th ed.). St. Louis: Mosby-Year Book.

STUDY QUESTIONS

1. Meniere's disease presents with a triad of symptoms that includes all of the following:
   a. vertigo, tinnitus, hearing loss
   b. pain, vertigo, bindness
   c. tinnitus, pain, hearing loss
   d. fever, inflammation, pain

2. The vitreous humor is normally:
   a. a firm mass
   b. where tears are formed
   c. below the retina
   d. jellylike

3. Early symptoms of retinal detachment may include:
   a. pain
   b. reddened eye
   c. floaters
   d. purulent discharge

4. Open-angle glaucoma differs from other types in that it is usually:
   a. congenital
   b. asymptomatic
   c. easily reversible
   d. a medical emergency

5. Which of the following symptoms would the nurse *not* expect to assess in a patient with glaucoma?
   a. pain
   b. blurred vision
   c. halo vision
   d. intraocular pressure of 15 mm Hg

6. Nursing interventions for the patient with cataracts would include:
   a. administering pilocarpine
   b. teaching the patient to avoid sunlight
   c. encouraging night driving to avoid sunlight
   d. administering pain medications

7. A nurse instructs the parents of a child with otitis media that this disorder occurs more frequently in children than in adults because a child's eustachian tube is:
   a. shorter and straighter
   b. longer and curved
   c. more porous
   d. undeveloped

8. Pathophysiologic processes involved in otitis media include all of the following *except:*
   a. aerotitis
   b. blockage of the eustachian tube
   c. an upper respiratory infection sequela
   d. nerve damage

9. Conductive hearing loss involves:
   a. nerve damage
   b. inability of sound to reach the inner ear
   c. perceptive hearing loss
   d. ototoxicity

10. Assessment of neurosensory hearing loss involves:
    a. use of a tuning fork
    b. use of an ophthalmoscope
    c. observation of signs of infection
    d. Rhinne test

11. Untreated tonsillitis can lead to:
    a. pharyngitis
    b. laryngitis
    c. abscess
    d. cancer

12. A nurse is caring for a patient with epistaxis. The bleeding is profuse. The nurse can expect to:
    a. Place tissue and cotton gauze in the nares to stop bleeding
    b. Spray the nose with 0.50% phenylephrine hydrochloride
    c. Have patient lay flat with nose pointing upward
    d. Instruct patient to sit up and point nose forward

13. Which disorder is associated with overuse of steroids?
    a. cataracts
    b. Meniere's disease
    c. retinal detachment
    ad sinusitis

14. Normal intraocular pressure is:
    a. 13–22 mmHg.
    b. 10–20 mmHg.
    c. 8–12 mmHg.
    d. 30–50 mmHg.

ANSWER KEY

Question	Correct answer	Correct answer rationale	Incorrect answer rationales
1.	a	The triad of symptoms seen in Meniere's disease includes vertigo, tinnitus, and hearing loss.	b, c, and d. These choices are incorrect because pain, fever, and blindness are not part of Meniere's disease.
2.	d	The vitreous humor is normally jellylike.	a, b, and c. These responses are incorrect.
3.	c	The patient with a retinal detachment may complain of flashing lights or floaters early in the process.	a, b, and d. These symptoms are not seen in early retinal detachment.
4.	b	Open-angle glaucoma is usually asymptomatic, which makes it difficult to diagnose.	a. Primary closed-angle glaucoma may be congenital. c. This response is incorrect. d. Pupillary block closed-angle glaucoma is a medical emergency.
5.	d	Normal intraocular pressure is 13 to 22 mm Hg; in glaucoma, this pressure rises.	a, b, and c. Pain, blurred vision, and halo vision are symptoms of glaucoma.
6.	b	Patients with cataracts should be encouraged to avoid sunlight and to wear dark glasses.	a. Pilocarpine is used to treat glaucoma. c. Patients with cataracts have poor night vision, so driving at night should be discouraged. d. This response is incorrect.
7.	a	In children, the eustachian tube is shorter and straighter than in adults, allowing for transmission of bacteria to the middle ear.	b, c, and d. These responses are incorrect.
8.	d	Nerve damage is not associated with otitis media.	a, b, and c. Pathophysiologic changes in otitis media may involve aerotitis and blockage of the eustachian tube; this disorder also may occur secondary to an upper respiratory infection.
9.	b	Conductive hearing loss involves the inability of sound to reach the inner ear.	a, c, and d. These are associated with neurosensory hearing loss.
10.	a	A tuning fork is used to assess neurosensory hearing loss.	b. An ophthalmoscope is used to assess the eyes. c. This response is incorrect. d. The Rinne test is used to diagnose conductive hearing loss.

Question	Correct answer	Correct answer rationale	Incorrect answer rationales
11.	c	Untreated tonsillitis can lead to peritonsillar abscess as the infection extends into the palate.	a, b, and d. These choices are incorrect. Laryngitis and pharyngitis are inflammation of these structures and is present when there is an infection in the area. Throat cancer is not a sequelae of tonsillitis.
12.	d	During a nosebleed the patient should be instructed to sit up and tilt the head forward.	a. This answer in incorrect because tissues, cotton or gauze in the nose must be avoided. These objects will cause further damage. b. The proper solution is 0.25% phenylephrine. c. This position will cause aspiration.
13.	a	Overuse of steroids is associated with cataracts.	b, c, and d. These disorders are not associated with use of steroids.
14.	a	Normal intraocular pressure is 13–22 mmHg.	b, c, and d. These pressures are either too high or too low.

11

Liver and Biliary Disorders

I. Overview of pathophysiologic processes

A. Infectious and inflammatory diseases

1. Infectious liver diseases include disorders that result from viruses, bacteria, or protozoa.
2. These types of disorders are marked by inflammation and destruction of liver cells.
3. Hepatitis is classified as a viral liver disease.
4. Hepatic abscess is classified as a bacterial or protozoan liver disease.
5. Cholecystitis is inflammation of the gallbladder; inflammation may be caused by stone formation, known as cholelithiasis, or from infections.
6. Risk factors for infectious and inflammatory diseases include:
    a. Exposure to the antigen
    b. Infection present elsewhere in the body

B. Chronic degenerative disease

1. Chronic degenerative disease is progressive and accompanied by significant complications such as portal hypertension, ascites, bleeding, high serum ammonia levels, and esophageal varices.
2. This disorder also adversely affects electrolytes, metabolism, vitamin and trace metal storage, plasma proteins, and other important liver functions.
3. Cirrhosis is a chronic degenerative disease.
4. Risk factors for chronic degenerative disease include:
    a. Hepatitis infection
    b. Chronic alcoholism
5. Portal hypertension is a common complication of cirrhosis; it may be life-threatening if the patient also has esophageal varices.

C. Liver trauma

1. Liver trauma refers to any injury that results in damage to the liver.
2. Resulting damage can include laceration from fractured xiphoid and ribs or blunt trauma from falls.
3. Types of liver trauma include:
    a. *Transcapsular injuries:* Glisson's capsule (a fibroelastic capsule containing blood vessels, lymphatics, and nerves covering the liver) ruptures; blood vessels and bile fill the peritoneal cavity.

      b. *Subcapsular injuries:* Blood collects between Glisson's capsule and the parenchyma in the form of a hematoma.

      c. *Central injuries:* Trauma results in an interruption in the parenchyma.

D. Cysts

  1. Liver cysts are usually asymptomatic and require no intervention.

  2. Cysts can be nonparasitic or hydatid.

  3. There are no specific risk factors for developing cysts.

E. Liver cancer

  1. Tumors may occur in the liver as primary lesions.

  2. Usually, they present as metastatic lesions.

II. Physiologic responses to liver and biliary dysfunction

A. Pruritus: itchy, irritated skin

B. Fatigue: tired, exhausted feeling resulting in decreased physical and mental abilities

C. Varices

  1. Varices refers to a hemorrhagic process of the esophagus, which is caused by the formation of collateral circulation secondary to portal hypertension.

  2. The collateral veins dilate and become distended, causing ulcerative areas that hemorrhage.

D. Anorexia: loss of appetite

E. Ascites

  1. Ascites is an accumulation of fluid within the peritoneal cavity; the fluid contains a high concentration of albumin.

  2. Ascites commonly occurs in patients with cirrhosis, portal hypertension, and malignancies.

F. Caput medusae: collateral veins occurring on the abdomen as a result of portal hypertension

G. Splenomegaly: an enlargement of the spleen resulting from increased pressure in the splenic vein; evident in patients with portal hypertension

H. Hepatic encephalopathy

  1. Hepatic encephalopathy is a neurologic symptom resulting from an accumulation of ammonia; it may be acute or chronic.

  2. Symptoms may range from minor mental disturbances to impaired thought processes and neuromuscular changes.

I. Jaundice

  1. Jaundice is a condition characterized by a yellowing of the skin, whites of the eyes, and mucous membranes; it occurs as the total bilirubin value rises above 2.5 mg/dL.

  2. Types include:

      a. *Hepatocellular jaundice,* which develops when the liver is unable to metabolize bilirubin; this results in excessive circulating bilirubin levels.

      b. *Obstructive jaundice,* which develops when hepatic bile channels and ducts become obstructed and the normal bile and bilirubin excretion process is blocked; this also may occur when the common bile duct is obstructed by gallstone or tumor.

      c. *Hemolytic jaundice,* which occurs as a result of excessive breakdown of red blood cells.

III. Hepatitis

A. Description

    1. Hepatitis is an inflammatory process that results in liver cell destruction.

    2. Classifications include viral hepatitis and toxic (or chemical) hepatitis.

    3. **Types of viral hepatitis include hepatitis A (HAV), hepatitis B (HBV), hepatitis C (HCV), and hepatitis D or delta hepatitis (HDV).**

B. Etiology

    1. *Hepatitis A,* the most common type of viral hepatitis, can be transmitted by way of fecal–oral contamination or from contaminated water or food; occasionally, it can be transmitted sexually.

    2. *Hepatitis B* can be transmitted sexually or from blood transfusions; contaminated syringes, needles, or instruments; or direct contact with infected body fluids or mucosa (eg, saliva, gastric juices, semen, and tears).

    3. *Hepatitis C* (also known as non-A, non-B hepatitis) can be transmitted by way of blood transfusions, direct contact with infected body fluids, or sexual contact with an infected person.

    4. *Hepatitis D* occurs in conjunction with hepatitis B and depends on it for replication; it occurs most commonly in parenteral drug users.

    5. *Toxic hepatitis* is associated with toxic reactions to drugs or hepatotoxins such as industrial toxins (yellow phosphorus and carbon tetrachloride), medications (halothane, aldomet, isoniazid, and dilantin), or alcohol.

C. Pathophysiologic processes and manifestations

    1. After exposure to a causative agent, the liver becomes inflamed, causing hepatocellular damage, local necrosis, hyperplasia of Kupffer's cells, and infiltration by mononuclear phagocytes.

    2. As the liver becomes edematous, the normal lobular pattern becomes distorted; bile channels may be obstructed, resulting in cholestasia and intrahepatic obstructive jaundice.

    3. Hepatocellular regeneration usually begins within 48 hours and is complete within 2 to 3 months.

    4. Hepatitis has three phases (see Display 11-1)

      a. Prodromal

      b. Icteric

      c. Recovery

    5. *HAV* has an incubation period of 14 to 42 days; it usually is a mild infection characterized by fatigue, low-grade fever, abdominal pain, rash, and enlarged, tender liver.

    6. *HBV* has an incubation period of 40 to 180 days; it is characterized by the

DISPLAY 11-1
Phases of Hepatitis

Phases of Hepatitis

Prodromal
- This highly infectious phase begins 2 weeks aftger exposure and progresses to jaundice.
- Symptoms incude nausea, vomiting, fatigue, headache, cough, low-grade fever, right upper-quadrant pain, and weight loss.

Icteric
- This phase, considered the actual illness, begins approximately 1 week after the prodromal phase and lasts up to 6 weeks.
- Symptoms commonly include fatigue and abdominal pain; other symptoms may include dark urine, clay-colored stool, and itching.

Recovery
- In this phase, jaundice subsides, symptoms diminish, and liver function tests return to normal.

---

same symptoms as HBA, but those symptoms tend to be more dramatic and severe. HBV may progress to fulminant hepatitis, chronic active hepatitis, or cirrhosis (see Section V for a discussion of cirrhosis).

7. Fulminant hepatitis is a rare but commonly fatal complication of HBV, especially with coinfection of HDV. It results from the failure of the liver cells to regenerate, causing massive hepatic necrosis.

8. Chronic active hepatitis is characterized by progressive liver damage and necrosis, inflammation, and fibrosis.

9. *HCV* has an incubation period of 40 to 100 days; its symptoms are similar to those of hepatitis A.

10. *HDV* causes additional damage to the liver and may lead to chronic hepatitis with symptoms more severe than in other forms of hepatitis.

11. Toxic hepatitis due to alcohol use is characterized by inflammation, degeneration, and necrosis of liver cells.

D. Overview of nursing interventions

1. Follow the protocol for use of universal precautions.

2. Provide adequate rest periods for the patient based on the severity of symptoms; increase activity as tolerated.

3. Administer medications such as antiemetics, as ordered, to combat nausea.

4. Assess the patient for nutritional needs, (eg, small frequent meals, vitamin supplements, or high carbohydrate and protein intake).

5. Instruct the patient to avoid close personal contact and sexual activity with others until test results are negative.

6. Educate the patient and family members about preventing transmission, including use of universal precautions, handwashing, and personal hygiene.

7. Emphasize the importance of rest to reduce the metabolic demands of the organ.

 8. **Take steps to protect infection of self and others.**

IV.   Hepatic abscesses

A.   Description

   1.   Hepatic abscesses result from invasion by bacteria or protozoa; the pathogen destroys tissue, causing necrosis.
   2.   Types are pyogenic and amebic abscesses.

B.   Etiology and incidence

   1.   Causative factors associated with pyogenic abscesses include:
      a.   Cholangitis (most common cause)
      b.   Ascending biliary tract infection
      c.   Transportation of pathogen from superior and inferior mesenteric vein into portal venous system
      d.   Septicemia through the hepatic arterial circulation
      e.   Direct invasion from intraperitoneal infection
      f.   Hepatic trauma
      g.   Carcinoma of extrahepatic bile duct system
   2.   *Escherichia coli* is the most prominent microbe that causes biliary tract infection. *Staphylococcus aureus* is the most prominent organism associated with systemic infection and septicemia.
   3.   Amebic abscesses are caused by the organism *Entamoeba histolytica* and are associated with amebic dysentery; they typically occur in middle-aged males.

C.   Pathophysiologic processes and manifestations

   1.   *Pyogenic abscesses* present with the following symptoms:
      a.   Fever
      b.   Chills
      c.   Nausea and vomiting
      d.   Anorexia
      e.   Leukocytosis
      f.   Hypoalbuminemia
   2.   *Amebic abscesses* form a single sac filled with reddish-brown fluid and commonly occur in the right lobe of the liver. Symptoms include:
      a.   Fever (not as high as with pyogenic abscesses)
      b.   History of diarrhea
      c.   Tender hepatomegaly
      d.   Chills and sweating
      e.   Right shoulder pain

D.   Overview of nursing interventions

   1.   Administer antibiotics, acetaminophen, and metronidazole, as prescribed, to combat and prevent further infection.
   2.   Provide comfort measures to relieve fever and chills.
   3.   Provide nutritional support.
   4.   Emphasize the importance of rest to reduce the metabolic activity of the organ.

V.   Cirrhosis

A.   Description

1.   Cirrhosis is an irreversible chronic inflammatory disease characterized by massive degeneration and destruction of hepatocytes, resulting in a disorganized lobular pattern of regeneration.

2.   Classifications of cirrhosis based on morphologic changes in regenerated nodules include micronodular cirrhosis, macronodular cirrhosis, and mixed cirrhosis.

   a.   *Micronodular cirrhosis* is characterized by an enlarged liver and small, thick connective tissue bands.

   b.   *Macronodular cirrhosis* is characterized by a small, shrunken, nonpalpable liver that is irregularly shaped and multilobular; connective tissue bands vary in thickness.

   c.   *Mixed cirrhosis* is characterized by micronodular and macronodular patterns of connective tissue bands.

3.   Types of cirrhosis include

   a.   Laennec's cirrhosis; also called alcoholic cirrhosis

   b.   Postnecrotic cirrhosis

   c.   Biliary cirrhosis (can be primary or secondary)

   d.   Cardiac cirrhosis

B.   Etiology and incidence

1.   *Laennec's cirrhosis,* the most common cirrhosis, is caused by the liver's toxic reactions to alcohol. It occurs primarily in middle-aged men, but incidence is increasing in women.

2.   *Postnecrotic cirrhosis* results from severe liver disease with widespread liver cell necrosis, usually as a result of acute viral hepatitis or chemical hepatitis.

3.   *Primary biliary cirrhosis* begins with inflammation and intrahepatic bile duct destruction, which leads to nodular regeneration and cirrhosis with resultant portal hypertension.

4.   *Secondary biliary cirrhosis* develops as a result of chronic partial or complete common bile duct obstruction due to gallstones, strictures, chronic pancreatitis, or tumors.

5.   *Cardiac cirrhosis* results from severe right-sided congestive heart failure (CHF).

C.   Pathophysiologic processes and manifestations

1.   In *Laennec's cirrhosis*

    a.   Alcohol causes metabolic changes in the liver that progress to fatty infiltration of the hepatocytes with liver cell necrosis and scarring between lobules.

   b.   As cirrhosis progresses, inflammation decreases and fibrosis increases; this causes the liver to become distorted, resulting in structural (biliary channel) and vascular changes.

   c.   Scar tissue forms, and irregular hepatocyte regeneration compresses branches of the portal vein, producing postsinusoidal obstruction and portal hypertension.

   d.   Inflammation causes excessive collagen formation, which increases connective tissue proliferation.

2. Manifestations of Laennec's cirrhosis may include:
    a. Decreased vitamin K absorption resulting in bleeding abnormalities
    b. Depletion of glycogen stores resulting in hypoglycemia
    c. Decreased serum albumin with increase in hydrostatic pressure resulting in edema and ascites
    d. Decreased bilirubin metabolism resulting in hyperbilirubinemia and jaundice
    e. Portal hypertension resulting from portal circulation obstruction
    f. Esophageal varices resulting from portal hypertension
    g. Encephalopathy
    h. Leukopenia and increased infection resulting from immune system disturbances
    i. Hematologic disorders including thrombocytopenia, anemia, splenomegaly, and disseminated intravascular coagulation (DIC)
    j. Elevated antidiuretic hormone (ADH) in serum and urine of cirrhotic patients with ascites; this may result in hyponatremia from water retention
3. Manifestations of *postnecrotic cirrhosis* are the same as for Laennec's cirrhosis.
4. In *biliary cirrhosis*
    a. Chronic obstruction leads to increased pressure in the hepatic bile duct, resulting in an accumulation of bile.
    b. Areas of necrosis appear, leading to edema, fibrosis, hepatocellular destruction, and regeneration of fine nodules.
    c. Scar tissue causes destruction of lobules and lobes.
    d. Hepatomegaly, an early sign of the disease, is replaced by a small, nonpalpable, macronodular liver.
5. Manifestations of biliary cirrhosis may include:
    a. Jaundice
    b. Pruritus
    c. Hyperbilirubinemia
    d. Clay-colored stools
    e. Right upper quadrant pain and low-grade fever (secondary biliary cirrhosis)
6. In *cardiac cirrhosis*
    a. The liver is enlarged, dark colored, and congested with venous blood that the heart is unable to pump into circulation.
    b. Congestion causes the liver to become anoxic, which results in necrosis and fibrosis.

7. **Hepatorenal syndrome, a major complication of cirrhosis, is characterized by renal failure in anatomically normal kidneys, resulting in progressive oliguria and azotemia.**
8. Other symptoms of hepatorenal syndrome include elevated serum urea nitrogen and creatinine levels, decreased urine sodium content, higher urine osmolarity, and elevated serum ammonia and bilirubin levels.
9. Ascites is a common finding in cirrhosis. It is caused by several physiologic changes. (Figure 11–1 illustrates factors contributing to ascites.)
    a. Decreased albumin formation causes a hypoproteinemic state which leads to edema (from decreased colloidal osmotic pressure).

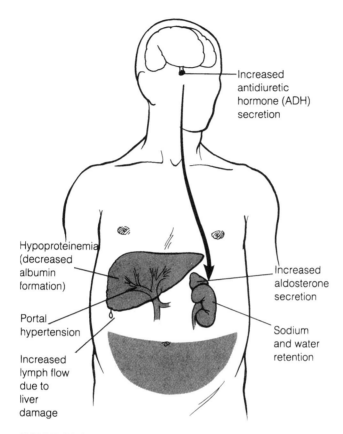

FIGURE 11-1.
Factors contributing to the development of ascites. (Bullock, B. L.
Pathophysiology: Adaptations and Alterations in Function [4th
ed.]. Philadelphia: Lippincott-Raven, 1996, p. 820)

     b.   Portal hypertension develops as the blood supply meets resistance to flow through the scarred liver.
     c.   This obstructive process causes increased lymph flow.
     d.   The liver can not metabolize hormones, resulting in increased sodium and water retention from the actions of aldosterone and antidiuretic hormone.

D. Overview of nursing interventions

    1. **Assess the patient for signs of bleeding.**
    2. Monitor vital signs and laboratory results (eg, platelets, prothrombin time, liver enzymes).
    3. Monitor intake and output.
    4. Monitor daily weight and abdominal girth to detect ascites formation.
    5. Administer medications (eg, vitamin K, vasopressin, diuretics, stool softeners), as prescribed, to combat symptoms of liver disease.

6. Assess the patient for changes in cardiac output, decreased renal function, and electrolyte imbalances.
7. Assess the patient for impaired skin integrity related to edema, ascites, and pruritus.
8. Use preventive measures to keep skin intact (eg, mild soaps or cleansers, skin sealants, frequent linen changes, soothing baths and lotions, and padding of bony areas).

9. **Assess the patient for signs of impaired breathing related to congestion or infection.**
10. Place the patient in a semi-Fowler's or Fowler's position to relieve breathing difficulty related to ascites; turn the patient from side to side often; monitor blood gases and vital signs.
11. Observe the patient for signs of encephalopathy, (eg, lethargy, confusion, personality changes, motor changes, depression, or irritability).
12. Teach the patient how to prevent injuries related to increased potential for hemorrhage (eg, use soft toothbrush and electric razor and avoid straining with bowel movements, blowing nose forcefully, and working with sharp objects).
13. Educate the patient and family members regarding:
    a. Nutritional needs (eg, small frequent meals, increased caloric intake, increased protein and carbohydrate intake, low-fat and sodium diets)
    b. Avoidance of alcohol
    c. Drug interactions related to decreased liver function
    d. Proper rest
    e. Signs and symptoms needing medical intervention (eg, rapid weight gain or loss, blood in urine or stool, nosebleeds, bleeding gums, coughing or vomiting blood, increased abdominal girth, increased difficulty in breathing, and mental changes)
14. Provide counseling for the patient and family members to reduce anxiety regarding the prognosis; make referrals to counselors or support groups as necessary.

VI. Portal hypertension

A. **Description: elevated pressure within the portal venous system caused by an increased resistance or obstruction of blood flow through the portal vein and its tributaries; as a result, blood seeks collateral pathways around the high pressure areas**
B. Etiology
1. Four causative conditions are associated with portal hypertension.
    a. Increased hepatorenal flow without obstruction (eg, hepatic arterial-portal venous fistula)
    b. Extrahepatic outflow obstruction (eg, Budd-Chiari syndrome, right-sided CHF) or obstruction of extrahepatic portal venous system (eg, congenital obstruction, infection, trauma)
    c. Intrahepatic obstruction (eg, cirrhosis, infiltrating lesions, parasitic infection)

2. **The most common intrahepatic cause of portal hypertension is obstruction from cirrhosis caused by thrombosis, inflammation, or fibrotic changes in the sinusoids.**

C. Pathophysiologic processes and manifestations

1. As blood backs up into the liver and spleen, it causes hepatomegaly and splenomegaly.
2. Increased pressure in the portal vein causes formation of collateral veins between the portal and systemic veins where pressure is lower, enabling blood to bypass obstructed areas.
3. Collateral veins appear in the esophagus, abdomen, and rectum causing varices, ascites, and hemorrhoids.
4. As pressure in the area increases, the veins become varicose (varices).

 5. **Bleeding, which may be fatal, occurs with time and increasing pressure from obstruction.**

6. Bleeding esophageal varices is the most common symptom of portal hypertension.

D. Overview of nursing interventions

1. Monitor intake and output.
2. Monitor daily abdominal girth measurement.
3. Administer Aldactone®, as prescribed, to relieve ascites.
4. Observe for fluid and electrolyte imbalances.
5. Use preventive measures for avoiding skin breakdown.
6. Provide psychological support for anxiety related to the disease's impact on body image.

VII. Esophageal varices

A. Description

1. Esophageal varices are enlarged, tortuous veins located in the lower esophagus.
2. This condition is associated with liver cirrhosis; liver cancer may also cause the same phenomenon in the liver as cirrhosis.

B. Etiology: cause is portal hypertension (see Section VI for more information)

C. Pathophysiologic processes and manifestations

1. Liver damage that occurs in cirrhosis causes scar tissue to replace normal liver tissue.
2. The portal veins carry blood from the gastrointestinal tract, pancreas, and spleen into the diseased and fibrous liver, but the fibrous scar tissue does not allow blood to easily enter the liver.
3. Eventually, blood backs up through the entire portal circulation and into the collateral esophageal veins. Pressure in the portal vessels is normally 3 mm Hg, but in portal hypertension those pressures may more than triple to 10 mm Hg.
4. The esophageal vessels then become dilated and torturous and are called varices (varicose veins; Fig. 11-2).
5. The more severe the liver disease, the worse the varices.
6. The varices may bleed. Bleeding may occur from irritation of the vessel wall

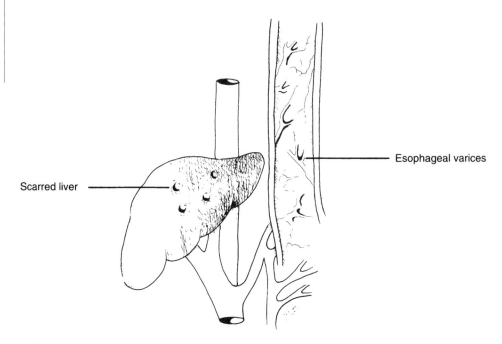

Scarred liver

Esophageal varices

FIGURE 11-2.
Esophageal varices.

with food, or it may occur spontaneously; it may be a massive rupture or a slow ooze.

 7. **Because the blood of patients with liver disease does not clot well, bleeding may be fatal even if it occurs in the form of a slow ooze.**

8. The same phenomenon can occur when there is pressure in the portal circulation for reasons other than cirrhosis, including cardiac disorders, hepatic vein thrombosis, hepatitis, or other inflammatory conditions.

D.   Overview of nursing interventions

1. Prevent bleeding if possible.

 2. **Administer fresh frozen plasma and other therapeutic agents aimed at increasing clotting time, as ordered.**

3. Assist with insertion of Sengstaken-Blakemore tube if bleeding occurs.

4. If sclerotherapy or shunt insertion is planned, provide appropriate pre- and postoperative care.

5. Provide a soft diet and adequate nutrition.

6. Manage the patient's symptoms, because there is no treatment to eliminate the varices.

VIII.   Liver trauma

A.   Description

1. Liver trauma includes any injury that results in liver damage; types include penetrating and blunt trauma.

2. Injuries are classified as:
   a. *Transcapsular* (usually associated with penetrating trauma)
   b. *Subcapsular* (usually associated with blunt trauma)
   c. *Central*

B. Etiology
   1. Penetrating trauma commonly results from gunshot wounds, stabbing wounds, or rib fractures.
   2. Blunt trauma commonly results from motor vehicle accidents or crushing injuries.

C. Pathophysiologic processes and manifestations
   1. In *transcapsular trauma,* Glisson's capsule (a fibroelastic capsule containing blood vessels, lymphatics, and nerves covering the liver) ruptures; blood vessels and bile fill the peritoneal cavity.
   2. *Transcapsular trauma* results in massive blood loss, leading to signs and symptoms of shock, including:
      a. Hypotension
      b. Tachycardia
      c. Diaphoresis
      d. Cool, clammy skin
      e. Tachypnea
      f. Confusion
      g. Abdominal pain, tenderness, distention, guarding, and rigidity
      h. Recurrent bleeding related to necrosis (may occur)
   3. In *subcapsular trauma,* blood collects between Glisson's capsule and the parenchyma in the form of a hematoma.
   4. In *central trauma,* a rupture results in an interruption in the parenchyma.

D. Overview of nursing interventions

   1. **Bleeding may be profuse because the liver is highly vascular.**
   2. Monitor vital signs frequently.
   3. Administer blood and blood products, as ordered, to replace lost volume.
   4. Maintain adequate hydration.
   5. Observe for signs of continued bleeding.
   6. Observe for signs of shock.
   7. Observe for signs of infection related to bile peritonitis.
   8. Administer pain medications and antibiotics, as ordered.

IX. Cysts

A. Description
   1. Cysts are sacs containing fluids or semisolids.
   2. Types of liver cysts include:
      a. Nonparasitic (blood, degenerative, dermoid, lymphatic, endothelial, retention, and proliferative cysts)
      b. Hydatid (unilocular and alveolar cysts)

B. Etiology and incidence
   1. Nonparasitic cysts result from the formation of cysts from body tissue, such as blood, lymph tissue, derm tissue, or endothelial tissue. Solitary nonparasitic cysts are most often seen in persons ages 40 to 60.

2. Unilocular hydatid cysts are caused by *Echinococcus granulosus* and alveolar hydatid cysts are caused by *Echinococcus multilocularis;* they commonly occur in regions with infected sheep, cattle, and pigs.

3. Polycystic liver disease is more common in women than in men; it is usually associated with polycystic disease of other organs, especially the kidneys.

C. Pathophysiologic processes and manifestations

1. *Nonparasitic cysts* may be singular, multiple, localized, diffuse, unilocular or multilocular; retention cysts may be solitary, polycystic, proliferative, or cystadenomas.

2. *Hydatid cysts* are most commonly superficial and consist of two membranes; alveolar hydatid cysts may become metastatic and invade blood vessels and the lymph system.

3. The most common symptoms of cysts (if any symptoms occur) are abdominal pain and tenderness.

D. Overview of nursing interventions

1. Provide supportive care if polycystic liver disease occurs.

2. Provide postoperative care as required if surgical intervention is treatment of choice.

X.   Cholelithiasis and cholecystitis

A. Description

1. Cholelithiasis is stone formation in the ducts that drain the gallbladder; common types of gallstones are cholesterol or pigmented.

2. Cholecystitis is inflammation of the gallbladder.

B. Etiology

1. Cholelithiasis results from the accumulation of metabolic precipitates in the small gallbladder ducts.

2. Cholecystitis may result from infectious disease or ingestion of high-fat foods that stimulate gallbladder contraction. It also may be caused by cholelithiasis.

C. Pathophysiologic processes and manifestations

1. Cholelithiasis

   a. Bile that becomes supersaturated with cholesterol forms very small stones (cholesterol stones) as crystals develop in the gallbladder.

   b. Unconjugated bilirubin in bile precipitates and, along with calcium, causes pigmented stones to form.

   c. Additional crystals form on top of these small stones.

   d. No symptoms will occur if the stones remain in the gallbladder or if they are ejected into the cystic duct with the bile and pass through the gastrointestinal tract.

   e. If the stones enlarge and become wedged in the cystic or common bile duct, symptoms of biliary obstruction will occur. These symptoms include pain (may include pain radiating to the upper back behind the shoulder), jaundice (as bile backs up through the biliary system), dyspepsia, flatulence, and fat intolerance.

   f. Stones may occur as one stone or may be multiple. The degree of obstruction varies with the size and location of the stone.

2. Cholecystitis
   a. This condition is characterized by the same symptoms as cholelithiasis, plus fever.
   b. Bile duct obstruction causes distention and inflammation.
   c. If the inflammation exerts excessive pressure on the surrounding vessels, ischemia and necrosis may occur.
   d. Gallbladder rupture may occur in the presence of ischemia. If this occurs, rebound tenderness, severe abdominal pain, and elevated bilirubin and alkaline phosphatase levels may be present.

D. Overview of nursing interventions
1. Educate the patient about the importance of following the prescribed diet therapy.

2. **Administer pain medications, as prescribed. Do *not* administer morphine for pain because it causes spasm of the sphincter muscle inside the gallbladder and can induce, rather than abate, an attack.**

XI. Liver cancer

A. Description
1. Liver carcinoma may be primary or metastatic.
2. Primary tumors can be benign or malignant.
3. Primary benign tumors include hemangiomas (most common), hamartomas, adenomas, and focal nodular hyperplasias.
   a. *Hemangiomas* must be differentiated from malignancies because there are similarities in their presentation.
   b. *Hamartomas* consist of cells normally found in the liver but arranged in a scattered pattern varying in size from small nodules to large tumors; they rarely are clinically significant.
   c. *Adenomas* are tumors that arise from gland tissue and are associated with the use of oral contraception.
   d. *Focal nodular hyperplasias* are nodule type growths that become enlarged.
4. Common primary malignant tumors include hepatocellular carcinomas and cholangiomas.
   a. *Hepatocellular carcinomas* develop in the hepatocytes and invade the portal vein and its branches as well as the hepatic vein. These types of tumors are very vascular and are identified by their trabecular cell structure.
   b. *Cholangiomas* develop in the bile duct and are identified by a columnar cell structure; they are difficult to distinguish from cancer of the gallbladder.
5. Other, less common primary malignant tumors include hepatoblastomas, sarcomas, and mesenchymomas.

B. Etiology
1. Hemangiomas, the most common benign nodules of the liver, are sometimes associated with cysts or focal nodular hyperplasia.
2. Hepatocellular carcinoma is the most common primary malignant tumor

and has been associated with cirrhosis, viral hepatitis, and exposure to my-
cotoxins produced by *Aspergillus flavus*.

3.   The specific etiology for the other tumor types is unknown.

C.   Pathophysiologic processes and manifestations

1.   *Primary benign tumors* are rarely symptomatic and usually need no intervention.

2.   *Primary carcinomas* may present as a single large nodule, with widespread
nodularity, or with diffuse permeation.

3.   Symptoms most commonly associated with *primary carcinomas* include:
a.   Weight loss
b.   Pain (dull and persistent)
c.   Nausea and vomiting
d.   Weakness
e.   Hepatomegaly
f.   Splenomegaly
g.   Jaundice
h.   Ascites

4.   *Metastatic carcinomas* are commonly associated with the following symptoms:
a.   Symptoms consistent with primary carcinoma
b.   Hepatic nodularity on examination
c.   Friction rub
d.   Portal hypertension
e.   Elevated serum alkaline phosphatase levels

5.   Hepatic tumors are spread by:
a.   Parasinusoidal invasion into the parenchyma
b.   Nodular invasion causing compression of surrounding hepatic tissue
c.   Venous invasion from the small branches of the portal system into
the main portal vein
d.   Invasion into the lymphatic and vascular systems to other sites

6.   Metastatic liver carcinoma is spread by:
a.   Portal venous circulation
b.   Lymphatic system
c.   Hepatic arterial system
d.   Direct extension from adjacent organs

D.   Overview of nursing interventions

1.   Provide supportive care to help the patient and family members cope with
the diagnosis and poor prognosis.

2.   Prepare the patient for possible treatment plans, including surgery,
chemotherapy, radiation, or transplantation.

3.   Monitor nutritional status and arrange for a consultation with a nutritionist.

4.   Observe for early signs of mental changes.

5.   Observe for signs of pressure sores and other skin breakdowns as a result of
poor nutrition and ascites.

6.   Assess for signs of respiratory difficulty as a result of ascites and for signs of
increased portal hypertension.

7.   Assess for signs of bleeding as a result of rupture.

8.   Assess for signs of infection.

9.   Manage pain and comfort needs.

Bibliography

Bullock, B. (1996). *Pathophysiology: Adaptations and alterations in function* (4th ed.). Philadelphia: Lippincott-Raven.

Ganong, William F. (1997). *Review of medical physiology* (18th ed.). Stamford, CT: Appleton and Lange.

Guyton, Arthur C., & Hall, John E. (1996). *Textbook of medical physiology* (9th ed.). Philadelphia: W. B. Saunders.

Ignatavicius, D., & Bayne, M. (1991). *Medical-surgical. A nursing process approach.* Philadelphia: W. B. Saunders.

Kinney, M., Packa, D., & Dunbar, S. (1993). *AACN's clinical reference for critical-care nursing* (3rd ed.). St. Louis: C.V. Mosby.

McCance, K., & Huether, S. E. (1994). *Pathophysiology: The biologic basis for disease in adults and children* (2nd ed.). St. Louis: Mosby-Year Book.

Porch, C. (1994). *Pathophysiology: Concepts of altered health states* (4th ed.). Philadelphia: Lippincott-Raven.

STUDY QUESTIONS

1. Which of the following are characteristics of viral hepatitis?
   a. hepatic cell atrophy
   b. Kupffer's cell hypoplasia
   c. Kupffer's cell hyperplasia
   d. absence of mononuclear phagocytes

2. Which of the following types of jaundice result from fibrosis or scarring of the hepatic bile channels and ducts?
   a. obstructive jaundice
   b. hepatocellular jaundice
   c. hemolytic jaundice
   d. all of the above

3. Which of the following is a malignant tumor of the liver?
   a. adenomas
   b. hamartomas
   c. hepatocellular carcinoma
   d. focal nodular hyperplasia

4. Metastatic carcinomas are spread by which of the following routes?
   a. lymphatic system
   b. portal venous circulation
   c. direct extension
   d. all of the above

5. Which of the following manifestations is *not* characteristic of cirrhosis?
   a. decreased vitamin K absorption
   b. increased serum albumin
   c. esophageal varices
   d. encephalopathy

6. Chronic obstruction in biliary cirrhosis may result from:
   a. necrosis
   b. edema and fibrosis
   c. chronic pancreatitis
   d. hepatocellular destruction

7. When assessing a patient with chronic alcoholism for cirrhosis, which of the following types of cirrhosis would the nurse expect to find?
   a. biliary cirrhosis
   b. Laennec's cirrhosis
   c. postnecrotic cirrhosis
   d. none of the above

8. When caring for a patient with cirrhosis, the nurse would do all of the following *except:*
   a. monitor intake and output
   b. place the patient in a supine position
   c. assess the patient for signs of bleeding
   d. observe for signs of encephalopathy

9. Portal hypertension resulting from intrahepatic obstruction may be seen in all of the following *except:*
   a. Addison's disease
   b. Cushing's disease
   c. Cirrhosis
   d. Budd-Chiari syndrome

10. Collateral veins observed on examination of the abdomen of a patient with portal hypertension are called:
    a. varices
    b. caput medusae
    c. pruritus
    d. ascites

11. A patient with cholelithiasis should *never* receive which of the following medications?
    a. demerol
    b. morphine
    c. aspirin
    d. Tylenol®

12. Which type of liver trauma results in hypovolemic shock:
    a. supracapsular
    b. subcapsular
    c. central
    d. transcapsular

13. Fresh frozen plasma is administered to patients with cirrhosis and esophageal varices in order to:

a. replace fluid volume
b. prevent hypotension
c. increase clotting time
d. balance electrolytes

14. A nurse conducting a physical examination on a patient with alcoholism dis-covers splenomegaly. This is significant because it reflects:

a. portal hypertension
b. cancer
c. HIV infection
d. hepatic cysts

ANSWER KEY

Question	Correct answer	Correct answer rationale	Incorrect answer rationales
1.	c	Kupffer's cell hyperplasia does occur in hepatitis.	a. Hepatic cell atrophy does not occur, rather it is hyperplasia that is present. b. Hypoplasia refers to shrinkage of liver cells, which is the opposite of what actually occurs, which is hyperplasia. d. Mononuclear phagocytes infiltrate during hepatitis, making this choice incorrect.
2.	a	Fibrosis and scarring compress the hepatic ducts, obstructing them and making it impossible for bile to flow out. As bile back flows into the blood stream, jaundice results.	b. Hepatocellular jaundice results from the liver's inability to metabolize bilirubin. c. Hemolytic jaundice results from an excessive breakdown of red blood cells. d. This response is incorrect.
3.	c	Hepatocellular carcinoma is a malignancy.	a, b, and d. These are benign tumors.
4.	d	Metastatic carcinoma may be spread by all of these routes; it also may be spread by the hepatic arterial system.	
5.	b	Serum albumin decreases with an increase in hydrostatic pressure, resulting in edema and ascites.	a, c, and d. These are characteristics of cirrhosis.
6.	c	Chronic pancreatitis can lead to obstruction of the common bile duct and may be the cause of secondary biliary cirrhosis.	a, b, and d. These are incorrect responses. Necrosis, edema, fibrosis, and hepatocellular destruction may be present in a variety of biliary diseases, but the question stem asks for the cause of biliary cirrhosis. Thus the only one correct answer, which is pancreatitis.
7.	b	Laennec's cirrhosis is caused by the liver's toxic reactions to alcohol.	a. Biliary cirrhosis is associated with inflammation in the bile canaliculi and ducts. c. Postnecrotic cirrhosis is associated with acute viral hepatitis or chemical hepatitis. d. This response is incorrect.
8.	b	The patient should be placed in semi-Fowler's or Fowler's position to relieve breathing difficulty related to ascites.	a, c, and d. These are recommended nursing actions.

Question	Correct answer	Correct answer rationale	Incorrect answer rationales
9.	c	Cirrhosis is associated with portal hypertension from intrahepatic obstruction.	a and b. Intrahepatic obstruction is not associated with Addison's or Cushing's diseases. d. Budd-Chiari syndrome is seen in patients with extrahepatic outflow obstruction.
10.	b	Caput medusae is the term used to describe collateral veins.	a. Varices are a hemorrhagic process in the esophagus. c. Pruritus is an area of itchy, irritated patches on the skin. d. Ascites is an accumulation of fluid in the peritoneal cavity.
11.	b	Morphine should never be administered to a patient with cholecystitis or cholelithiasis because it causes spasms in the Sphincter of Oddi, which intensifies pain.	a, c, and d. These drugs are not contraindicated in this condition. Demerol is preferred to morphine in these conditions.
12.	d	Transcapsular trauma (rupture of Glisson's capsule) results in massive blood loss leading to signs of shock.	a. There is no category known as supracapsular. b and c. These describe types of traumatic injury not associated with hypovolemia.
13.	c	Fresh frozen plasma is given to increase clotting time. Plasma may help restore volume in hypovolemic patients, but it is the presence of clotting factors in the plasma that make it valuable in situations of liver cirrhosis and esophageal varices.	a, b, and d. These choices may be secondary benefits that result from administration of plasma. The stem asks for the purpose which is to increase clotting time.
14.	a	Splenomegaly is an enlargement of the spleen resulting from increased pressure in the splenic vein, and is often evident in persons with portal hypertension. This patient's history leads to this as the most likely answer choice.	b. Splenomegaly may be present in certain types of cancer, but there is not enough information in this question to lead to this conclusion. c and d. Splenomegaly is not necessarily associated with HIV or hepatic cysts.

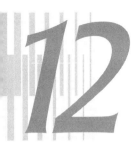

Endocrine Disorders

I.   Overview of pathophysiologic processes

A. Hypersecretion disorders

1. Hypersecretion disorders are those in which the bloodstream contains an oversecretion of hormones.
2. The abundant hormones exert their effect on the target cells, causing an exaggerated response.
3. Hyperthyroidism, hyperparathyroidism, Cushing's syndrome, and syndrome of inappropriate antidiuretic hormone (ADH; SIADH) are hypersecretion disorders.
4. Risk factors for hypersecretion disorders include autoimmune factors and tumor formation.

B. Hyposecretion disorders

1. Hyposecretion disorders are those in which the bloodstream contains an undersecretion of hormones.
2. The hormone deficiency causes some of the target cells to function abnormally.

3. Hypothyroidism, hypoparathyroidism, adrenal hypofunction, hypopituitarism, diabetic ketoacidosis (DKA), and hyperglycemic hyperosmolar nonketotic coma (HHNK) are hyposecretion disorders.

4. Risk factors for hyposecretion disorders include autoimmune factors, tumor formation, and certain medications.

II. Physiologic responses to endocrine system dysfunction

A. Fatigue: tired, exhausted feeling resulting in decreased physical and mental functioning

B. Polydipsia: excessive thirst

C. Polyuria: excessive urine excretion

D. Nocturia: excessive urination at night

E. Anorexia: loss of appetite

F. Hypomenorrhea: uterine bleeding of less than normal amounts occurring at regular intervals

G. Amenorrhea: absent menses

H. Gynecomastia: mammary gland overdevelopment in men

I. Change in libido: increase or decrease in the instinctual energy or drive related to the desire for sexual activity

J. Myxedema: condition resulting from advanced hypothroidism or thyroxin deficiency

K. Exophthalmos: abnormal eyeball protrusion

L. Impotence: partial or complete inability of a man to perform the sexual act or to achieve orgasm

M. Nephrolithiasis: presence of renal calculi

N. Nephrosclerosis: hardening of the kidney associated with hypotension

O. Hypotonia: abnormally decreased muscle tonicity or strength

P. Anxiety: feeling of uneasiness, apprehension, or dread

Q. Tetany: continuous tonic muscle spasms or steady muscle contraction without distinct twitching

R. Trousseau's sign: sign for hypercalcemia in which carpal spasm can be elicited by compressing the upper arm and causing ischemia to the nerves distally

S. Chvostek's sign: facial muscle spasm resulting from tapping the muscles or the branches of the facial nerve; seen in hypercalcemia.

T. Integumentary changes

1. In hyposecretion disorders, skin may be cool, pale, yellowish, dry, coarse, and scaly; nails may be brittle and thick; hair may be dry, brittle, and coarse.

2. In hypersecretion disorders, the skin, nails, and hair display characteristics opposite those found in hyposecretion disorders.

U. Cardiovascular changes

1. Common changes include bradycardia or tachycardia with atrial arrhythmias.

2. In hyposecretion disorders, changes may include decreased activity or exercise tolerance with hypotension and an enlarged heart.
3. In hypersecretion disorders, changes may include chest pain and palpitations with tachycardiac arrhythmias.

V. Gastrointestinal changes

1. Anorexia with weight loss or increased appetite with weight gain may be present, depending on the disease.
2. Constipation and abdominal distention or diarrhea may also occur, depending on the disease.

III.   Hyperthyroidism

A. Description:

1. Hyperthyroidism refers to oversecretion of thyroid hormone.
2. Thyroid gland enlargement (goiter) occurs in hyperthyroid, hypothyroid, and euthyroid states.

B. Etiology

1. Hyperthyroidism can result from a number of diseases.

2. Causes may include:
    a. **Graves' disease (toxic diffuse goiter): familial autoimmune disease that affects the thyroid**
    b. **Struma ovarii: dermoid tumor of the ovary that secretes thyroid hormone**
    c. **Thyroiditis: transient inflammation of the thyroid that occurs with thyroxin and triiodothyronine secretion.**
    d. **Toxic multinodular goiter: occurs when multiple thyroid nodules result in thyroid hyperfunctioning**
    e. **Thyroid cancer: uncommon, but can occur with large follicular carcinomas**

C. Pathophysiologic processes and manifestations (Fig. 12-1)

1. Because the normal regulatory controls of thyroid hormone secretion are lost, a state of hypermetabolism with increased sympathetic nervous system activity exists.
2. Physiologic responses occur as the body attempts to compensate for the hypermetabolic state.
3. Elevated thyroid hormone levels stimulate the heart, resulting in:
    a. Increased heart rate and stroke volume, causing increased cardiac output and peripheral blood flow
    b. An increase in adrenergic responsiveness at the betaadrenergic receptor sites in the heart, which may increase heart rate or cause arrhythmias
4. Elevated thyroid hormone levels also increase:
    a. **Protein, carbohydrate, and lipid metabolism**
    b. **Vitamin metabolism, leading to decreasing tissue stores of vitamins**
    c. **Peristaltic activity, leading to diarrhea**
    d. **Appetite (as metabolism increases)**

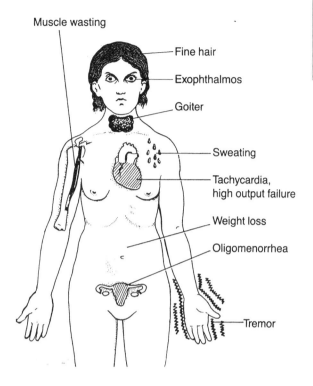

Muscle wasting

Fine hair

Exophthalmos

Goiter

Sweating

Tachycardia, high output failure

Weight loss

Oligomenorrhea

Tremor

FIGURE 12-1.
The major clinical manifestations of hyperthyroidism. (*Source:* Rubin, E., and Farber, J. L. *Pathology* [2nd ed.]. Philadelphia: J.B. Lippincott, 1994.)

5. Increased metabolism leads to weight loss.

6. Excessive sweating, flushing, and heat intolerance occur.

7. Hair may become fine and soft; alopecia may occur.

8. Nails may grow away from the nail beds.

9. The central nervous system may react with agitation, nervousness, anxiety, and insomnia.

10. The eyelids become elevated, and exophthalmos and edema of the orbital structure occur. Itching, pain, lacrimation, photophobia, and eventually corneal ulceration may occur because the eyelids may not close properly.

11. Menstrual irregularities occur in women.

12. In Graves' disease, thyroid-stimulating immunoglobulin (TSI) overrides normal regulatory mechanisms.

    a. Thyroid hypersecretion leads to pituitary suppression of thyroid-stimulating hormone (TSH) and hypothalamic suppression of thyrotropin-releasing hormone (TRH).

    b. Iodine uptake increases, and the gland has an increased metabolic rate.

13. When Graves' disease is the cause of hyperthyroidism, there may be subcutaneous swelling on the anterior part of the leg (pretibial myxedema) and erythematous skin. Palmar erythema may also occur.

14. In nodular goiter, the gland increases in size in response to an increased thyroid hormone demand resulting from other conditions (eg, pregnancy or iodine deficiency). Hypertrophy resolves when the condition abates (Fig. 12-2).

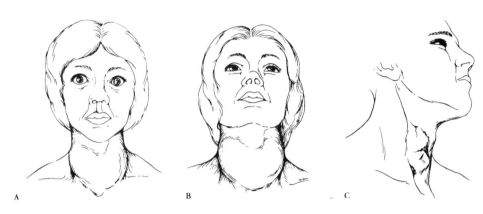

A   B   C

FIGURE 12-2.
Thyroid abnormalities. **A.** Diffuse toxic goiter (Graves' disease) with exophthalmos. **B.** Diffuse nontoxic goiter. **C.** Nodular goiter. (Judge, R. D., Zuidema, G. D., and Fitzgerald, F. T. [eds.]. *Clinical Diagnosis* [4th ed.]. Boston: Little, Brown, 1982.)

       a.   The thyroid may return to normal or some of the thyroid cells may continue to secrete independently, resulting in thyroid hormone oversecretion.

       b.   The term *toxic nodular goiter* is used to describe the resultant hyperthyroidism.

  15.   Thyroid storm (thyrotoxicosis) occurs when hyperthyroidism worsens to such an extent that tachycardia, hypertension, and heat intolerance become life-threatening. It may happen spontaneously, may result from insufficient treatment, or may be induced by stress due to illness, surgery, or emotions.

  D.   **Overview of nursing interventions**

     1.   Administer antithyroid medications, as prescribed., because cardiac symptoms are life-threatening.

     2.   Monitor cardiac status, because cardiovascular complications can be fatal.

     3.   Administer medications, as ordered, for cardiac dysrhythmias.

     4.   Provide comfort measures such as a cool environment and cold fluids to combat heat intolerance.

     5.   Administer nonsalicylate antipyretics, as prescribed, for fever.

     6.   Monitor vision changes or eye injuries related to ophthalmopathy.

     7.   Elevate the head of bed to decrease eye pressure.

     8.   Evaluate nutritional status and intervene to improve it.

IV.   **Hypothyroidism**

  A.   **Description: condition resulting from insufficient secretion of thyroid hormone to the peripheral tissues; may be primary or secondary**

  B.   **Etiology**

     1.   Primary hypothyroidism may result from:

    a.   Congenital defects due to poor thyroid development or absent thyroid development *in utero* (cretinism)

    b.   Hashimoto's disease (an autoimmune process in which circulating thyroid antibodies and lymphocytes destroy thyroid tissue)

    c.   Thyroiditis (due to a bacterial or viral infection)

  2. Secondary hypothyroidism results from the suppression of TSH due to pituitary tumors.

  3. In post-thyroidectomy patients and those with known hypothyroidism, secondary hypothyroidism results from inadequate medication therapy.

  4. A hypothyroid condition that develops after birth is known as *Myxedema* or mucinous edema.

C. **Pathophysiologic processes and manifestations (Fig. 12-3)**

  1. To compensate for inadequate thyroid hormone production, the thyroid gland enlarges.

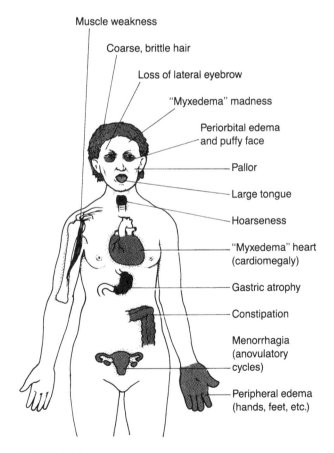

FIGURE 12-3.
The dominant clinical manifestations of hypothyroidism.
(*Source:* Rubin E., and Farber, J. L. *Pathology* [2nd ed.].
Philadelphia: J.B. Lippincott, 1994.)

2. Thyroid tissue loss due to any cause reduces thyroid hormone production and concomitantly elevates TSH, leading to goiter (simple or nontoxic).

3. **Low thyroid hormone levels result in a decreased basal metabolism, causing body system changes directly opposite those that occur in hyperthyroidism. Such changes may include:**
    a. **Bradycardia with reduced blood flow to vital organs**
    b. **Cardiomegaly with pericardial effusion**
    c. **ECG changes**
    d. **Constipation**
    e. **Cold intolerance**
    f. **Reduced sweat gland secretion**
    g. **Reduced metabolic rate leading to low energy**

4. When proteins and other substances accumulate in the interstitial space, interstitial fluid increases and the myxedema (mucinous edema) occurs. Symptoms of myxedema include changes in the composition of the dermis and other tissues.

5. Myxedema coma is a life-threatening state characterized by severely decreased level of consciousness, temperature, blood pressure, respirations, and metabolism.

D. Overview of nursing interventions

1. Administer replacement hormones, as prescribed, because symptoms (especially cardiac symptoms) are life-threatening.
2. Provide comfort measures to alleviate the above symptoms.
3. Evaluate nutritional status and intervene to improve it.
4. Keep alert for life-threatening complications.
5. Teach the patient how to recognize and prevent disease complications and how the disease is treated.

V.   Hyperparathyroidism

A. Description: excess parathyroid hormone (PTH) secretion; may be primary, secondary, or tertiary

B. Etiology

1. Primary hyperparathyroidism results when one or more hyperfunctioning glands do not respond to the normal feedback of serum calcium and secrete autonomously. The most common presentation is a benign, autonomous adenoma in one of the glands; in the remainder of the cases, hyperplasia in all four of the glands is present.
2. Secondary hyperparathyroidism is a parathyroid response to hypocalcemia. PTH levels are secreted in excess, but the target organ (kidney) has failed and calcium levels remain low.
3. Tertiary hyperparathyroidism commonly occurs in renal failure. Autonomous PTH secretion occurs as hyperplastic parathyroid cells lose their sensitivity to circulating calcium levels.

C. Pathophysiologic processes and manifestations

1. **Hyperparathyroidism results in hypercalcemia and bone demineralization, because the bone is overstimulated to release calcium into the serum.**

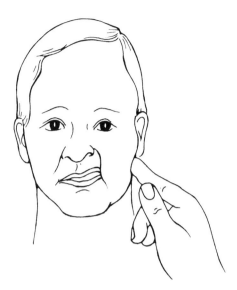

FIGURE 12-4.
Tapping of the facial nerve approximately 2 cm anterior to the earlobe elicits the Chvostek sign (unilateral twitching of the facial muscles) in some patients with hypocalcemia or hypomagnesemia. (*Source:* Metheny, N. M. *Fluid and Electrolyte Balance* [2nd ed.] Philadelphia: J.B. Lippincott, 1992.)

    2.   If this process continues, bone deformities (compression fractures) can occur.

    3.   Hypercalcemia causes an increased amount of calcium to be delivered to the kidneys, resulting in hypercalciuria and kidney stones.

    4.   Renal tubules respond by producing an alkaline urine, which sometimes causes metabolic acidosis, because bicarbonate is eliminated to make the urine alkaline.

    5.   Hypophosphatemia occurs in the presence of hypercalcemia.

    6.   Hypercalcemia results in positive Chvostek's and Trousseau's signs—hallmark traits (Fig. 12-4 and Fig. 12-5).

D.   **Overview of nursing interventions**

    1.   Monitor for cardiac arrhythmias and decreased cardiac output.

    2.   Provide a safe environment to ensure against complications related to potential osteoporosis and joint and bone pain.

    3.   Monitor calcium levels.

    4.   Teach the patient how to recognize and prevent hypercalcemia.

    5.   If applicable, follow hospital protocol for care of the post-thyroidectomy patient.

VI.   **Hypoparathyroidism**

A.   **Description**

    1.   Hypoparathyroidism, an uncommon endocrine disorder, is directly related to deficient PTH secretion or to decreased effectiveness of PTH on target tissues.

    2.   It is also considered a metabolic crisis when occurring with hypocalcemia.

 B.   **Etiology: most common cause is damage to the parathyroid glands secondary to thyroid surgery.**

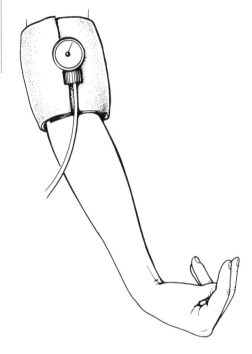

FIGURE 12-5.
Carpopedal spasm (Trousseau's sign) elicited when blood supply is occluded to the arm for 3 minutes. It is a characteristic sign of hypocalcemia. (*Source:* Bullock, B. L. [1996]. *Pathophysiology: Adaptations and Alterations in Function* [4th ed.]. Philadelphia: Lippincott-Raven, p. 724.)

C. Pathophysiologic processes and manifestations

1. Lack of PTH activity results in decreased serum calcium with a concomitant increased serum phosphate level.
2. Absent PTH hinders calcium reabsorption from the renal tubules and the bone, allowing phosphates to be reabsorbed and causing hyperphosphatemia.
3. Hypomagnesemia (from any cause) may be a contributing factor in hypoparathyroidism, but the parathyroids usually return to normal when magnesium levels are restored.
4. Hypocalcemia may cause symptoms such as:
   a. Muscle spasms
   b. Hyperreflexia
   c. Altered sensorium (in severe cases)
5. Hypocalcemia and hyperphosphatemia in the absence of renal or gastrointestinal disease suggest the diagnosis of hypoparathyroidism.

D. Overview of nursing interventions

1. Administer calcium replacements, as ordered, to treat hypocalcemia.
2. Note that as calcium levels are restored, phosphorus levels will return to normal by way of urinary elimination.
3. Closely monitor serum levels for phosphorus and calcium; their ratio must be in adequate proportions to prevent bone demineralization and tissue calcification.

VII. Cushing's disease and syndrome

A. Description

1. Cushing's *disease* is characterized by hypersecretion of adrenal hormones due to excess secretion of adrenocorticotropic hormone (ACTH) by the pituitary gland or by extrapituitary tumors.

2. Cushing's *syndrome* is hypercorticism resulting from Cushing's disease or due to administration of steroid hormones.

3. Steroid medications given to reduce inflammation have the same effect as hormones secreted from the adrenal cortex (hence, the term *corticosteroid*).

4. Because the hormone is given exogenously, the negative feedback loop between the adrenal and pituitary glands is turned off, and steroid levels stay at a constant high.

5. So as time goes on, the person develops Cushing's syndrome.

B. Etiology: Causes of Cushing's disease include tumor formation outside the endocrine system (such as in the lungs) and adrenal gland neoplasms.

C. Pathophysiologic processes and manifestations

1. Elevated levels of cortisol and other steroid hormones have exaggerated effects, causing symptoms in almost every body system.

 2. **Because steroids antagonize insulin, their excessive presence causes increased serum glucose levels and a possible diabetic state; polyuria is sometimes present.**

3. Fat metabolism is affected, so adipose tissue accumulates in the abdomen and behind the shoulders (buffalo hump); the arms and legs become thinner.

4. Accelerated protein catabolism leads to muscle wasting, which causes weakness and difficult movement.

5. Protein loss also leads to:
   a. Osteoporosis (over time this can cause pathologic fractures)
   b. Thinning skin and hair and increased facial and body hair in women
   c. Weakened blood vessel support (making bruising easier as smaller vessels rupture)

6. Other manifestations can include:
   a. Mood changes (from euphoria to depression)
   b. Amenorrhea
   c. Immunosuppression
   d. Changes in skin pigmentation (as ACTH stimulates melanocytes)
   e. Appearance of a moon face (characteristic sign) (Fig. 12-6)

D. Overview of nursing interventions

1. Monitor vital signs.
2. .Monitor serum laboratory values.
3. Administer antihypertensive drugs, as prescribed, to control hypertension.
4. Provide adequate nutrition.
5. Teach the patient about prevention and early detection of complications.

 6. **Warn the patient on steroids about the dangers of sudden withdrawal from this medication.**

7. Adjust the insulin dosages for diabetic patients.

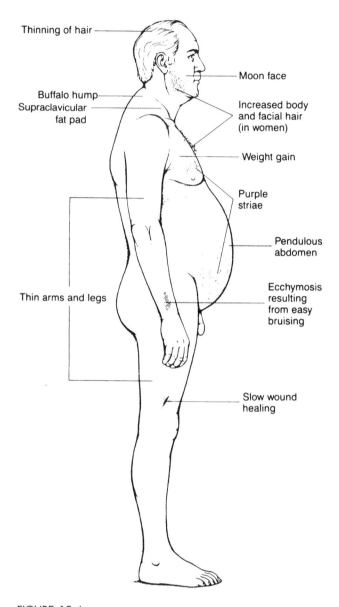

Thinning of hair

Moon face

Buffalo hump
Supraclavicular
fat pad

Increased body
and facial hair
(in women)

Weight gain

Purple
striae

Pendulous
abdomen

Thin arms and legs

Ecchymosis
resulting
from easy
bruising

Slow wound
healing

FIGURE 12-6.
The major clinical manifestations of Cushing syndrome. (*Source:*
Smeltzer, S. C. and Bare, B. G. *Brunner and Suddarth's Text-
book of Medical-Surgical Nursing.* [7th ed.]. Philadelphia: J.B.
Lippincott, 1992.)

VIII. **Adrenal hypofunction**

A. Description

1. Adrenal hypofunction refers to insufficient hormone secretion due to adrenal gland abnormality. As a result, adrenal cortex destruction occurs, impairing glucocorticoid and mineralocorticoid production.
2. It may be primary (Addison's disease) or secondary.

B. Etiology

1. Primary adrenal hypofunction may result from:
   a. Atrophy or autoimmune destruction of the adrenal cortex
   b. Tumors
   c. Suppressed pituitary functioning from any reason (for example, head injuries or craniocerebral disorders that affect the hypothalamic pituitary mechanisms)
2. Secondary adrenal hypofunction results from an impairment in the hypothalamic–pituitary–adrenal axis; insufficient ACTH stimulation causes adrenal hypofunction.
3. Rapid withdrawal of long-term steroid administration may also cause adrenal hypofunction.

C. Pathophysiologic processes and manifestations

1. **Adrenal cortex dysfunction results in deficient mineralocorticoid and glucocorticoid secretion.**
2. Two hormones, aldosterone and cortisol, are deficient.
3. Decreased levels of aldosterone lead to reduced sodium absorption and increased sodium excretion.
4. Water is excreted along with sodium, leading rapidly to hypovolemia and hypotension.
5. **Because potassium moves in the opposite direction of sodium, sodium excretion results in hyperkalemia.**
6. If left untreated, hyperkalemia and hypotension may be life-threatening.

D. Overview of nursing interventions

1. Administer replacement therapy of small amounts of mineralocorticoid and glucocorticoid, as ordered.
2. Restrict the patient to a low-potassium, high-sodium diet.
3. Prepare the patient for surgery, if a tumor is the causative factor.
4. Monitor for sleep disturbances.
5. Assess skin turgor for signs of dehydration.
6. Assess vital signs frequently to detect any changes in peripheral tissue perfusion.
7. **Be aware that this condition can be fatal, because vascular collapse and hypotension are severe conditions**

IX. **Hyperpituitarism**

A. Description

1. Hyperpituitarism is a chronic, progressive disease marked by excess growth hormone (GH) secretion and tissue overgrowth.

2. It appears in two forms.
    a. Gigantism
    b. Acromegaly
3. Gigantism is caused by an excess of growth hormone secretion that occurs before puberty and is characterized by excessive skeletal growth.
4. Acromegaly occurs in adults when excessive growth hormone is secreted after epiphyseal fusion.
5. Growth hormone cannot stimulate skeletal growth

B. **Etiology: usual cause is an anterior pituitary adenoma**

C. **Pathophysiologic processes and manifestations (Fig. 12-7)**
1. The progression of acromegaly is usually slow with an insidious onset.
2. Local expansion of a pituitary adenoma (when present) causes both neurologic and secretory effects.
3. Optic and trigeminal nerve involvement causes visual disturbances.
4. While skeletal growth is not possible, soft tissues are influenced by the excess of growth hormone.
5. The skeletal structures of the small and membranous bones of the hands, feet, face, and skull enlarge from growth hormone. This causes a characteristic enlargement of the hands, feet, and nose; slanting of the forehead; protrusion of the jaw; and widening of the teeth.
6. Nutrition may be effected if changes in teeth make eating difficult.
7. The respiratory cartilage becomes enlarged making the patient prone to respiratory diseases.
8. Soft tissue changes increase the size of every body organ, leading to dangerous conditions like cardiomegaly and hepatomegaly.
9. High-risk metabolic conditions, such as atherosclerosis, are accelerated.
10. Growth hormone is an insulin antagonist, causing the beta cells of the pancreas to work hard to produce enough insulin. If the cells eventually burn out, diabetes may occur.
11. Hypogonadism, hypothyroidism, and adrenal insufficiency may occur.
12. Other symptoms include hypertension, fatigue, weight gain, oily skin, heat intolerance, and muscle weakness.
13. Pressure from the tumor results in hyposecretion of follicle-stimulating hormone (FSH) and luteinizing hormone (LH), causing menstrual irregularities and decreased libido. Pressure from the tumor also causes headaches, visual field defects, optic nerve compression, and palsy of cranial nerves III, IV, VI.
14. Paresthesias, kyphosis, arthralgias, and arthritis cause pain and discomfort.

D. **Overview of nursing interventions**
1. Provide counseling to help the patient deal with feelings about changed body image.
2. Assist with range-of-motion exercises to maximize joint movement.
3. Monitor for visual disturbances.
4. Prepare the patient for surgery, if indicated.
5. Administer Octreotide®, a growth hormone analogue that suppresses growth hormone production, if prescribed.

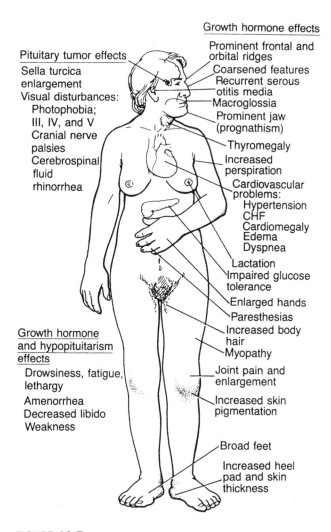

Growth hormone effects

Pituitary tumor effects
- Prominent frontal and orbital ridges
- Coarsened features
- Recurrent serous otitis media
- Macroglossia
- Prominent jaw (prognathism)
- Thyromegaly
- Increased perspiration
- Cardiovascular problems:
  - Hypertension
  - CHF
  - Cardiomegaly
  - Edema
  - Dyspnea
- Lactation
- Impaired glucose tolerance
- Enlarged hands
- Paresthesias
- Increased body hair
- Myopathy
- Joint pain and enlargement
- Increased skin pigmentation
- Broad feet
- Increased heel pad and skin thickness

Pituitary tumor effects
- Sella turcica enlargement
- Visual disturbances:
  - Photophobia;
  - III, IV, and V Cranial nerve palsies
- Cerebrospinal fluid rhinorrhea

Growth hormone and hypopituitarism effects
- Drowsiness, fatigue, lethargy
- Amenorrhea
- Decreased libido
- Weakness

FIGURE 12-7.
Appearance of acromegaly. Clinical manifestations relate to growth hormone secretion and effects from tumor encroachment in small pituitary space. (Bullock, B. L. [1996]. *Pathophysiology: Adaptations and Alterations in Function* [4th ed.]. Philadelphia: Lippincott-Raven, p. 691.)

X. Hypopituitarism

A. Description: deficient secretion of the anterior pituitary hormones (GH, TSH, FSH, LH, ACTH) secreted by the anterior pituitary gland; condition is marked by dwarfism, metabolic dysfunction, sexual immaturity, and growth retardation

B. Etiology: causes can include tumors, congenital defects, pituitary ischemia, partial or total hypophysectomy, radiation therapy, chemical agents, or head injury

C.   Pathophysiologic processes and manifestations

1. The gland must be at least 75% dysfunctional before manifestations become apparent.
2. Glandular dysfunction is caused by pressure from basophil adenoma; it is marked by excessive fat deposition and the persistence (or acquisition) of adolescent characteristics.
3. Pituitary gland infarction results in tissue necrosis followed by edema, which further impedes the blood supply.
4. If the pituitary undersecretes hormones, then the entire gland affected by its targets also undersecretes.
5. These include the adrenal glands, which are stimulated by the pituitary adrenocorticotropic hormone (ACTH). Too little ACTH results in insufficient adrenal secretion and Addison's disease.
6. The pituitary secretes TSH, so hypopituitarism causes hypothyroid states.
7. FSH and LH are not secreted, so sexual development is delayed or absent.
8. The skeletal system lacks the influence of growth hormone resulting in short stature.
9. If ADH secretion is reduced, diabetes insipidus results.

D.   Overview of nursing interventions

1. Institute thyroid and cortisol replacement therapy, as ordered.
2. Monitor for and treat diabetes insipidus.
3. Monitor for gonadal failure and loss of secondary sex organs.
4. Monitor for signs of gastrointestinal disturbance.
5. Closely observe the patient's overall health, because many metabolic functions are affected by the pituitary gland.

XI.   Syndrome of inappropriate ADH (SIADH)

A.   Description

1. **SIADH involves continuous secretion of ADH when plasma osmolarity is low (dehydration); normally, dehydration inhibits ADH secretion.**
2. SIADH is one of the most common causes of hyponatremia.
3. It is the direct opposite of diabetes insipidus (see Section XII, Diabetes insipidus, for more information).

B.   Etiology

1. SIADH results from a central nervous system disorder that interferes with the hypothalamic–pituitary mechanisms.
2. Pharmacologic agents also may cause SIADH.

C.   Pathophysiologic processes and manifestations

1. SIADH is characterized by plasma hypotonicity and hyponatremia resulting from the aberrant or sustained secretion of ADH.
2. The negative feedback system fails, because ADH secretion continues in spite of low plasma osmolality and expanded volume.
3. Excessive secretion of ADH causes excessive water reabsorption.

4. This extra water that is reabsorbed dilutes plasma, lowering serum sodium and making the plasma hypotonic.
5. Eventually the dysfunction results in water intoxification.
6. Display 12-1 describes nursing assessment for a patient with SIADH.
7. Display 12-2 describes clinical manifestations of SIADH.

D. Overview of nursing interventions

1. Assess for signs and symptoms of water intoxication, closely monitoring serum sodium levels.
2. Maintain strict fluid limitations.
3. Monitor weight daily.
4. Monitor the environment to control access to fluids.
5. Assess for changes in mentation.
6. Monitor vital signs, hemodynamic parameters, and breath sounds (Display 12-3).

XII. Diabetes insipidus

A. Description

1. Diabetes insipidus is a permanent or transient deficiency in ADH synthesis or release or osmoreceptor dysfunction, or a decrease in kidney responsiveness to ADH; it results in large-volume excretion of dilute urine.
2. It may be pituitary, nephrogenic, or psychogenic in nature.

B. Etiology

1. Diabetes insipidus may be familial or idiopathic.

DISPLAY 12-1
Nursing Assessment for SIADH

1. Identify patients at risk
2. Maintain accurate I&O.
   - Look for fluid intake greatly exceeding output; I&O should be totaled and the overall picture observed for several consecutive days.
3. Maintain daily body weight records.
   - Look for sudden weight gain (recall that 1 L of fluid weighs approximately 2.2 lb).
   - Although there will be an acute weight gain, do not expect to detect peripheral edema because most (approximately two thirds) of the excess fluid will be retained inside the cells, not in the interstitial space.
4. Monitor serum sodium concentrations.
5. Observe for gastrointestinal symptoms, which usually occur early.
   - Be alert for anorexia, nausea, vomiting, and abdominal cramping.
6. Observe the neurologic status carefully.
   - Be particularly alert for lethargy because this is usually the first symptom. Also, look for personality changes, decreased or absent deep tendon reflexes, headache, convulsions, and coma.

(*Source:* Metheny, N. M. *Fluid and Electrolyte Balance: Nursing Considerations* [3rd ed.]. Philadelphia: Lippincott-Raven, 1996.)

DISPLAY 12-2
Clinical Manifestations of SIADH

Water retention
- Intake of fluid greatly exceeds urinary output (as evidenced by I&O records)
- Weight gain (reflecting water retention)
- No significant peripheral edema (water is primarily retained inside the cells, not the interstitium)
- Fingerprint edema over sternum (reflecting cellular edema)
- Signs of cerebral edema (see neurological symptoms below)

Gastrointestinal symptoms
- Anorexia
- Nausea
- Vomiting
- Abdominal cramps

Neurologic symptoms
- Lethargy
- Headaches
- Personality changes
- Seizures
- Pupillary changes
- Coma

Laboratory findings
- Hyponatremia
  - Symptoms usually do not appear unless serum sodium level is <125 mEq/L
  - Plasma osmolality below normal (reflecting low serum sodium level)
- Low BUN and creatinine
  - Reflecting state of overhydration
- Urinary signs
  - Urinary sodium >20 mEq/L (As opposed to hyponatremia due primarily to sodium loss, where much lower sodium levels are expected due to renal conservation of the needed cation.)
  - Urinary SG >1.012
  - Urine osmolality is usually higher than plasma osmolality (urine contains important amounts of sodium and plasma is diluted with water)

SG, specific gravity: SIADH, syndrome of inappropriate antidiuretic hormone secretion.
(*Source:* Metheny, N. M. *Fluid and Electrolyte Balance: Nursing Considerations* [3rd ed.]. Philadelphia: Lippincott-Raven, 1996.)

    2.   Other possible causes include:
        a.   Traumatic injury
        b.   Neoplasms (craniopharyngioma, leukemia, breast cancer)
        c.   Infections (meningitis)
        d.   Vascular disorders (aneurysm)
     e.   Infiltration disorders
     f.   Renal disease
     g.   Pharmacologic agents
     h.   Pathology to the hypothalamic/pituitary area from brain surgery, brain trauma, or tumor formation
   C. **Pathophysiologic processes and manifestations**

DISPLAY 12-3
Nursing Interventions Related to Therapy for SIADH

1. Restrict fluids to the prescribed level.
   - Consider all routes of intake (eg, oral fluids, "keep-open" IV, piggyback medications).
   - Gain the patient's cooperation, if he or she is rational, by explaining the need for fluid restriction.
   - Place "fluid restriction" signs at the bedside.
   - Remove the water pitcher.
   - Explain the need for fluid restriction to visitors.
   - Space the allotted fluid allowance over the 24-hour period.
   - Minimize the risk of accidental overadministration of IV fluids by using a volume-controlled device.
2. Maintain an accurate I&O record and study its pattern.
   - A greater urinary output than fluid intake is desired because it indicates a negative water balance. (Remember, the excessive water load must be excreted before significant improvement occurs.)
3. Maintain an accurate body-weight record.
   - With proper therapy, expect to see an acute decline in body weight due to excretion of excess water. Recall that a liter of fluid is equivalent to 2.2 lb; for example, a weight loss of 6.6 lb over a period of 1 to 2 days indicates a loss of approximately 3 L.
4. Assess neurologic signs.
   - With appropriate therapy, an increased level of consciousness and increased muscle strength is hoped for. Unfortunately, neurological damage induced by SIADH is not always reversible, particularly if treatment is delayed.
5. Initiate safety precautions.
   - Elevate siderails for the patient with a decreased level of consciousness; be prepared for seizure activity; modify other aspects of the patient's environment as indicated.
6. Monitor serum sodium levels.
   - With appropriate therapy, the sodium concentration should elevate slowly toward normal. It is important that the correction not take place too rapidly.
7. Administer hypertonic saline, when prescribed, with great caution.
   - Review the facts regarding administration of hypertonic saline (Table 4-5).

SIADH, syndrome of inappropriate antidiuretic hormone secretion.
(*Source:* Metheny, N. M. *Fluid and Electrolyte Balance: Nursing Considerations.* [3rd ed.]. Philadelphia: Lippincott-Raven, 1996.)

1. The mechanism for water balance is mediated between the hypothalamus, pituitary, and kidney. Osmoreceptors in the hypothalamus sense the need for water to be either excreted or reabsorbed in the kidney.
2. When dehydration occurs, the hypothalamus sends a message to the pituitary, which releases ADH and sends it to the kidney. There, it acts on the distal and collecting tubules to reabsorb water.
3. When overhydration occurs, the osmoreceptors turn off pituitary secretion of ADH, allowing the kidneys to balance water by excretion.
4. ADH deficiency results in the body's inability to conserve water. An adequate thirst mechanism and readily available fluids will ensure only minor fluid balance alterations result, although extreme polydipsia and polyuria will occur.
5. The patient cannot concentrate urine, so large volumes of dilute urine are excreted (Displays 12-4 and 12-5).

DISPLAY 12-4
Assessment for Diabetes Insipidus

1. Be aware of patients at risk for DI
   Central DI
   - Head trauma (particularly with fractures at the base of the skull or surgical procedures near the pituitary)
   - Cerebral infections
   - Brain tumors
   Nephrogenic DI
   - Hypokalemia
   - Hypercalcemia
   - Certain drugs (such as lithium and demeclocycline)
2. Maintain an accurate I&O record for at-risk patients.
   - Look for a significantly greater output than intake (a danger signal of impending hypernatremia). Fortunately, many patients keep themselves "in balance" by drinking approximately as much as they urinate. It is helpful to calculate and record cumulative amounts for several days to obtain a more accurate account of the patient's fluid balance status, particularly if onset of polyuria was insidious.
3. Be alert for polyuria in at-risk patients.
   - It is frequently necessary to measure hourly urine volumes in such individuals to foster early detection. For example, a frequent directive in the care of postoperative neurosurgical patients is to report a urine volume greater than 200 mL in each of 2 consecutive hours or more than 500 mL in a 2-hr period.
4. Monitor urinary SG in at-risk patients.
   - A persistently dilute urine is a hallmark of DI. (The SG may be as low as 1.005.)
5. Monitor serum sodium levels at least once a day (more often as indicated) in at-risk patients.
   - Look for hypernatremia (serum sodium >145 mEq/L). Once vasopressin therapy has been initiated, look for hyponatremia (a possible rebound effect).
6. Monitor body weights.
   - Look for weight loss paralleling polyuria. Maintaining a weight chart helps detect excessive fluid loss, particularly when I&O records are in doubt (as may occur in incontinent patients).

DI, diabetes insipidus; SG, specific gravity.
(*Source:* Metheny, N. M. *Fluid and Electrolyte Balance: Nursing Considerations.* [3rd ed.]. Philadelphia: Lippincott-Raven, 1996.)

   D. Overview of nursing intervention
      1. Tailor your interventions to the cause of the disease.
      2. Assess for signs and symptoms of dehydration.
      3. Monitor intake and output.
      4. Measure urine glucose.
      5. Measure plasma osmolarity.
      6. Administer replacement hormones.

XIII.   Diabetes mellitus

   A. Description
      1. Diabetes is a metabolic disorder resulting from failure of the pancreas (beta

DISPLAY 12-5
Clinical Manifestations of Diabetes Insipidus

Excessive urinary output regardless of fluid intake:
- Urinary output usually ranges between 3 to 20 liters per 24 hr (depending on the severity of the pathologic process)
- Urinary output often exceeds 200 mL/hr
- In complete DI, urinary specific gravity <1.010, urine osmolality <300 mOsm/L
- In partial DI, urinary specific gravity and urinary osmolality are somewhat higher (such as 1.010 to 1.023 and 300 to 800 mOsm/L, respectively)
- Inability of kidneys to concentrate urine by fluid restriction (a common test for this disorder)

Intense thirst in the alert patient, resulting in an intake that corresponds to the urinary volume

Serum osmolality and sodium levels greater than normal if water intake does not match urinary losses (severe hypovolemia may occur with inadequate fluid intake)

(*Source:* Metheny, N. M. *Fluid and Electrolyte Balance: Nursing Considerations.* [3rd ed.]. Philadelphia: Lippincott-Raven, 1996.)

cells in the islets of Langerhans) to secrete adequate insulin, the hormone responsible for glucose utilization. The major result is chronic hyperglycemia.

2. Types include:
   a. Type I: insulin-dependent diabetes mellitus (IDDM)
   b. Type II: noninsulin-dependent diabetes mellitus (NIDDM)

B. Etiology and incidence
1. The exact cause of diabetes mellitus is unknown.
2. Possible causative factors include:
   a. Obesity
   b. Family tendency
   c. Age
   d. Autoimmunity
3. Type I usually affects persons under age 30.
4. Type II is the most common type; it usually affects persons over age 40.

C. Pathophysiologic processes and manifestations
1. In type I diabetes mellitus:
   a. Nearly 80 to 90% of the islet cells in the pancreas are destroyed before hyperglycemia occurs. The destruction is caused by islet cell antibodies (IgG classification), which are found at the time of diagnosis.
   b. As a result, there is insufficient insulin and excess glucagon.
   c. Glucose accumulates in the serum, causing hyperglycemia; blood that is delivered to the kidneys has a high glucose concentration, leading to osmotic diuresis and glycosuria.
   d. Osmotic diuresis causes water loss, resulting in polydipsia.
   e. Lack of insulin makes the body unable to use its primary source of energy, carbohydrates; instead, it uses fats and proteins for energy, which results in ketosis and weight loss.
   f. Polyphagia (excessive hunger) and fatigue result from the breakdown of nutritional stores.

2.   In type II diabetes mellitus
  a.   Beta cell weight and number decreases for unknown reasons.
  b.   In obesity, the ability of insulin to foster glucose uptake and metabolism in the liver, skeletal muscles, and adipose tissue is decreased.
  c.   Symptoms may be similar to those of type I diabetes mellitus; some nonspecific symptoms (pruritus, recurrent infections) may also occur.

D.   Overview of nursing interventions
  1.   Monitor blood glucose, and teach the patient how to do so.
  2.   Prevent complications such as ketoacidosis, and teach the patient how to do so.
  3.   Provide patient teaching covering:
    a.   Dietary and lifestyle changes
    b.   All aspects of self-care (especially foot care)
    c.   Administration and management of insulin (for the patient with IDDM)
    d.   Use of oral hypoglycemic medications (for the patient with NIDDM)

XIX.   Diabetic ketoacidosis (DKA)

A.   Description: an acute insulin deficiency resulting in metabolic acidosis from ketone bodies (acid end-products of fat breakdown)

B.   Etiology: causes may include inadequate secretion of endogenous insulin, insufficient exogenous insulin, increased insulin requirements (due to physical or emotional stress), or medications that interfere with insulin secretion or action

C.   Pathophysiologic processes and manifestations
  1.   Normally, insulin breaks down glucose. In diabetes there is inadequate insulin, so glucose is not metabolized properly and subsequently builds up in the serum (hyperglycemia).
  2.   Exogenous insulin is the only way to metabolize glucose.
  3.   Eventually, the body uses fat for energy because it is unable to use glucose, the body's primary energy source.

  4.   **Fat metabolism yields ketone bodies, an acid end-product; the person is then in a state of ketosis.**
  5.   As ketones build up in the serum, acidosis occurs.
  6.   Acidosis worsens as serum glucose levels rise and more ketones accumulate.

  7.   **Symptoms of acidosis include:**
    a.   **Polyuria (as osmotic diuresis occurs from renal perfusion with hyperglycemic blood)**
    b.   **Polydipsia (as extracellular dehydration occurs)**
    c.   **Hypokalemia**
    d.   **Kussmaul's respirations**
    e.   **Ketonuria**
    f.   **Dizziness**

D.   Overview of nursing interventions
  1.   Administer regular insulin, as ordered.
  2.   Monitor serum glucose levels as insulin is given.

3. Monitor potassium levels, because potassium shifts effect the heart.
4. Monitor respirations, because respiratory distress can occur.
5. Replace fluids.
6. Monitor blood gas studies to check the progression of acidosis.

XV.   Hyperglycemic hyperosmolar nonketotic coma (HHNK or HHNC)

A. **Description: severe hyperglycemia and hypertonic dehydration without significant ketoacidosis; results from reactive insulin deficiency**
B. **Etiology**
   1. HHNK may result from several causes, including:
      a. Inadequate insulin secretion or action
      b. Increased insulin requirements associated with stress
   2. HHNK also has been associated with high-caloric parenteral and enteral feedings and ingestion of the following medications:
      a. Thiazide diuretics
      b. Glucocorticoid
      c. Phenytoin
      d. Sympathomimetics
      e. Diazoxide
      f. Chlorpromazine
C. **Pathophysiologic processes and manifestations**
   1. Serum glucose levels rise; although some insulin is present, there is not enough to bring serum glucose levels to normal.
   2. Acidosis does not occur because the body secretes enough insulin to avoid fat metabolism (therefore there are no ketones present), but not enough to use glucose properly.
   3. As a result of hypergylcemia, glycosuria and polyuria (from osmotic diuresis) occur.
   4. Polyuria causes dehydration of the extracellular and intracellular spaces, leading to neurologic changes.
D. **Overview of nursing interventions**
   1. Monitor for rapid, thready pulse and cool extremities.
   2. Monitor vital signs, checking for low blood pressure and orthostatic hypotension.
   3. Monitor intake and output.
   4. Assess gastrointestinal status for abdominal pain and cramping.
   5. Assess fluid and electrolyte balance by monitoring laboratory values.
   6. Administer insulin as prescribed.
   7. Replace fluids as ordered.

Bibliography

Bullock, B. (1996). *Pathophysiology: adaptations and alterations in function* (4th ed.). Philadelphia: Lippincott-Raven.

Davidson, J. K. (1991). *Clinical diabetes mellitus: A problem oriented approach* (2nd ed.). New York: Theme.

Ganong, W. F. (1997). *Review of medical physiology* (18th ed.). Stamford, CT: Appleton & Lange.

Greenspan, F., & Strewler, G. (Eds.) (1997). *Basic and clinical endocrinology* (5th ed.). Stamford, CT: Appleton & Lange.

Guyton, A. C., & Hall, J. E. (1996). *Textbook of medical physiology* (9th ed.). Philadelphia: W.B. Saunders.

Ignatavicius, D., & Bayne, M. (1991). *Medical-surgical. A nursing process approach.* Philadelphia: W. B. Saunders.

Kinney, M., Packa, D., et al. (1993). *AACN's clinical reference for critical-care nursing* (3rd ed.). St. Louis: C.V. Mosby.

McCance, K. L., & Huether, S. E. (1994). *Pathophysiology: The biologic basis for disease in adults and children* (2nd ed.). St. Louis: Mosby-Year Book.

Peragallo-Dittko, V. (1993). *Core curriculum for diabetes education* (2nd ed.). Chicago: American Association of Diabetes Educators.

Porth, C. (1994). *Pathophysiology: Concepts of altered health states* (4th ed.). Philadelphia: Lippincott-Raven.

Thelan, L., Davie, J., et al. (1994). *Critical care nursing diagnosis and management* (2nd ed.). St. Louis: C. V. Mosby.

Wilson, J. D., & Foster, D. W. (Eds.) (1997). *Williams textbook of endocrinology* (9th ed.). Philadelphia: W. B. Saunders.

STUDY QUESTIONS

1. When assessing a patient for symptoms of Graves' disease, the nurse would expect to see:
   a. dehydration
   b. cyanosis
   c. cold intolerance
   d. palmar erythema

2. Pathophysiologic processes found in hyperthyroidism include:
   a. decreased cardiac output
   b. decreased heart rate
   c. decreased bowel sounds
   d. increased vitamin metabolism

3. Which of the following is *not* an etiology of primary hypothyroidism?
   a. thyroid cancer
   b. thyroiditis
   c. Hashimoto's disease
   d. congenital defects

4. While caring for a patient with secondary hypothyroidism, the nurse would monitor for the life-threatening complication of:
   a. thyroid storm
   b. myxedema coma
   c. Cushing's syndrome
   d. Graves' disease

5. The body's normal pathophysiologic response to elevated serum calcium is:
   a. decreased PTH secretion by the parathyroid
   b. increased PTH secretion by the parathyroid
   c. calcium retention in the bone
   d. decreased release of calcium to the kidneys

6. When assessing a patient for serum calcium abnormalities, the nurse is aware that classic symptoms include:
   a. seizures
   b. Chvostek's sign
   c. Hoffman's sign
   d. Hashimoto's disease

7. Pathophysiologic processes involved in Cushing's disease include:
   a. hyperglycemia from excessive steroids
   b. decreased levels of cortisol
   c. hyperreflexia in the nervous system
   d. decreased protein catabolism

8. Ketosis in diabetes mellitus results from:
   a. protein gain
   b. water retention
   c. fat metabolism
   d. insulin excretion

9. Patient teaching for the client with diabetes mellitus should focus on:
   a. glucose testing, medication administration, diet
   b. avoidance of exercise and food
   c. skin care, urine testing, rest
   d. daily weights, blood pressure measurements

10. Diabetes insipidus involves a dysfunction of:
    a. glucose metabolism
    b. antidiuretic hormone (ADH)
    c. insulin production
    d. follicle-stimulating hormone (FSH)

11. Which of the following medications can cause signs of Cushing's disease?
    a. penicillin
    b. aspirin
    c. Indocin
    d. prednisone®

12. Which life-threatening situation occurs with Addison's disorder?
    a. hyponatremia
    b. hypervolemia
    c. hypernatremia
    d. hyperkalemia

13. A nurse caring for a patient with diabetic ketoacidosis should monitor blood gas studies because which of the following may develop:

a. respiratory acidosis
b. respiratory alkalosis
c. metabolic acidosis
d. metabolic alkalosis

a. hyponatremia
b. metabolic acidosis
c. respiratory alkalosis
d. hyperkalemia

14. When caring for a patient with SIADH, the nurse assesses carefully for:

ANSWER KEY

Question	Correct answer	Correct answer rationale	Incorrect answer rationales
1.	d	Palmar erythema is present during Grave's disease.	a, b, and c. These are not manifestations of Graves' disease.
2.	d	In this hypermetabolic condition, increased protein, carbohydrate, lipid, and vitamin metabolism occurs.	a. Cardiac output is increased, not decreased. b. Tachycardia (rapid heart rate) is present. c. Bowel sounds increase in hyperthyroidism.
3.	a	Thyroid cancer may lead to hyperthyroidism, not hypothyroidism.	a, c, and d. Thyroiditis, Hashimoto's disease, and congenital defects are etiologies of hypothyroidism.
4.	b	Myxedema coma is a life-threatening state characterized by severely decreased level of consciousness, heart rate, blood pressure, and metabolism.	a. Thyroid storm is a complication of hyperthyroidism. c. Cushing's disease is associated with adrenal glands. d. Graves' disease is a hyperthyroid state.
5.	a	The normal feedback response to increased levels of serum calcium is decreased PTH secretion; hyperparathyroidism may result.	b, c, and d. These responses are incorrect; none of these occurs in response to calcium imbalances.
6.	b	Chvostek's sign, Trousseau's sign, and tetany are associated with serum calcium abnormalities.	a, c, and d are not signs of calcium abnormalities.
7.	a	Because steroids antagonize insulin, their excessive presence causes increased serum glucose levels.	b. Steroids increase levels of cortisol. c. Hyperreflexia is not a symptom associated with Cushing's disease. d. Steroids increase protein catabolism.
8.	c	In diabetes, the body is unable to use glucose due to lack of insulin. Because it is unable to use glucose as a primary source of energy, it begins to metabolize fat for energy. Fat metabolism yields ketone bodies, an acid end-product. This results in ketosis.	a, b, and d. These are incorrect; none of these occurs in association with diabetes.
9.	a	Patient teaching for diabetes mellitus should focus on the need for exercise, medication administration, dietary adjustment, and a balance between exercise and rest. Prevention of long-term	b, c, and d. These choices are not accurate with regard to diabetes teaching.

Question	Correct answer	Correct answer rationale	Incorrect answer rationales
		complications should also be included in the teaching.	
10.	b	Diabetes insipidus involves a dysfunction of ADH synthesis or release.	a and c. These are involved in diabetes mellitus. d. FSH is associated with reproduction.
11.	d	Prednisone is a steroid preparation, and administering large amounts will mimic the effects of steroids.	a, b, and c. These medications will not exert a steroid-like effect on the body.
12.	d	Hypovolemia and hyperkalemia are two life-threatening disorders that occur with Addison's disease.	a, b, and c. These are not associated with mortality from Addison's disease.
13.	c	Metabolic acidosis is a consequence of DKA.	b, c, and d. These disorders do not result from DKA.
14.	a	Excessive amounts of ADH cause water reabsorption, which results in hypotonicity of the ECF space and hyponatremia.	b, c, and d. These alterations are not a result of SIADH.

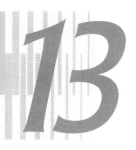

Gastrointestinal Disorders

I.   Overview of pathophysiologic processes

A.   Disorders of food intake

1.   Disorders of food intake can affect the mouth or esophagus, compromising a person's ability to ingest food.

2.   These disorders usually occur secondary to a primary disease (eg, cancer, acquired immunodeficiency syndrome [AIDS], diabetes) or result from poor dentition.

3.   Stomatitis, esophagitis, achalasia, esophageal hiatal hernia, and oral and esophageal cancers are disorders of food intake (Fig. 13-1).

4.   **Risk factors include:**
    a.   **Presence of primary disease**
    b.   **Malnutrition**
    c.   **Use of tobacco**

5.   Some disorders, such as hiatal hernia and achalasia, have no specific risk factors.

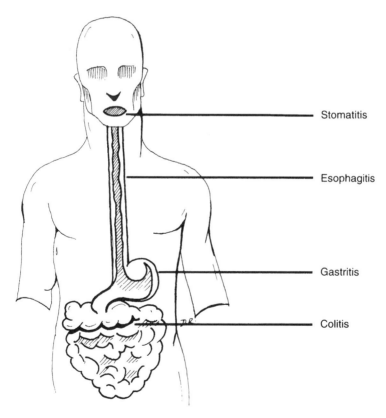

FIGURE 13-1.
GI tract. Inflammatory conditions of the GI tract can affect the mouth, esophagus, stomach, and bowel.

B. Disorders of digestion and absorption

1. Disorders of digestion and absorption affect the stomach and small intestine, hindering the body's ability to break down food and absorb essential nutrients.

2. Gastritis, peptic ulcer disease, gastroenteritis, malabsorption syndrome, stomach cancer, and cancer of the small intestine are disorders of digestion and absorption.

3. Ulcerative colitis and regional enteritis (Crohn's disease) are considered disorders of digestion and absorption as well as elimination.

4. **Risk factors include:**
    a. **Genetic predisposition**
    b. **Stress**
    c. **Administration of certain drugs**
    d. **Use of tobacco**

C. Disorders of elimination

1. Disorders of elimination affect the large intestine, rendering a person unable to maintain a normal elimination pattern.

2. These disorders may occur alone, as a sequela to another disease, or as a result of administering certain drugs.

3. Disorders in elimination result in abnormal amounts or constituents of stool.

4. Ulcerative colitis, regional enteritis (Crohn's disease), irritable bowel syndrome, diverticulitis, and cancer of the large intestine are disorders of elimination.

5. **Risk factors include:**
    a. **Presence of cancer**
    b. **Genetic predisposition**
    c. **Stress**
    d. **Ingestion of foods that do not agree with the individual.**
    e. **Administration of certain drugs**
    f. **Use of tobacco**

D. Inflammatory disorders

1. Inflammatory disorders include appendicitis, peritonitis, and pancreatitis

2. **These disorders are always made worse by the use of tobacco and alcohol. Avoiding these substances is part of the treatment for any gastrointestinal disorder.**

II. Physiologic responses to gastrointestinal dysfunction

A. Halitosis: foul-smelling or malodorous breath; may indicate a periodontal or an oral infectious process

B. Dysphagia: difficulty swallowing; may result from a mechanical problem (eg, neoplasm, surgery) or occur secondary to neurologic damage or dysfunction (eg, cerebral vascular accident)

C. Odynophagia: painful swallowing; an important marker for infection or disease

D. Pyrosis (heartburn): a burning sensation usually in the midsternal area caused by reflux of gastric contents into the esophagus

E. Dyspepsia (indigestion): feeling of discomfort during the digestive process, or the inability to digest food secondary to a gastrointestinal (GI) disorder

F. Anorexia: loss of appetite, a common complaint associated with GI disease; causes can include a neoplastic process, anxiety, pain, depression, infection, or constipation

G. Satiety: feeling of fullness, at times beyond the point of satisfaction

H. Nausea: feeling of gastric uneasiness characterized by the urge to vomit

I. Vomiting: expulsion of gastric contents, usually following a feeling of nausea; most commonly an involuntary response

J. Abdominal cramping: involuntary spasmodic muscular contraction that causes discomfort and pain

K. Abdominal distention: expansion of the abdomen noted by observation, percussion, or palpation; commonly indicates increased amounts of air or fluid, or the presence of an abdominal mass

L. Malabsorption: inability to absorb nutrients secondary to a GI disorder or surgery

M. Pain: sensation of discomfort varying in severity; indicates an underlying injury, disease, or emotional disorder

N. Diarrhea: excessive expulsion of watery stool in high volume or increased frequency

O. Constipation: decreased or diminished frequency of fecal evacuation, leading to bowel impaction; stool consistency is most commonly dry and hardened, however it may be formed and soft if motility disorders are present

P. Altered bowel sounds

    1. Bowel sounds heard on auscultation indicate the passage of air and fluid in the GI tract; normal frequency range is approximately 5 to 25 sounds per minute.

    2. Bowel sounds may be diminished or absent after abdominal surgery or may be hyperactive or high-pitched (borborygmi) as a result of hypermotility of the GI tract.

Q. Melena: black or tarry stools indicating the presence of blood; results from bleeding or hemorrhage within the digestive tract

R. Weight loss: common symptom usually denoting inadequate enteral intake or related to hypermetabolic processes or malabsorption of nutrients; severe weight loss over a particular time frame usually indicative of malnutrition

III.   **Stomatitis**

A. Description

    1. Stomatitis is an inflammation of the oral cavity (excluding dental disease); it may be primary or secondary.

    2. *Primary stomatitis* includes:

        a. Aphthous stomatitis or canker sores (most common type)

        b. Herpes simplex virus (HSV) type I and HSV type II lesions

3. *Secondary stomatitis* includes:
    a. Candidiasis or thrush (yeast infection or overgrowth of an organism normally present in the flora of the oral cavity)
    b. Lichen planus (see Chapter 9, Skin Disorders, for a discussion of lichen planus)

B. Etiology
1. *Primary stomatitis*
    a. Aphthous stomatitis (canker sore) results from unknown causes; however, it may be associated with autoimmune disorders or emotional stress. It is more prevalent in young adults, especially females.
    b. HSV type I and type II lesions result from exposure to, or recurrent infection from HSV.
2. Secondary stomatitis
    a. Candidiasis is caused by Candida albicans.
    b. *Secondary stomatitis* commonly occurs in a compromised host (eg, an immunosuppressed or malnourished patient or one with allergy, systemic diseases, or emotional distress).

C. Pathophysiologic processes and manifestations
1. Severity of symptoms depends on the type of stomatitis.
2. *Canker sores*
    a. Appear as recurrent circular lesions anywhere within the oral cavity, with well-defined, indurated margins measuring 2 to 5 cm in diameter
    b. Remain approximately 1 week and usually heal within 2 weeks
3. *HSV type I lesions*
    a. Are uniform-size vesicles commonly occurring on buccal and labial mucosa, tongue, and palate
    b. Rupture and form painful ulcerations
    c. May be accompanied by gingivitis with or without additional lesions on gingiva
    d. Are manifested by halitosis, malaise, and fever
    e. Heal usually within 2 weeks
4. *HSV type II lesions*
    a. Manifest as a cold sore or fever blister on the lip or labial mucosa
    b. Occur as a single vesicle or a group of vesicles circumscribed with erythema
    c. Rupture and form crustation
    d. Heal usually within 1 to $1\frac{1}{2}$ weeks
5. *Candidiasis*
    a. Presents as white patchy milk-curdlike lesions on the tongue, palate, and buccal and labial mucosa
    b. Lesions are firmly secured, but may be removed with a tongue blade
    c. Requires continued antimicrobial therapy for approximately 1 week after disappearance of patches

D. Overview of nursing interventions
1. Administer analgesics and antibiotics as ordered, to reduce or alleviate inflammation and discomfort and to treat underlying causative factors.
2. Explain the importance of diet therapy.

       a.   Instruct the patient to eliminate irritating foods.

       b.   Provide soft or pureed diet if indicated.

3.   Promote good oral hygiene.

4.   Instruct the patient in medication-intake methods (eg, oral washings) and observe for efficacy.

5.   Provide emotional support and discuss the patient's concerns.

IV.   Esophagitis

A.   **Description: inflammation of the esophagus; may be acute or chronic**

B.   **Etiology**

   1.   Esophagitis is most commonly caused by gastroesophageal reflux disease (GERD), a syndrome caused by a reflux of gastric contents into the esophagus.

       a.   Reflux occurs when the lower esophageal sphincter (LES) tone is decreased or relaxed.

       b.   Hiatal hernia is a contributing factor.

       c.   Reflux also can result from emesis, depending on frequency and duration.

       d.   Reflux also may be related to a delayed gastric emptying time (eg, gastroparesis), which is common in diabetics.

   2.   Esophagitis can also result from an infectious process (eg, herpes or monilial invasion); this usually occurs in immunosuppressed patients.

   3.   May also result from ingestion of hot or corrosive substances or from radiation therapy (dose related).

C.   **Pathophysiologic processes and manifestations**

   1.   Clinical manifestations vary with severity.

   2.   The severity of inflammation in GERD is related to the frequency of reflux, the acidic concentration of gastric contents, and the duration of exposure of esophagus to acidic irritant.

   3.   Pyrosis is a hallmark symptom; if severe, it may radiate to the back, neck, or jaw.

   4.   Pain after eating and at night when in a supine position may indicate esophagitis, particularly if a hiatal hernia exists.

   5.   Pain also may be aggravated by activities that increase intraabdominal pressure (eg, straining, lifting).

   6.   Epithelial cells are damaged by the acidic stomach contents.

   7.   In severe cases, erosion may occur all the way through the muscularis, causing motor dysfunction; this results in dysphagia, or esophageal "fullness."

   8.   Other common symptoms, which are usually precipitated by ingestion of fatty foods, include:

       a.   Regurgitation

       b.   Increased salivary secretion secondary to esophageal reflux

       c.   Belching

       d.   Flatulence

   9.   Permanent strictures may develop as esophageal walls may adhere together.

  10.   Bleeding may occur because acids are erosive in nature.

D.   Overview of nursing interventions

1.   Administer medications (eg, antacids, H_2-receptor antagonists) to neutralize irritating gastric materials, as ordered.
2.   Reinforce the importance of a low-fat diet—with six small feedings per day and no alcohol, caffeine, and spices—to reduce LES pressure.
3.   Make sure the patient completely understands the diet and the importance of avoiding food that causes discomfort or brings on an attack.
4.   Teach the patient about proper positioning (high Fowler's) during mealtime and hour after mealtime; instruct the patient to refrain from eating for several hours before bedtime.
5.   Stress the importance of weight reduction, in the absence of malnutrition.
6.   Encourage the patient to stop smoking, if applicable.
7.   Instruct the patient to avoid wearing tight, restrictive clothing.
8.   Encourage the patient to avoid activities that increase intraabdominal pressure.
9.   Prepare the patient for antireflux surgery, if indicated, to support the esophagus and increase LES pressure.

V.   Achalasia (cardiospasm)

A.   Description

1.   Achalasia is an esophageal motility disorder marked by progressively worsening dysphagia.
2.   It may be accompanied by regurgitation of ingested food, particularly if the patient is supine.
3.   Achalasia is also known as cardiospasm because the clinical manifestation of radiating substernal pain may resemble that of a myocardial infarction.

B.   Etiology

1.   Achalasia is idiopathic in nature; however, it is thought to be related to neuromuscular factors and inadequate relaxation of the LES.
2.   It has been associated with a familial tendency.

C.   Pathophysiologic processes and manifestations

1.   Lack of peristalsis, relaxation or spasm of the muscle dilates the esophagus and slows down digestive transport; precipitating causes include esophageal cell degeneration and vagal tone alterations.
2.   This chronic condition progresses slowly, so symptoms may worsen in time.

3.   Common manifestations may include:
   a.   Dysphagia, with a feeling of food getting "stuck" in the esophagus
   b.   Substernal pain of varying degree (from mild to excruciating) radiating to the back, neck, and jawline
   c.   Halitosis from food remnants retained in the esophagus (this may result in esophagitis secondary to stagnant undigested food)
   d.   Weight loss related to decreased dietary intake (which, in many cases, is related to a fear of eating)

5. Symptoms may be exacerbated with emotional stress, indiscriminate over-intake, or hurried-ingestion practices.

D. Overview of nursing interventions

1. Assess the patient for pain.
2. Administer medications, as ordered, to relieve pain.
3. Instruct the patient to eat six small meals consisting of low-fat, high-protein foods and to avoid chocolate and citrus juices; suggest consuming liquids or semisolid foods during the acute phase. Make sure that the patient is able to identify and avoid food in the diet that exacerbates the condition.
4. Educate the patient about the importance of chewing foods well and about proper positioning (usually high-Fowler's) during mealtimes and at night (semi-Fowler's) to avoid nocturnal regurgitation.
5. Provide frequent oral hygiene.
6. Tell the patient to avoid wearing tight-fitting or restrictive clothing.
7. Discourage alcohol or cigarette use.
8. Prepare the patient for surgery to dilate the unrelaxed LES (balloon dilatation) or to enlarge the sphincter opening (myotomy), if drug and dietary management are unsuccessful; afterward, provide appropriate postoperative care.

VI. Esophageal hiatal hernia

A. Description

1. Esophageal hiatal hernia refers to herniation or displacement of a portion of the lower esophagus or the stomach into the thoracic cavity.
2. Two major types include:
    a. *Sliding esophageal hernia* (accounts for approximately 90% of occurrences): herniated portion of the stomach slides back and forth upward through the hiatus secondary to positional changes
    b. *Rolling esophageal hernia:* fundus and possibly the greater curvature of the stomach herniate alongside the esophagus into the thorax; although this type occurs less commonly, complications are high and include gastric volvulus, strangulation, or obstruction.

B. Etiology

1. *Sliding esophageal hernia* results from weakening of the muscles of the esophageal hiatus due to the aging process (more than 60% of these types of hernias occur in the aged), trauma, surgery, or hereditary factors.
2. *Rolling esophageal hernia* is theorized to result from improper anchoring of the stomach below the diaphragm secondary to an anatomic defect.

C. Pathophysiologic processes and manifestations

1. In *sliding esophageal hernia*

   a. **Clinical manifestations are associated with gastro-esophageal reflux.**
   b. **Dysphagia, pyrosis, regurgitation, and bloating are common symptoms.**
2. In *rolling esophageal hernia*
   a. Symptoms are related to increased intrathoracic pressure secondary to displacement of the thoracic contents by hernia.

        b.   Symptoms may include chest pain, shortness of breath, and tachycardia with subsequent impaired gas exchange.

        c.   Chest pain is characteristic because it mimics anginal pain and usually is not relieved when the patient is recumbent.

D. Overview of nursing interventions

1. Administer medications (eg, antacids, H_2-receptor antagonists), as ordered; note that drug therapy is consistent with that for esophagitis (see Section IV).
2. Instruct the patient to follow the same dietary guidelines as for esophagitis (see Section IV).
3. Prepare the patient for surgery (hiatal hernia repair), if indicated (rolling esophageal hernia nearly always requires surgical intervention); afterward, provide appropriate postoperative care.
4. Provide emotional support to allay anxiety and encourage compliance with drug and dietary regimen.
5. Provide pain relief by teaching the patient to position himself in semi-Fowler's during sleep or to use analgesics if needed.
6. Institute a weight-loss regimen, if applicable.
7. Promote frequent oral hygiene.
8. Teach the patient to avoid wearing tight-fitting or restrictive clothing.
9. Discourage alcohol or cigarette use.
10. Assess the patient for recurrent dysphagia (which may suggest the need for dilatation).

VII. Gastritis

A. Description: inflammation of the stomach mucosa; may be acute (transient intermittent inflammation) or chronic

B. Etiology

1. *Acute gastritis*
   a. May be caused by local irritants (eg, drugs, alcohol, corrosive substances), allergy, and bacterial endotoxin invasion (eg, *Salmonella*, *Escherichia coli*).
   b. Is typically associated with mucosal hemorrhages and erosions.
2. *Chronic gastritis*
   a. Is associated with atrophy of the gastric glands and achlorhydria
   b. May occur secondary to bile acid reflux (after gastrojejunal surgery) or to peptic ulcer disease
   c. May be related to chronic use of local irritants (eg, alcohol, drugs)

C. Pathophysiologic processes and manifestations

1. Severity of symptoms depends on the type, etiology, and extent of the disorder.
2. Symptoms may include:
   a. Mild to severe abdominal discomfort or pain, which may or may not be accompanied by nausea, vomiting, and diarrhea
   b. Intolerance of spicy or high-fat foods
   c. Diarrhea (if intractable, this may result in dehydration, which has severe implications in the pediatric or frail elderly population)

3. If symptoms are unabated, gastric ulceration (developed by about 50% of patients with gastritis) and hemorrhage can result.
4. As the disorder progresses, hemorrhage (as hematemesis or melena) and subsequent anemia and vitamin B_{12} deficiency may occur.

D. Overview of nursing interventions

1. Administer antacids, antiemetics, H_2 antagonists (to inhibit gastric acid formation), and sucralfate (to provide a protective coating for gastric mucosa), as ordered.
2. Administer antidiarrheal agents, as prescribed, if diarrhea is persistent.
3. Administer antibiotic therapy, as ordered, if etiology is related to an infectious agent.
4. Administer anticholinergics (antispasmodics), analgesics, and supplementary vitamin B_{12}, if indicated.
5. Correct fluid and electrolyte disorders.
6. Institute diet therapy.
   a. Avoid oral feeding until emesis subsides.
   b. Avoid foods contributing to gastric distress.
   c. Initiate parenteral nutrition if diarrhea is unresponsive.
7. Teach the patient about diet and lifestyle changes to prevent exacerbation.
   a. Avoid cigarette smoking and alcohol consumption.
   b. Avoid foods considered to be at high risk for bacterial contaminants (eg, eggs, rare red meat, pork), spicy foods, and caffeine.

VIII. Peptic ulcer disease

A. Description

1. Peptic ulcer disease is most commonly a chronic condition characterized by an ulceration of the gastric mucosa, duodenum, or less frequently, of the lower esophagus and jejunum (Fig. 13-2).
2. Occasionally, peptic ulcer disease is an acute response to medical or surgical stress (stress ulcer).

B. Etiology and incidence

1. Peptic ulcer disease results from unknown causes; however, possible contributing factors include:
   a. Mucosal breakdown secondary to infection (*Campylobacter pylori*)
   b. Genetic predisposition
   c. Tobacco use
   d. Ingestion of food or drugs that injure or alter gastric mucosa or increase hydrochloric acid production (eg, acetylsalicylic acid [ASA], corticosteroids, caffeine, spicy foods).
   e. Stress
   f. Presence of diseases that alter gastric secretion (eg, pancreatitis, Crohn's disease, Zollinger-Ellison syndrome)
2. Gastric ulcers are thought to occur secondary to an injury or break in gastric mucosa, either from an excess or an imbalance of hydrochloric acid (HCl) relative to natural gastric protective barriers.
3. Duodenal ulcers are three times more prevalent than gastric ulcers and usually occur between the second and fifth decades of life.

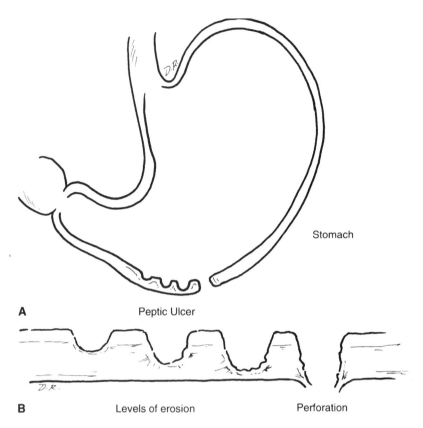

A   Peptic Ulcer

B   Levels of erosion   Perforation

FIGURE 13-2.
Peptic ulcer disease. If the ulcer is left untreated, it becomes deeper and eventually perforates, leaking gastric contents into the peritoneum. **(A)** Location of peptic ulcer in stomach, showing different degrees of erosion. **(B)** Detailed view of perforation.

C.   Pathophysiologic processes and manifestations

   1.   *Gastric ulcers*

   a.   In response to injury to the gastric mucosa, histamine is released; this results in further increased HCl production, adding to injury potential.

   b.   Histamine release may also occur as a result of pyloric sphincter dysfunction, causing increased diffusion of gastric acid back into stomach.

   c.   Hematemesis and melena can occur secondary to erosion of the ulcer into blood vessels.

   d.   Other complications include pyloric obstruction and perforation.

   e.   Gastric ulcers are slow to heal, in part because of poor circulation to the ulcerative site.

   2.   *Duodenal ulcers*

   a.   An increased rate of gastric acid secretion, either related to an increased number of parietal cells or secondary to vagal stimulation, affects gastric release.

 b.   An increased rate of gastric emptying reduces the buffering effects of food.

 c.   Subsequent gastric acid secretion causes duodenal irritation and ulceration.

 d.   High gastric acid secretion is indicated by low pH levels in the duodenum.

 e.   Complications include hemorrhage, obstruction, or perforation.

3.   *Stress ulcers*

 a.   Upper GI bleeding (coffee-ground aspirate) is commonly the hallmark indicator of stress ulcers.

 b.   Multiple ulcerations felt to be erosions develop secondary to gastric ischemia.

4.   Common manifestations of all types of peptic ulcer disease may include:

 a.   Bloating

 b.   Belching

 c.   Nausea

 d.   Vomiting

 e.   Pain (usually described as burning or aching) located in the upper abdomen and occurring between mealtimes or at night

5.   At times, pain may be associated with ingestion of specific foods (spicy or fried), alcohol, or medications known to irritate gastric mucosa (eg, ASA).

D.   **Overview of nursing interventions**

1.   Administer medications (eg, antacids, H_2 antagonists, anticholinergics, antimuscarinics, and mucosal barrier protectants) to neutralize stomach acid, reduce acid secretion, decrease vagal stimulation, inhibit gastric acid secretion, and provide a protective coating over the ulcerative site.

2.   **Instruct the patient to avoid foods or substances that provoke symptoms or stimulate gastric acid secretion (eg, spicy or fried foods, coffee [caffeinated and decaffeinated], caffeinated beverages, and alcohol).**

3.   Teach the patient stress-reduction techniques if the ulcer etiology is suspected to be related to high-stress situations.

4.   Instruct the patient to stop smoking, if applicable.

5.   Explain potential complications and advise the patient when to seek medical assistance.

6.   If medication therapy and diet and lifestyle changes are unsuccessful—or if complications such as hemorrhage, pyloric obstruction, or perforation occur—prepare the patient for surgery; possible procedures include:

 a.   Antrectomy, Billroth I, or Billroth II (depending on surgery)

 b.   Vagotomy (severing of the vagus nerve); this may be performed to eliminate acid-secreting stimuli and decrease parietal cell stimulation

 c.   Pyloroplasty, which may be performed to sever both right and left vagus nerves and to widen the pyloric outlet

7.   After surgery, provide appropriate postoperative care, including:

 a.   Pain management

 b.   Gastric drainage system management

 c.   Nutritional support

8. When the patient is ready to begin oral intake, explain how to prevent dumping syndrome (secondary to rapid delivery of nutrients into jejunum); suggest a high-fat diet of frequent small feedings, separation of liquids from solids, and avoidance of concentrated hyperosmolar foods.

IX. Gastroenteritis

A. Description

1. Gastroenteritis is an inflammation of the GI tract; it most commonly affects the small intestine.
2. The term *gastroenteritis* is used to describe a variety of GI disorders (eg, traveler's diarrhea, dysentery).
3. A thorough patient history is extremely important in differentiating gastroenteritis from other intestinal disorders (eg, appendicitis, colitis).

B. Etiology and incidence

1. Bacterial gastroenteritis is caused by a variety of bacteria, including *Escherichia coli* and *Campylobacter* (traveler's diarrhea) and Shigellosis (bacillary dysentery); it typically is transmitted by ingesting contaminated water or food, by way of fecal-oral route, or by way of fomites.
2. Viral gastroenteritis is caused by various types of viruses including the rotavirus and parvovirus-type organisms; it may be transmitted by way of the respiratory system.
3. Outbreaks of gastroenteritis may be of epidemic proportions in areas where there is a lack of sanitation and unclean housing conditions.
4. *E. coli* and *Campylobacter* affect all ages, particularly in warm climates.
5. Infants and the aged are particularly prone to *Shigellosis,* especially in crowded living situations.

C. Pathophysiologic processes and manifestations

1. The severity of symptoms depends on the organism and extent of exposure.
2. Symptoms common to all types of gastroenteritis include:
   a. Nausea
   b. Vomiting
   c. Diarrhea
3. In gastroenteritis caused by *Campylobacter,* stool specimens are positive for high white blood cell count (WBC) and possibly high red blood cell count (RBC).
4. High WBC and the presence of pus indicate *Shigella.*
5. Isolation of *E. coli* is the determining factor for that pathogen.
6. Degree of temperature elevation depends on the specific organism and the severity of infection.
7. Manifestations of viral gastroenteritis include symptoms associated with headache, weakness, muscle aches and pains; abdominal distention and tenderness may be identified, but no rebound tenderness exists.
8. Infection can last anywhere from 2 to 7 days.
9. If diarrhea and vomiting become severe, complications such as dehydration, orthostatic hypotension, oliguria, and shock can result.

D. Overview of nursing interventions

1. Administer anti-infective agents, analgesics, and electrolyte replacement medications (eg, potassium, acetate), as ordered. Note that drugs that suppress intestinal motility *are contraindicated* to avoid further absorption of the suspected microbe.

 2. **Monitor and manage fluids and electrolytes.**

3. Instruct the patient about dietary changes (eg, intake of clear liquids initially, lactose-free foods for 1 to 2 weeks after symptoms subside).

4. For severe cases in which emesis or diarrhea is unresolved and the patient is at actual or potential nutritional risk, institute parenteral nutritional support, as prescribed.

5. Observe intake and output.

6. Monitor daily weight if assessment of fluid shifts is essential for fluid management; monitor weekly weight to identify need for changes in nutritional methodology.

7. Collect stool specimens.

8. Provide meticulous perianal skin care.

9. Monitor blood pressure to identify orthostatic hypotension.

10. Provide patient teaching covering:
    a. Adherence to medication regimen
    b. Appropriate sanitary methods for cooking and personal hygiene

X. Malabsorption syndrome

A. Description

1. Malabsorption syndrome refers to impaired absorption or digestion of nutrients secondary to altered digestion or nutrient transport, or to surgical interventions within the GI tract.

2. If untreated, it may lead to varying degrees of malnutrition.

B. Etiology

1. Malabsorption syndrome results from either impaired digestion or impaired absorption.

2. Impaired digestion can result from:
   a. Surgery (eg, gastrectomy)
   b. Deficiency of digestive enzymes (eg, bile salts, pancreatic or gastric enzymes)

3. Impaired nutrient transport across cell membranes of villi can result from:
   a. Genetic disorders (eg, lactase deficiency)
   b. Small bowel disease (eg, inflammatory bowel disease, celiac disease, tropical and nontropical sprue)
   c. Drug therapy
   d. Short bowel syndrome

4. Impaired nutrient transport from villi into lymphatic or circulatory systems can result from radiation enteritis or obstructive lymphatic disease.

C. Pathophysiologic processes and manifestations

1. Nutrient malabsorption is specific to each particular etiology.

2. Gastric surgery results in elimination of intrinsic factor secretion, which is necessary for vitamin B_{12} absorption.
3. Intestinal surgery, particularly the ileum, results in bile salt, vitamin, and nutrient malabsorption.
4. Bile salt deficiency results in malabsorption of fats and fat-soluble vitamins.
5. Pancreatic insufficiency results in carbohydrate, protein, fat, and vitamin B_{12} malabsorption.
6. Lactase deficiency (either from genetic predisposition or disease process) results in carbohydrate malabsorption.
7. Decreased intestinal peristalsis may result in bacterial overgrowth and subsequent breakdown of bile salts, which results in impaired fat and vitamin B_{12} absorption.
8. Intestinal mucosal alterations from sprue (tropical and nontropical) and inflammatory bowel disease result in the malabsorption of most nutrients.

9. **The degree of protein malabsorption correlates with degree of inflammatory bowel disease.**
10. Both protein and mineral loss occur with lymphatic obstruction.
11. Clinical manifestations depend on the type and etiology of malabsorption.

12. **Symptoms of malabsorption syndrome may include:**
    a. **Increased number of daily bowel movements**
    b. **Weight loss without a decrease in oral intake**
    c. **Decreased serum levels of vitamins, minerals, or albumin or total protein**
    d. **Signs associated with vitamin deficiencies (eg, easy bruising, anemia, bone pain) or protein loss (eg, edema)**

D. Overview of nursing interventions
   1. Administer enzyme replacements, antibiotics, vitamins, minerals, antidiarrheal agents, anticholinergics, or anti-inflammatory medications, as ordered.
   2. Institute dietary therapy to avoid or control symptoms (eg, lactose or gluten-free foods) and to supplement deficiencies (eg, high-protein or low-fat foods).
   3. Explain appropriate methods of oral intake to avoid dumping syndrome (eg, eat small, frequent meals; separate solids from liquids).
   4. Assess intake and output, particularly frequency, volume, and consistency of stools.

XI.   Ulcerative colitis

A. Description
   1. Ulcerative colitis is an inflammatory process affecting the mucosa and submucosa of the colon and rectum.
   2. The chronic condition is characterized by exacerbations and remissions of varying degrees of severity.

B. Etiology and incidence
   1. Although the cause of ulcerative colitis is unknown, factors associated with the disease include:
      a. Infection (bacterial, fungal, or viral)

      b.   Autoimmune dysfunction

      c.   Genetic predisposition

      d.   Psychological stressors

  2. Incidence is higher in young adults, ages 15 to 30.

  3. The disorder is more prevalent in Jewish population.

C. **Pathophysiologic processes and manifestations**

  1. Diffuse inflammation of the intestinal mucosa (commonly beginning in the rectosigmoid region) leads to swelling of epithelial cells, necrosis, and crypt formation.

  2. Crypts formed in the mucosa become the site for abscess formation, leading to mucosal ulceration and bleeding.

  3. Chronic condition leads to fibrous tissue deposition and narrowing of lumen.

  4. The most common symptom is bloody diarrhea (15 to 20 times daily), with or without the presence of pus; it is typically associated with abdominal pain and tenderness.

  5. Symptoms may also include:

      a.   Nausea

      b.   Vomiting

      c.   Fever

      d.   Loss of appetite

      e.   Weight loss

  6. Complications can range from chronic anemia and coagulation defects (secondary to poor absorption of vitamin K), to bowel perforation, fissure and fistula formation, and subsequent life-threatening peritonitis.

D. **Overview of nursing interventions**

  1. Administer medications (eg, antiinflammatory agents [corticosteroids], antimicrobial agents [Azulfidine, Flagyl], antidiarrheal agents, and antispasmodics), as ordered, to reduce inflammation, treat infection, and alleviate symptoms.

  2. Institute dietary alterations, depending on symptom severity, to provide bowel rest; changes may include:

      a.   Low-residue, lactose-free diet

      b.   Elemental-type diet (absorbed higher up in GI tract)

      c.   Parenteral nutrition (if diarrhea is severe)

  3. Observe intake and output, particularly bowel movement frequency and volume; facilitate collection of stool specimens.

  4. Monitor weight.

  5. Provide emotional support and instruct the patient in stress reduction activities, particularly if the patient associates oral intake with diarrhea.

  6. Prepare the patient for surgery (bowel resection), if the disease is severe and medical management has been unsuccessful or if complications occur (eg, obstruction, perforation, and peritonitis); nursing responsibilities include:

      a.   Administering antibacterial bowel preparation (eg, neomycin enemas)

      b.   Administering antibiotics, as ordered.

      c.   Monitoring vital signs

      d.   Managing fluids and electrolytes

      e.   Managing care of gastric drainage system

7. After surgery, provide appropriate postoperative care.
    a. Provide aseptic wound care.
    b. Manage fluids and electrolytes.
    c. Institute oxygenation.
    d. Provide pain management.
    e. Assess for return of normoactive bowel function or for abdominal complications (eg, paralytic ileus, wound evisceration).
    f. Instruct the patient in relaxation techniques.
    g. Manage ileostomy or colostomy; provide a referral to home health care services and local stomal support groups.
    h. Provide emotional support to help the patient cope with altered body image.

XII.   Regional enteritis (Crohn's disease)

A. Description
1. Regional enteritis is a chronic inflammatory bowel disease affecting segmental areas along the entire wall of the GI tract.
2. It most commonly is noted within the terminal ileum; lymphatics and the mesentery system may also be involved.
3. Similar to ulcerative colitis, it is characterized by repeated bouts of exacerbation and remission of varying degrees of severity.

B. Etiology and incidence

1. **Although the etiology is unknown, factors associated with the disorder include:**
    a. **Infectious process**
    b. **Allergy or immune disorder**
    c. **Lymphatic obstruction**
2. A genetic predisposition has been identified.
3. Incidence is higher in the Jewish population, affecting persons in the second through the fourth decades of life.

C. Pathophysiologic processes and manifestations
1. Characteristic cobblestone granulomas along the segment of involved GI tract assist in differentiating this disorder from ulcerative colitis.
2. Thickening and inflammation of the bowel also are present.

3. **Advanced disease can result in ulcerations and fistula tracts, which extend to the skin or to other organs (eg, bladder, vagina).**
4. Healing lesions result in scar tissue formation and subsequent obstruction of GI tract.
5. Diarrhea (approximately three to five times daily) occurs, usually without blood.
6. If the upper portion of the small intestine is involved, steatorrhea and subsequent fat-soluble vitamin deficiency may result.
7. Abdominal pain, if acute, may resemble the clinical picture of appendicitis and thus requires careful assessment. Pain may be colicky in nature and may precede (and be relieved by) a bowel movement.

8. Symptoms may also include:
   a. Weakness
   b. Malaise
   c. Nutritional alterations
   d. Weight loss
   e. Fever with leukocytosis (if abscess or fistula formation has occurred)

D. Overview of nursing interventions
   1. Administer drug therapy similar to that for ulcerative colitis (see Section XI, D); administer specific antibiotic therapy for patients with abscess or fistula formation.
   2. Institute diet therapy, ranging from avoiding foods that provoke symptoms to restricting oral intake to an elemental formula; with fistula formation, parenteral nutrition is usually indicated.
   3. Provide rigorous vitamin supplementation (eg, vitamin B_{12}, folic acid) if there is extensive small bowel involvement.
   4. Observe fluid and nutritional status.
   5. Monitor bowel movement consistency, frequency, and volume; facilitate collection of stool specimens, if applicable.
   6. Prepare the patient for surgery, if indicated (eg, presence of obstruction secondary to stricture formation, occurrence of perforation or peritonitis); afterward, provide appropriate postoperative care (refer to pre- and postoperative nursing interventions for ulcerative colitis, Section XI, D).
   7. Provide wound management with meticulous skin care; note that fistulas may necessitate placement of drains, skin barriers (eg, stomahesive or Duo-Derm®), or collection pouches.

 XIII. **Irritable bowel syndrome (IBS)**

A. Description
   1. IBS is a common digestive disorder also known as spastic bowel or mucus colitis.
   2. It is differentiated from ulcerative bowel disease because no inflammation or ulceration is present.

B. Etiology and incidence
   1. Although the cause of IBS is unknown, it is associated with such factors as:
      a. Emotional stress or anxiety
      b. Diverticulitis
      c. Intolerance to specific food substances such as gastric stimulants (eg, caffeine, spicy foods) or lactose
   2. Incidence of IBS is twice as common in women as in men; incidence also is higher among Caucasians and in the Jewish population.
   3. Onset commonly occurs in adolescence.

C. Pathophysiologic processes and manifestations
   1. Alterations in gastric motility and transit time in the absence of organic dis-

ease support the suggested etiologies of emotional stress and anxiety or food intolerance.

2. Affected persons can typically associate the oral intake of specific food types or an emotional situation with an exacerbation of symptoms.

3. Alterations in bowel function may fluctuate between constipation and diarrhea.

4. Diarrhea may be accompanied by abdominal cramps or pain, most commonly in the left lower quadrant; abdominal pain or cramping usually dissipates after elimination of gas or stool.

 5. **Other symptoms may include:**
   a. **Anorexia**
   b. **Fatigue**
   c. **Headache**

D. Overview of nursing interventions

1. Administer antidiarrheal agents, antispasmodics, and bulkforming laxatives, as ordered.

2. Encourage a high-fiber diet and avoidance of fatty foods and foods that produce bloating or gas (eg, carbonated beverages, cauliflower, beans).

 3. **Instruct the patient to avoid alcohol and tobacco.**

4. Encourage the patient to drink six to eight glasses of water daily to prevent constipation.

5. Help the patient identify an association between stressors and bowel changes.

 6. **Emphasize the importance of lifestyle changes (eg, exercising regularly, resting adequately, avoiding smoking, and using stress reduction techniques).**

XIV.   Diverticulitis

A. **Description: inflammation of diverticula or herniations within the wall of the intestinal tract**

B. **Etiology and incidence**

1. Diverticulitis results from increased intraluminal pressure (secondary to such factors as chronic constipation and obesity), which causes formation of diverticula (pocketing) or herniation through a muscular weakness in the intestinal wall. Note: diverticula refers to one pocket, diverticulosis refers to the condition, and diverticulitis is present when the diverticula are inflamed.

 2. **Inflammation of diverticula results from bacteria formed from trapped, undigested food particles.**

3. Increased incidence is associated with ulcerative colitis and Crohn's disease.

4. Diverticula occurs more commonly in the elderly, affecting less than 5% of persons younger than 40 years of age.

5. Diverticulitis develops in approximately 25% of persons with diverticula.

C. **Pathophysiologic processes and manifestations**

1. Diverticulitis most commonly occurs within the sigmoid colon.

2. Inflammation of diverticula may subsequently lead to local abscess development and/or perforation (Fig. 13-3).
3. Inflammatory processes lead to intraluminal wall thickening, which can also result in bowel obstruction.
4. The disorder may progress to intraabdominal perforation or to generalized peritonitis.

5. **Symptoms include:**
   a. **Pain or tenderness in left-lower quadrant**
   b. **Constipation**
   c. **Intermittent rectal bleeding**
   d. **Diarrhea (less common)**
   e. **Fever with an elevated WBC count (may be present)**
6. The danger of this condition is that rupture of a diverticula can occur and intestinal contents spill into the peritoneum, requiring temporary colostomy as the treatment. This is associated with ingestion of high-residue foods.

D. Overview of nursing interventions
   1. Administer medications (eg, broad-spectrum antibiotics, analgesics, antispasmodics) to treat infection, alleviate symptoms, and reduce inflammation.
   2. Institute dietary regimen.
      a. Provide low-fiber diet for acute inflammation.
      b. Gradually introduce high-fiber diet for asymptomatic patient.
      c. Eliminate foods with seeds, nuts, and popcorn, because seeds may deposit in the diverticula and cause rupture.
   3. Prevent increased intraluminal pressure in patients with chronic constipation by increasing dietary fiber and bran and encouraging intake of six to eight glasses of water daily.
   4. Observe fluid status, particularly frequency, volume, and consistency of stools; facilitate collection of stool specimens, if indicated.

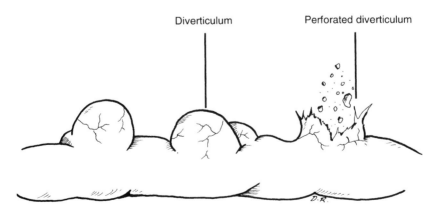

FIGURE 13-3.
Diverticulitis. Perforated diverticulum leaks bowel contents into the peritoneal cavity.

5. Prepare the patient for surgery (colostomy), if indicated, to divert fecal flow, particularly if diverticula perforation or advanced inflammatory process exists; afterward, provide appropriate postoperative care (refer to pre- and postoperative nursing interventions for ulcerative colitis, Section XI, D).

XV.   Appendicitis

A.   Description: inflammation of the vermiform appendix (near ileocecal valve); may lead to obstruction or perforation with subsequent peritonitis

B.   Etiology and incidence

1. Although the exact etiology of appendicitis is unknown, precipitating factors include:
    a. Fecal impaction
    b. Kinking of the appendix
    c. Parasites
    d. Infections

C.   Pathophysiologic processes and manifestations

1. Severity of symptoms is related to the degree of inflammation present.
2. The inflammatory process ranges from mild appendiceal swelling to severe appendiceal swelling and obstruction.
3. Concurrent infection can cause mucosal ulceration and subsequent development of abscess, necrosis, or rupture.
4. Typically, abdominal pain is present; it usually is described as being in the lower right quadrant, localized at McBurney's point.
5. Other common symptoms include anorexia, nausea, and vomiting; fever (usually low grade) and elevated white blood cell count (>10,000).

D.   Overview of nursing interventions

1. Prepare the patient for surgical removal of appendix (appendectomy) to avoid life-threatening complications of perforation and peritonitis; nursing responsibilities include:
    a. Administering antibiotics, as ordered
    b. Monitoring vital signs
    c. Managing fluids and electrolytes
    d. Managing care of gastric drainage system
2. Note that preoperative laxatives or enemas *are contraindicated* because they may precipitate appendix perforation.
3. After surgery, provide appropriate postoperative care.
    a. Provide aseptic wound care (postoperative incisional drains may be in place if abscess or perforation occurs).
    b. Manage fluids and electrolytes.
    c. Institute oxygenation.
    d. Provide pain management.
    e. Assess for return of normoactive bowel function or for abdominal complications (eg, paralytic ileus, wound evisceration).
    f. Instruct the patient in relaxation techniques.
4. If the diagnosis is not definitive, prepare the patient for an exploratory laparotomy.

XVI. Peritonitis

A. Description

    1. Peritonitis is an inflammation of the peritoneum that may be localized (eg, an abscess) or generalized.

    2. It may be primary or secondary.

B. Etiology

    1. *Primary peritonitis*

        a. Is an acute bacterial infection that invades the peritoneum by way of the vascular system

        b. May be associated with alcoholic cirrhosis and ascites, or with tuberculosis

    2. *Secondary peritonitis*

        a. **Occurs either from bile released into the peritoneum or secondary to trauma or perforation of the abdominal viscus from bacteria or chemical reactions to digestive enzymes; perforation may also be from trauma (penetrating wound), appendicitis, diverticulitis, peptic ulcer disease, mesenteric thrombosis, or small bowel disease (eg, volvulus, ileitis, gangrene)**

        b. Can also occur secondary to a ruptured bladder, ovary, or fallopian tube

C. Pathophysiologic processes and manifestations

    1. Manifestations are related to the specific etiology, extent of peritoneal involvement, and immunocompromised condition of the host.

    2. The inflammatory process, in conjunction with the body's natural defense mechanisms, causes the body to attempt to isolate the contaminants or irritants (eg, abscess or adhesion formation).

    3. If the defense mechanisms fail, diffuse peritonitis may result.

    4. **Symptoms may include:**

        a. **Nausea**

        b. **Vomiting**

        c. **Abdominal tenderness (commonly noted as rebound tenderness) and rigidity**

    5. Decreased peristalsis can lead to accumulation of gas and fluid (up to 8 L/day) and subsequent development of paralytic ileus.

    6. Bacterial translocation into the bloodstream and subsequent septicemia and septic shock may occur.

    7. Increased vascular permeability and fluid shifts may result in decreased circulatory fluid volume leading to decreased kidney perfusion and subsequent renal failure.

    8. Associated abdominal pain and increased abdominal distention can also result in respiratory complications.

    9. Elevated temperature and high WBC are prominent symptoms, unless the host is immunocompromised.

    10. The patient is often in the intensive care unit as this is a life threatening illness.

D.   Overview of nursing interventions

1.   **Administer medications (eg, broad-spectrum antibiotics, analgesics), as prescribed.**
2.   Institute intravenous electrolyte replacement therapy, as ordered.
3.   Prepare the patient for paracentesis (removal of peritoneal fluid by needle aspiration), if indicated, to determine the infectious process.
4.   Prepare the patient for surgery (eg, appendectomy, colostomy), if indicated; note that antibiotic irrigation of the peritoneum and placement of irrigation and drainage catheters may be performed.
5.   After surgery, provide appropriate postoperative care, including:
    a.   Providing aseptic wound care
    b.   Positioning the patient in semi-Fowler's to aid peritoneal drainage
    c.   Managing pain
6.   Monitor fluids and electrolytes.
7.   Monitor weight.
8.   Provide nutritional support, most likely parenteral nutrition.
9.   Provide meticulous oral hygiene.
10.   Provide patient teaching covering:
    a.   Dietary recommendations (depending on surgery and food tolerances)
    b.   Physical limitations (eg, lifting) and need to avoid straining of abdominal muscles for approximately 6 weeks postoperatively

XVII.   Pancreatitis

A.   Description: inflammation of the pancreas; may be acute or chronic
B.   Etiology: results from alterations in the structure or function of the pancreas, commonly caused by chronic alcohol abuse
C.   Pathophysiologic processes and manifestations

1.   **A disruption of the pancreatic ducts occurs, allowing pancreatic enzymes to spill out into the pancreatic tissues.**

2.   **The enzymes then work on the pancreatic tissues the way they work on food intended for digestion, resulting in autodigestion—the hallmark pathophysiologic process involved in pancreatitis.**
3.   Autodigestion causes edema, hemorrhage, and possibly necrosis in acute cases.
4.   Autodigestion may be so severe at times that the pancreatic enzymes spill over into the peritoneum and affect diaphragmatic excursion, causing adult respiratory distress syndrome (ARDS).
5.   During acute attacks, the process of autodigestion causes extreme incapacitating pain in the left upper quadrant.
6.   In chronic situations, this type of pain (although less severe) may be present after meals because eating triggers the digestive process; pain may radiate to the back.
7.   Pancreatic cysts containing pancreatic juices and blood may form on or around the pancreas.

8. Many symptoms depend on the disease's severity and progression; common manifestations can include:
   a. Fever
   b. High WBC
   c. Nausea
   d. Vomiting
9. Serum amylase levels are always high; this is the characteristic indicator of pancreatitis.
10. As the disease progresses, less functional pancreatic tissue is left.
11. As enzymes are released, fluid is lost; subsequent hypotension and shock may occur.
12. Pancreatitis may be life threatening as pancreatic juices spill on to the diaphragm making breathing impossible.

D. Overview of nursing interventions

1. **Prevent autodigestion by avoiding oral food intake (Oral intake stimulates the pancreas to secrete enzymes).**
2. Insert nasogastric tube during an acute attack, because oral intake precipitates an attack.
3. Relieve pain with Demerol; note that morphine *is contraindicated* because it causes spasm in the Sphincter of Oddi.

4. **Administer IV fluids and antibiotics, as ordered, to replace lost fluid volume and prevent infection.**
5. Monitor for signs of complications such as hypotension, tachycardia, tachypnea, and respiratory distress.

 XVIII. Oral cancer

A. Description
1. Oral cancer consists of cancer of the lips (most common site) and pharynx, including the tongue, soft palate, and uvula.
2. Classification of tumors is determined according to the extent of the tumor, lymph node involvement, and distant metastasis.

B. Etiology
1. Oral cancer is most commonly associated with overuse of tobacco (smoking or chewing) and alcohol.

   a. **Tobacco is the most significant factor associated with cancer of the tongue.**
   b. Chronic irritation from cigarette and pipe smoking is associated with lip cancer; approximately 90% of all lip cancers occur in the lower lip.
2. Malnourished and immunocompromised persons are also at higher risk.

C. Pathophysiologic processes and manifestations
1. Cancer of the lip usually manifests as a nonhealing blister or induration within an area of leukoplakia; the ulcerated lesion recurs and commonly develops into a secondary infection and necrosis. As the lesion advances in size, it may metastasize to the local and regional lymphatic system.

    2.   Tumors of the tongue are either papillary (exophytic) or infiltrative; infiltrative tumors will quickly spread to cervical lymph nodes, which are abundant in this area. Early lesions cause local irritation; if they become infected, pain and tenderness occur.

    3.   Advanced tumor involvement of the pharynx (including the tongue) leads to dysphagia, odynophagia, slurring of speech, and voice changes.

    4.   If the lesion involves blood vessels, bleeding occurs.

    5.   Weight loss is common because oral intake is typically compromised.

D.   **Overview of nursing interventions**

    1.   Prepare the patient for radiotherapy, if indicated (eg, superficial lip cancer).

    2.   Prepare the patient for surgery, if indicated (eg, extensive tumor involvement of oral cavity); radical neck dissection, modified according to the extent of the disease process, is performed in the presence of cervical lymph node metastasis.

    3.   Prepare the patient for other treatment modalities, including:

        a.   Combination radiotherapy with surgery (if metastasis has been identified)

        b.   Chemotherapy in combination with surgery and radiotherapy

    4.   Maintain patent airway.

    5.   Provide oral hygiene.

    6.   Provide pain management.

    7.   Ensure adequate nutrition.

    8.   Administer antibiotic therapy, as prescribed.

    9.   Provide supportive care, including emotional support to help the patient cope with an altered body image.

   10.   Provide patient teaching covering

        a.   Use of sunscreen and limiting sun exposure

        b.   Avoidance of tobacco and alcohol

        c.   Proper oral hygiene

XIX.   Esophageal cancer

A.   **Description**

    1.   Esophageal cancer is a malignant tumor of the esophagus; it is the most common cause of obstruction in the esophagus.

    2.   It is rarely detected early enough to respond successfully to medical or surgical intervention.

B.   **Etiology and incidence**

    1.   Esophageal cancer is associated with excessive alcohol and tobacco consumption.

    2.   It also is linked to a diet deficient in protein, fruits, and vegetables and high in contaminants such as nitrosamine.

    3.   It accounts for about 2% of all cancer deaths.

    4.   The risk for developing esophageal cancer increases in persons with a history of esophageal disorders, including achalasia and hiatal hernia.

    5.   Occurrence is twice as common in men as in women, particularly in those over age 40.

C. **Pathophysiologic processes and manifestations**
1. The earliest warning signal is dysphagia, initially to solids, then progressing to liquids.

 2. **Common tumor site is in the lower two thirds of esophagus.**
3. Common tumor type is squamous epidermoid; less commonly, adenocarcinoma.
4. The tumor quickly encircles the esophagus, invading the lymphatics, which are richly supplied within esophageal mucosa.

 5. **Progressive obstruction leads to pulmonary complications secondary to regurgitation, aspiration, or fistula formation.**

D. **Overview of nursing interventions**
1. Administer chemotherapeutic agents, analgesics, and antacids, as prescribed.
2. Prepare the patient for surgery, if indicated; esophagogastrostomy is the most common procedure, involving both thoracotomy and laparotomy incisions. After surgery, provide appropriate postoperative care, including:
    a. Managing wound care
    b. Observing for signs of complications (anastomosis leakage), including elevated temperature and symptoms of shock
3. Prepare the patient for radiation therapy if tumor involvement is in the upper third of the esophagus (usually nonresectable).
4. Prepare the patient for esophageal dilatation, which is usually necessary to decrease dysphagia.
5. Institute diet therapy, including a high-protein, high-calorie diet modified in texture and consistency as appropriate.
6. Institute tube feeding if dysphagia is significant; if enteral feeding is contraindicated, parenteral nutritional support is usually prescribed.
7. Provide emotional support and education to allay anxiety and encourage compliance to drug and dietary regimen.

XX. **Stomach cancer**

A. **Description: malignant tumor of the stomach**
B. **Etiology**
1. Although the etiology of stomach cancer is unknown, it is associated with conditions involving alterations in gastric mucosa (eg, pernicious anemia, achlorhydria, chronic gastritis, gastric polyps)
2. Other predisposing factors include:
    a. Genetic predisposition
    b. Diet rich in gastric irritants, such as spicy foods and alcohol
C. **Pathophysiologic processes and manifestations**
1. Adenocarcinoma is the most common type of carcinoma, usually manifesting within pyloric and antral regions of stomach.
2. The disease usually is asymptomatic until the advanced stage, at which point it spreads within the regional lymphatics and adjacent organs, or within the peritoneum via seeding.

3. Initial symptoms are vague and include:
   a. Weakness
   b. Loss of appetite
   c. Weight loss
   d. Gastric discomfort (eg, belching, nausea)
4. Pain usually indicates advanced disease.

D. Overview of nursing interventions

1. Prepare the patient for surgery (subtotal gastrectomy or total gastrectomy [esophagojejunostomy], if tumor involvement is in the upper cardia); nursing responsibilities include:
   a. Providing nutritional support
   b. Managing gastric drainage system
   c. Providing meticulous oral hygiene
2. After surgery, provide appropriate postoperative care including:
   a. Assessing and monitoring for complications
   b. Managing gastric drainage system
   c. Monitoring fluids and electrolytes
   d. Instituting oxygenation
   e. Administering analgesics, antiemetics, and vitamin and mineral supplements, as ordered.
   f. Providing nutritional support
   g. Assessing for signs of fat malabsorption
3. Prepare a patient with metastases for radiation and chemotherapy.
4. Provide pain management for a patient with the advanced stage of the disease.

XXI.   Intestinal cancer

A. Description

1. Intestinal cancer refers to a malignancy of either the small or large intestine (Fig. 13-4).
2. *Cancer of the small intestine*
   a. Tumor type is most commonly adenocarcinomas; less frequently carcinoids, lymphomas, and sarcomas
   b. Small intestine malignancies account for approximately 1.5% of GI neoplasms.
3. *Cancer of the large intestine*
   a. Tumor type is nearly always (95%) adenocarcinoma; infrequently carcinoid, lymphoma, and leiomyosarcoma
   b. Large intestine malignancies account for approximately one third of all GI neoplasms.

B. Etiology

1. *Cancer of the small intestine*
   a. Etiology is unknown.
   b. Incidence is low compared to other cancers.
2. *Cancer of the large intestine*
   a. Etiology is unknown.

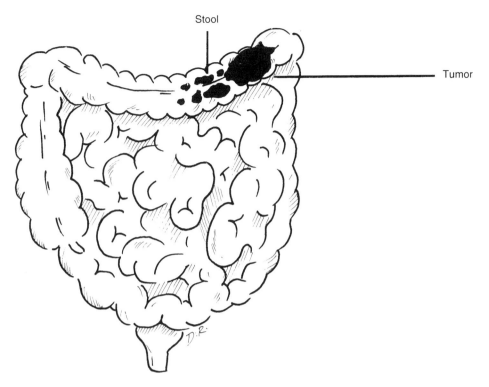

FIGURE 13-4.
Intestinal cancer. Cancer of transverse colon with bowel contents obstructed by tumor.

    b.   A strong correlation exists between this type of cancer and a low-fiber, high-fat diet.

    c.   Increased incidence is found in persons with a history of ulcerative colitis, Crohn's disease, adenomas, or polyps (particularly familial polyposis) and a history of breast or genital cancer.

C.   **Pathophysiologic processes and manifestations**

    1.   Both small and large intestinal carcinomas grow slowly; symptoms usually are absent until the tumor is extensive.

    2.   Metastasis of small intestinal carcinoma will most likely affect the peritoneum and mesentery.

    3.   Metastasis of large intestinal tumor is likely to involve the lymphatics, liver, and lung tissue.

    4.   Staging of the tumor (according to extent, lymph node involvement, and distant metastasis) is an important determinant of treatment and prognosis.

    5.   Severity of symptoms depends on the location and extent of tumor involvement.

    6.   Small intestine and ascending colonic masses rarely show clinical manifestations (because intestinal contents are in liquid form) unless obstruction occurs.

7. The most common symptom is rectal bleeding; consistency (frank bleeding with the presence of clots or occult bleeding) depends on the tumor location.

 8. Progressive constipation with a change in stool shape (eg, flattened, ribbon-shaped) may be noted.

 9. Other symptoms include anemia, nausea, anorexia, and weight loss.

10. Abdominal distention, discomfort, or pain occurs with tumor advancement.

11. When the flow of intestinal fluid through the bowel is obstructed by tumor growth, the fluid backs up.

12. Intestinal destruction is evidenced by abdominal distention, reduced or absent bowel sounds, and fecal-smelling vomitus.

D. Overview of nursing interventions

1. Administer medications (analgesics, chemotherapeutic agents, antiemetics, stool softeners, and preoperative antibiotic therapy, if indicated), as prescribed.

2. Prepare the patient for chemotherapy, if indicated, to reduce symptoms and limit metastasis; may be used in conjunction with surgery.

3. Prepare the patient for radiation therapy, if indicated; may be used pre- and postoperatively or as a palliative measure to alleviate pain, reduce hemorrhage and obstruction, or limit metastasis.

4. Prepare the patient for surgery, if indicated; procedures may include:
   a. Small bowel resection, which may necessitate an ileotransverse colostomy
   b. Colonic resection and anastomosis, which usually result in continuation of natural defecation functions; a temporary colostomy may be performed if colonic obstruction or perforation occurs

5. Provide appropriate pre- and postoperative care (refer to nursing responsibilities for appendicitis, Section XV, D).

6. Provide nutritional support.

7. Observe frequency, volume, and consistency of stools.

8. Provide emotional support to help the patient cope with changes in body image and ostomy care needs.

9. Instruct the patient to observe for signs of tumor reoccurrence (eg, blood in the stool, changes in bowel habits) and to seek medical attention, if indicated.

Bibliography

Bullock, B. (1996). *Pathophysiology: Adaptations and alterations in function* (4th ed.). Philadelphia: Lippincott.

Champion, G. L., & Richter, J. E. (1993). Atypical presentation of gastroesohageal reflux disease: chest pain, pulmonary, and ear nose and throat manifestations. *Gastroenterologist*, Mar 1(1):18–33.

Ganong, William F. (1997). *Review of medical physiology* (18th ed.). Stamford CT: Appleton and Lange.

Gaynor, E. B. (1991). Otolaryngologic manifestations of gastroesophageal reflux. *American Journal of Gastroenterology*. 86(7):801–8.

Guyton, Arthur C. and Hall John E. (1996). *Textbook of medical physiology*. (9th ed.). Philadelphia: W. B. Saunders.

Ignatavicius, D. D., & Bayne, M. V. (1991). *Medical surgical nursing: A nursing process approach*. Philadelphia: W. B. Saunders.

Kinney, M., Packa, D., & Dunbar, S. (1993). *AACN's clinical reference for critical-care nursing* (3rd ed.). St. Louis: C. V. Mosby.

McCance, K. L., & Huether, S. E. (1994). *Pathophysiology: The biologic basis for disease in adults and children* (2nd ed.). St. Louis: Mosby-Year Book.

Patrick, M. P., Woods, S. L., Craven, R. F., Rokolsky, J. S., & Bruno, P. M. (1991). *Medical surgical nursing: pathophysiologic concepts* (2nd ed.). Philadelphia: J. B. Lippincott.

Phipps, W. J., Long, B. C., Woods, N. F., & Cassmeyer, V. L. (1991). *Medical surgical nursing: concepts and clinical practice* (4th ed.). St. Louis: Mosby-Year Book.

Porth, C. (1994). *Pathophysiology: Concepts of altered health states* (4th ed.). Philadelphia: Lippincott.

Saxton, D. F., Nugent, P. M., & Pelikan, P. K. (1993). *Mosby's comprehensive review of nursing* (14th ed.). St. Louis: Mosby-Year Book.

STUDY QUESTIONS

1. A dietary regimen that includes a high-protein and high-fat diet, avoidance of concentrated sweets, separation of solids from liquids, and six frequent small feedings is most likely to be recommended for clients with which of the following disorders?
   a. Crohn's disease
   b. dumping syndrome after gastrectomy
   c. esophageal diverticulitis
   d. stomatitis

2. Follow-up care for a patient after total gastrectomy should include assessment for signs of pernicious anemia because:
   a. absorption of B complex takes place in the stomach
   b. the extrinsic factor is no longer produced by the gastric mucosa
   c. absence of hydrochloric acid prevents folic acid absorption
   d. the intrinsic factor necessary for absorption of vitamin B_{12} is diminished or no longer secreted

3. After gastrectomy, a vagotomy is performed to:
   a. decrease hydrochloric acid secretion and decrease gastric motility
   b. decrease hydrochloric acid secretion and increase gastric motility
   c. increase hydrochloric acid secretion and decrease gastric motility
   d. increase hydrochloric acid secretion and increase gastric motility

4. Crohn's disease is differentiated from other inflammatory bowel disorders by which characteristic finding?
   a. diarrhea
   b. malabsorption of nutrients
   c. bowel segments that are cobblestonelike in appearance
   d. absence of inflammation or ulceration

5. Symptoms of an esophageal hiatal hernia include all of the following *except:*
   a. malabsorption
   b. dysphagia, or difficult swallowing
   c. pyrosis, or heartburn
   d. chest pain, with shortness of breath

6. Mr. Edgegrove, a 46-year-old traveling salesman, has been admitted for upper GI bleeding secondary to a gastric peptic ulcer. When taking his patient history, the nurse should note which important etiologic clue?
   a. recent foreign travel
   b. less-than-adequate intake during traveling periods
   c. medications currently consumed
   d. high-fat diet

7. Mr. Edgegrove is being discharged on medication and diet specific for peptic ulcer disease. The nurse would instruct him to report any stools that appear:
   a. tarry or black
   b. floating
   c. clay colored
   d. frothy

8. Drugs such as neomycin and sulfasuxidine are administered before a surgical colostomy to:
   a. prevent electrolyte depletion
   b. reduce bacterial count in the colon
   c. promote a laxative effect
   d. elicit an antiinflammatory response

9. An elemental diet is primarily prescribed for a patient with inflammatory bowel to promote:
   a. repletion of protein stores via a high-protein diet
   b. supplementation of vitamins and minerals (increased losses are associated with diarrhea)
   c. nutrient absorption within the upper GI tract
   d. nutrient absorption by way of the lower intestinal tract

10. The *primary* reason to position a patient with peritonitis in semi-Fowler's position is to:
    a. encourage coughing and deep breathing:

    b. facilitate drainage of the peritoneal cavity

    c. reduce the likelihood of decubitus ulcer formation

    d. aid in gastric suction

11. Gastrointestinal disorders worsen when alcohol and/or tobacco are used. Avoidance of these substances is part of the treatment for:

    a. Crohn's disease

    b. ulcerative colitis

    c. diverticulitis

    d. all of the above

12. Physiological and inflammatory processes such as canker sore, HSV lesion, and candidiasis are manifestations of:

    a. gastritis

    b. stomatitis

    c. achalasia

    d. peptic ulcer disease

13. Which of the following patients identified by the nurse is at greatest risk for colon cancer?

    a. Crohn's disease

    b. low-fiber/high-fat diet

    c. ulcerative colitis

    d. all of the above

14. Preoperative interventions for the patient undergoing appendectomy for appendicitis include all of the following *except:*

    a. administer antibiotics

    b. monitor vital signs and laboratory studies

    c. administer preoperative laxatives or enemas

    d. provide IV fluids and electrolytes, as ordered.

ANSWER KEY

Question	Correct answer	Correct answer rationale	Incorrect answer rationales
1.	b	Patients who exhibit dumping syndrome after gastrectomy require this type of dietary regimen to avoid the physiological responses (eg, weakness, flushing, sweating, and faintness) secondary to the rapid emptying of gastric contents into the small bowel. A high fat diet is necessary for energy requirements and to delay transit time. High-protein intake is necessary for energy and tissue repair.	a. Crohn's disease, if acute, may necessitate an elemental diet. c. Avoidance of spicy foods and nuts or seeds is usually advocated with a diagnosis of esophageal diverticulitis. d. The dietary regimen for stomatitis is as tolerated.
2.	d	Intrinsic factor is present in stomach mucosa and is responsible for vitamin B_{12} absorption in the small bowel.	a. B-complex is not absorbed in stomach. b. Extrinsic factor is not present in stomach mucosa, but is present in food. c. The presence or absence of hydrochloric acid does not affect folic acid absorption.
3.	a	A vagotomy is performed to negate the effects of the vagal nerve, which stimulates hydrochloric acid secretion and gastric motility.	b, c, and d. These responses are incorrect.
4.	c	A cobblestone-like inflammatory process interspersed throughout sections of the bowel mucosa is a significant finding and serves to diagnose Crohn's disease.	a and b. Diarrhea and malabsorption of nutrients are common to all inflammatory bowel diseases. d. The absence of inflammation or ulceration is consistent with the diagnosis of irritable bowel syndrome.
5.	a	Malabsorption is not associated with an esophageal hiatal hernia; it is characteristic of disorders of the gastric or intestinal tract.	b, c, and d. Dysphagia, pyrosis, and chest pain that mimics angina are commonly noted complaints in a person with an esophageal hiatal hernia.
6.	c	The patient's current medication regimen, particularly if it includes drugs such as ASA and corticosteroids, can cause damage to the stomach lining and be a causative factor for upper GI bleeding.	a. A history of recent foreign travel might provide etiologic information for a patient with an inflammatory intestinal process. b. A poor intake does not predispose a person to peptic ulcer disease. d. A high-fat diet is not associated with gastric irritation.

Question	Correct answer	Correct answer rationale	Incorrect answer rationales
7.	a	Tarry or black stools (melena) suggest bleeding of the upper GI tract.	b and d. Floating or frothy stools may result from steatorrhea (high fecal fat content). c. Clay-colored stools may be related to biliary disease and decreased bile in the stool.
8.	b	The administration of drugs such as neomycin or sulfasuxidine before a surgical colostomy is primarily to reduce the bacterial count in the colon, which, in turn, reduces the likelihood of postoperative infection.	a, c, and d. Neither of these two drugs prevents electrolyte depletion, produces a laxative effect, or elicits an anti-inflammatory response.
9.	c	Although an elemental diet provides adequate protein, vitamins, and minerals, it is primarily prescribed for a patient with inflammatory bowel disease for nutrient absorption higher up in the GI tract, thus placing the colon at rest and allowing the lower GI tract to heal.	a. An elemental diet is not considered to be a particularly high-protein diet b. Supplementation of vitamins and minerals is not the optimal rationale of diet choice. d. Nutrient absorption by way of the lower intestinal tract would not place the colon at rest.
10.	b	The primary reason to position a person with a diagnosis of peritonitis in semi-Fowler's position is to localize infection in the pelvic area.	a. The ability to cough and deep-breathe is not limited to semi-Fowler's position. c and d. These responses are incorrect.
11.	d	Crohn's, ulcerative colitis, diverticulitis, irritable bowel, Cancer of the large intestine, and GI disorders are always made worse by the use of alcohol and tobacco.	
12.	b	Stomatitis is an inflammatory disorder of the oral cavity characterized by canker sores, type I and II HSV and oral candidiasis.	a, c, and d. These are not conditions related to these manifestations.
13.	d	Increased incidence found in persons with Crohn's disease, history of ulcerative colitis, adenomas or polyps, and history of breast or genital cancer. A strong correlation exists between the type of intestinal cancer and low-fiber/high-fat diets.	
14.	c	Laxatives and enemas are contraindicated because they may precipitate appendix perforation.	a, b, and d. These statements are true.

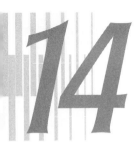

Renal Disorders

I. Overview of pathophysiologic processes

A. Infectious disorders

1. Infections of the kidney are disorders that result from hematogenous spread of bacteria or from organisms that ascend from the urethra.

 2. **Infections can alter the metabolic functions of the renal system.**

3. Glomerulonephritis and pyelonephritis are examples of infectious renal disorders.

4. The most common causative organism is *Escherichia coli; Pseudomonas* and *Staphylococcus* also are causative agents.

 5. **Risk factors for renal infection include:**
   a. **Immunosuppression**
   b. **Infections of the reproductive tract or lower urinary tract (more likely to occur if the urinary tract is prone to any abnormality in structure [ie, insertion of Foley catheter, instrumentation, congenital defects]).**

B. Nephrotic syndrome

1. Nephrotic syndrome is a group of symptoms associated with increased glomerular permeability.

 2. **The primary symptoms are proteinuria, hypoproteinemia, and edema.**

3. Many different types of kidney disease, such as glomerulonephritis, present as nephrotic syndrome.

4. There are no risk factors for nephrotic syndrome.

C. Renal failure

1. Renal failure occurs when the kidneys are unable to filter and excrete wastes, regulate blood pressure, and balance fluids, electrolytes, and acids and bases.

2. Renal failure may be acute or chronic.

3. Some forms of acute renal failure are reversible, but many are not. Chronic renal failure is not reversible.

4. Causes of renal failure are classified into three categories:
   a. *Pre-renal* causes result from pathology to the renal blood supply. Examples include aortic surgery, renal vascular stenosis, blood clots or tumors that obstruct renal blood flow, blood loss, shock from any cause. Pre-renal azotemia refers to the accumulation of nitrogenous wastes from pre-renal causes. Pre-renal pathology may be reversible.
   b. *Intra-renal* (also known as renal parenchymal or "renal" causes) describes pathology to the actual renal tissue from a disease process. Examples include diabetes (known as diabetic nephropathy), hypertension, polycystic disease, and amyliodosis, secondary to other diseases (such as systemic lupus erythematosus).
   c. *Post-renal* causes or obstructive uropathy, describe disorders that occur in the genitourinary tract below the level of the kidneys effecting urine flow. As the urinary stream is obstructed urine stays in the renal pelvis causing hydronephrosis. The occurrence of renal failure depends upon the actual cause and severity of the obstructive process. Causes of obstruction include renal stones, tumors, congenital defects, and inflammation. Uremic syndrome describes the group of symptoms present in every body system associated with waste products.

D. Fluid and electrolyte disorders
1. Fluid and electrolyte disorders are imbalances of the body's electrolytes in which either excesses or deficiencies exist.
2. Electrolyte disorders may result from diseases of the renal, cardiac, gastrointestinal, pulmonary, endocrine, and integumentary systems.
3. Electrolyte disorders are significant because electrolytes play a crucial role in cardiac, nerve and muscle cell contraction.
4. Normal electrolyte balance is required to maintain normal acid-base balance.
5. The balance of fluids and electrolytes is required for a state of homeostasis to exist.
6. Risk factors for fluid and electrolyte disorders in general include:
   a. Conditions in which electrolyte intake is either excessive or insufficient
   b. Conditions in which electrolyte elimination is either excessive or insufficient

E. Kidney cancer
1. Renal cell carcinoma refers to cancer of the kidney.
2. Like all cancers, the severity depends on the size of the tumor and presence of metastases.
3. Although tumors occur in one kidney, metastases may be rapid because the kidney is a highly vascular organ.
4. Renal cell carcinoma tends to occur in the fifth and sixth decade.
5. There are no particular risk factors for kidney cancer.

II. Physiologic responses to renal dysfunction

A. Pain
1. Pain may or may not be present; it can be described as dull or constant (when present in the flank).

2. Pain in other areas, such as the joints, may result from kidney disease if metabolic processes are affected.

B. Hematuria (bloody urine)
1. Hematuria with red blood cell casts indicates that blood has passed through the tubule; this condition is considered an emergency.
2. High-grade proteinuria (3 to 4+) suggests a glomerular pathologic process.

C. Uremia: presence of abnormal levels of urea and other nitrogenous products in the blood; results from renal failure. Every body system is effected.

D. Muscle weakness: may occur secondary to electrolyte imbalances, atrophy, and collection of uremic toxins.

E. Electrolyte and acid–base imbalances: occur in renal failure; most common ones are metabolic acidosis and hyperkalemia.

F. Fluid imbalances
1. Excessive fluid retention may cause systemic and pulmonary edema.
2. Salt and water retention from reduced glomerular filtration rate (GFR) leads to hypertension and edema.

G. Neurologic alterations
1. Neurologic alterations include decreased level of consciousness, somnolence, coma, changes in cognitive function and behavior, asterixis, and seizures.
2. These alterations result from electrolyte imbalances and emotional factors.

H. Gastrointestinal disturbances
1. Uremia manifests as gastrointestinal signs and symptoms, most commonly nausea and vomiting.
2. Other symptoms may include hematemesis, anorexia, melena, uremic fetor, and stomatitis.

I. Integumentary responses
1. The skin may appear sallow yellow due to urochrome retention.
2. Pruritus may also be associated with hyperphosphatemia that results from renal failure.

J. Cardiovascular responses: may include extracellular volume expansion (causing hypertension, and later, pulmonary edema), pericarditis with fever, chest pain, and pericardial rub. Dysrhythmias often occur from electrolyte imbalances (especially potassium and calcium), or coexisting cardiac disease.

K. Dyspnea (difficult breathing)
1. Dyspnea that results from pulmonary edema represents an emergency that may require hemodialysis for effective fluid removal.
2. Alterations in the respiratory system (sputum changes, depressed cough reflex, and altered white blood cell response) make the lungs susceptible to infection, causing dyspnea due to pneumonia.

III. Glomerulonephritis

A. Description
1. Glomerulonephritis is an inflammatory disorder involving the glomerulus.
2. Types of glomerulonephritis include:
    a. Acute poststreptococcal: Onset is abrupt, typically occurring 7 to 10 days after a streptococcal throat or skin infection.

  b. Chronic glomerulonephritis: Occurs when glomerular disease leads to chronic renal failure

3. Glomerular lesions may assume any shape or form; the type of lesions present often determines the course and severity of the disease.

B. **Etiology: glomerulonephritis is caused by an immune reaction to the presence of an infectious organism, usually group A beta-hemolytic *Streptococcus***

C. **Pathophysiologic processes and manifestations**

1. An antigen (usually group A beta-hemolytic *Streptococcus*) enters the blood, and an antigen–antibody complex is formed.

 2. **This complex deposits in the glomerulus, forming anti-GBM (glomerular basement membrane) antibodies.**

3. The extent of damage and subsequent symptoms depend on the location and length of exposure the glomerulus has to the antigen–antibody complexes.

4. When the antigen–antibody complex is formed, inflammation and activation of chemical mediators (complement and leukocytes) occur.

5. **Complement, leukocytes, and lysosomal enzymes migrate to the area and attack the glomerular basement membrane.**

6. As a result, membrane permeability is altered, permitting red blood cells and protein to pass through the glomerulus into the urine, but making normal glomerular filtration impossible (Fig. 14-1).

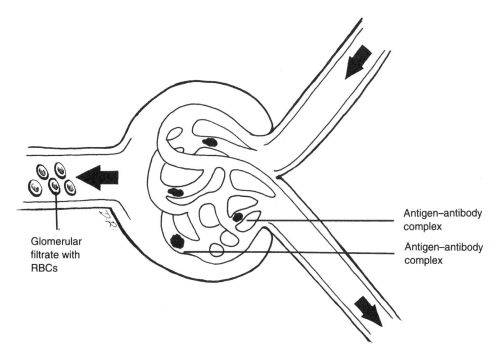

FIGURE 14-1.
Glomerulonephritis. Antigen–antibody complexes obstruct glomerular blood flow allowing red blood cells (RBCs) to leave the filter and enter the tubule.

7. These changes lead to acute or chronic renal failure, which could result in chronic renal failure.
8. Manifestations include
    a. Acute onset of hematuria
    b. Red blood cell casts
    c. Proteinuria
    d. Decreased glomerular filtration rate (GFR)
    e. Oliguria
    f. Edema (commonly occurs around the eyes, but may involve dependent areas such as the feet and ankles)
    g. Hypertension
9. Other symptoms depend on the original disease.

D. **Overview of nursing interventions**
1. Assess and monitor renal functions to determine the severity of renal disease; assess results from serum creatinine and blood urea nitrogen (BUN) tests.
2. Determine treatment by noting the degree of renal failure and severity of symptoms.
3. Observe for signs and symptoms of infection; avoid exposing the patient to persons with infections.
4. Limit sodium, potassium, fluid, and protein intake.
5. Prepare the patient with acute renal failure for dialysis, as indicated.
6. Measure fluid retention by daily weights.

IV. Pyelonephritis

A. **Description: infection of the kidney tissue and pelvis that occurs from several sources; may be acute or chronic**

B. **Etiology**
1. Pyelonephritis typically is caused by bacteria, but may result from fungi or viruses.
2. *Acute pyelonephritis* results from bacterial contamination by way of the urethra or from instrumentation. Bacterial invasion may also occur as organisms travel through the blood from another infected area to the kidneys; this is known as hematogenous spread.

 3. *Chronic pyelonephritis* **may be idiopathic or may occur in association with obstruction or reflux due to kidney stones or neurogenic bladder.**

C. **Pathophysiologic processes and manifestations**
1. The onset of symptoms is usually acute. Symptoms result from infection of the renal parenchyma and can include:
    a. Fever
    b. Chills
    c. Groin or flank pain
    d. Urinary frequency
    e. Dysuria
    f. Costovertebral tenderness
2. Bacteriuria may or may not be associated with these symptoms.
3. Infection of the renal parenchyma triggers an inflammatory response.

4. Because metabolic function is disturbed and infection is present, fatigue occurs.
5. The presence of a urinary tract obstruction will prevent bacteria elimination in the normal urine flow, resulting in progressive inflammation that causes fibrosis and scarring. The more inflammation that is present, the worse the symptoms are.
6. Diagnosis of chronic pyelonephritis is commonly established by intravenous pyelogram and ultrasound, which reveal a small density with a characteristic "clubbing" of the affected calyx.
7. Obstructive uropathy, glomerulonephritis, diabetes mellitus, polycystic kidney disease and renal calculi appear to lower the kidney's resistance to infection, making the person at high risk for infection.

D. Overview of nursing interventions
1. Administer antimicrobial agents, as ordered, and observe the patient for side effects.
2. Encourage high-normal fluid intake, 2 to 3 L daily (when possible).
3. Encourage bedrest during the acute phase to reduce the metabolic rate and rest the kidneys.
4. Assess the patient's need for analgesics to relieve pain.
5. Monitor the patient's intake, output, weight, temperature, pulse, respirations, and blood pressure to assess volume status.

V. Nephrotic syndrome

A. Description: a group of symptoms associated with the protein loss that occurs with various renal disorders

B. Etiology: results from the presence of other primary diseases, such as diabetes, amyloidosis, and systemic lupus erythematosus

C. Pathophysiologic processes and manifestations

1. **Injury to the glomerular membrane results in plasma protein loss by way of leakage from the blood through the glomerulus into the urine. Protein loss often exceeds 3.0 to 3.5 g/day.**
2. Because albumin is plentiful and of a low molecular weight, it is the primary protein lost.
3. Immunoglobulins, which also are proteins, are lost, lowering resistance to infection.
4. Hypoalbuminemia and hyperlipidemia result from protein loss.

5. **Protein loss also facilitates third spacing of fluid because blood vessels become more porous. This leads to soft, pitting edema, which may be noted in the feet, legs, sacrum, or in the periorbital area.**
6. Protein loss may also lead to vitamin D deficiency because the hormone required for its activation (25-hydroxycholecalciferol) is usually bound to protein.

D. Overview of nursing interventions
1. Determine treatment by noting the actual cause and severity of disease.
2. Provide the patient with a high-protein, low-salt, diet.
3. Administer diuretics, as ordered.

4. Observe carefully for signs of hypovolemia and hypokalemia.
5. Observe for and treat symptoms of renal failure.

VI. Acute renal failure (ARF)

A. Description

1. Acute renal failure is a sudden and almost complete loss of kidney function associated with azotemia (an accumulation of nitrogenous wastes in the blood) that is not due to extrarenal factors.
2. ARF can be acute or chronic; the acute syndrome, unlike the chronic syndrome, is usually reversible. The creatinine clearance (a measure of glomerular filtration) drops suddenly.
3. Classifications of ARF are:
   a. Prerenal
   b. Intrarenal
   c. Postrenal

B. Etiology

1. Prerenal ARF results from a prolonged deficit in renal blood flow for any reason (hypovolemia, aortic stenosis, hypotension, renal artery disease).
2. Intrarenal ARF refers to damage to the renal parenchyma (glomerulonephritis, acute tubular necrosis [ATN], diabetic nephropathy, pyelonephritis, drug induced).
3. Diagnostic tests requiring the use of dye may precipitate ARF because the dye is nephrotoxic.
4. Postrenal ARF is caused by an obstruction to urine outflow (renal stones, tumors, ureteral kinks, instrumentation).

C. Pathophysiologic processes and manifestations

1. The condition that most commonly causes ARF is ATN; it can be grouped into five phases:
   a. Onset phase: the period from the precipitating event to the onset of oliguria or anuria
   b. Oliguria-anuria phase: the period (usually 8 to 15 days) during which output is less than 400 mL/day (30 mL/hour). A longer duration leads to a poor prognosis. This is the phase where toxins (which are acids) accumulate, measured by the rising BUN and creatinine. Metabolic acidosis occurs from accumulation of acid end-products
   c. Early diuretic phase: extends from the time daily output is greater than 400 mL/day to the time that BUN values stop rising
   d. Late diuretic or recovery phase: extends from the first day BUN falls to the day it stabilizes or is in the normal range
   e. Convalescent phase: extends from the day BUN is stable to the day urine volume is normal and the patient returns to normal activity
2. The pathologic changes in dye-induced ARF are similar to those for ATN.
3. In intrarenal ARF, BUN and creatinine rise in a 10:1 to 15:1 ratio (eg, BUN 30: creatinine 3.0; BUN 40: creatinine 4.0).
4. In prerenal ARF, BUN levels rise in a proportion far greater than 10:1 to 15:1 (eg, BUN 60: creatinine 2.0).

D. Overview of nursing interventions

1. Prepare the patient for dialysis.

2. Monitor fluids, electrolytes, and acids and bases. (Hyperkalemia and metabolic acidosis is often fatal.)
3. Observe patient for fluid overload (common and can result in pulmonary edema).
4. Control by fluid balance delivering vital medications and nutrition through fluid administration.
5. Monitor cardiac status.
6. Administer medications to control symptoms, as ordered.
7. Note that uremic toxins are hard to control if conditions of cellular destruction are present (burns, surgery, bleeding).

VII. **Chronic renal failure**

A. **Description**
1. Chronic renal failure is a slow, insidious, and irreversible impairment of renal function.
2. Various processes that occur in the course of renal disease permanently destroy nephrons.
3. As excessive amounts of nitrogenous wastes (BUN, creatinine) accumulate in the blood, the kidneys are unable to maintain homeostasis.
4. Chronic renal failure progresses in three stages:
   a. Diminished renal reserve
   b. Renal insufficiency
   c. Endstage renal disease

B. **Etiology: causes include glomerular disorders, tubular disorders, vascular diseases, infectious or interstitial disorders, ureter obstruction, collagen-related diseases, metabolic disorders, congenital disorders, and nephrotoxicity (Display 14-1).**

C. **Pathophysiologic processes and manifestations**
1. Renal dysfunction causes numerous metabolic disruptions, such as pH changes and fluid and electrolyte imbalances.
2. Because vitamin D cannot be converted to its biologically active form (needed for calcium reabsorption), calcium levels drop from poor absorption.
3. Phosphorus excretion is lowered with poor renal excretory capabilities, leading to hyperphosphatemia.

4. **In the first stage of renal failure,** *diminished renal reserve,* **renal function is reduced, but no metabolic wastes accumulate. The healthier kidney compensates for the diseased one.**
5. In the second stage, *renal insufficiency,* metabolic wastes accumulate in the blood because the affected nephrons can no longer compensate. The degree of insufficiency, determined by decreasing GFR, is classified as mild, moderate, or severe. As GFR decreases, symptoms of renal failure increase.
6. In the final stage, *end-stage renal disease,* excessive amounts of metabolic wastes accumulate in the blood. The kidneys are unable to maintain homeostasis—a life-threatening condition.

D. **Overview of nursing interventions**
1. Institute dialytic therapies.
2. Teach the patient about drugs and therapies that will be used.

DISPLAY 14-1
Causes of Chronic Renal Failure

Glomerular diseases
- Can involve a single histologic alteration or a combination of alterations
- Include cellular proliferation, basement thickening, leukocyte exudation, sclerosis, and hyalinization.

Tubular disorders
- Can affect proximal tubules, altering the kidneys' reabsorption capabilities
- Can affect distal tubules, altering secretion and excretion

Vascular diseases
- Involve changes in the renal vessels, primarily the arteries and arterioles `
- Occlude the renal vessels as a result of thrombus formation, emboli, or from progressive vessel narrowing

Infectious or interstitial diseases
- Are characterized by inflammation of the interstitium, with accompanying cellular exudate, which progresses toward renal tissue destruction

Ureter obstruction
- Can result in hydronephrosis
- May be caused by tumors, renal calculi, inflammation associated with infection, fibrous bands that obstruct the ureteropelvic junction, or prostatic valves

Collagen-related diseases
- Are multisystem diseases
- Cause renal damage as the result of antigen-antibody complex disposition (as in systemic lupus erythematosus) and vascular changes such as inflammation, arterial narrowing, and necrosis

Metabolic disorders
- Can cause changes in one or all of the renal structures
- Include diabetes mellitus (which can cause structural changes in the blood vessels and tubular system) and amyloidosis (which primarily affects the glomeruli by causing basement membrane thickening)

Congenital disorders
- May be fatal, or may not cause renal dysfunction until later in life
- Result in structurally nonfunctional tissue, leading to diminished renal reserves and, eventually, altered renal status

Nephrotoxicity
- Causes renal problems as a result of exposure to nephrotoxic agents, most commonly radiographic contrast media and aminoglycosides
- May also be iatrogenic

3. Monitor fluids, electrolytes, intake, and output carefully.
4. Manage symptoms as they occur.
5. Recognize the severity of the disease and understand that the psychological treatment is as important as the medical management.

VIII.   Uremic syndrome

A. Description: a group of symptoms that occur in association with renal failure

B. **Etiology: results from the accumulation of metabolic waste products due to renal failure**

C. **Pathophysiologic processes and manifestations**

　　1.　Acid waste products accumulate from lack of excretion, and the buffering mechanisms fail due to renal failure.

　　2.　Waste accumulation also is coupled with the inability to balance fluids and electrolytes.

　　3. **The severity of symptoms depends on the extent of renal failure and the rise of uremic toxins; the higher the toxins the more severe the symptoms (Fig. 14-2).**

　　4.　Symptoms can include:

　　　　a.　Altered central nervous system function (dizziness, vertigo, and poor concentration)

　　　　b.　Neuropathy of the lower extremities (due to middle molecule accumulation on the peripheral nerves)

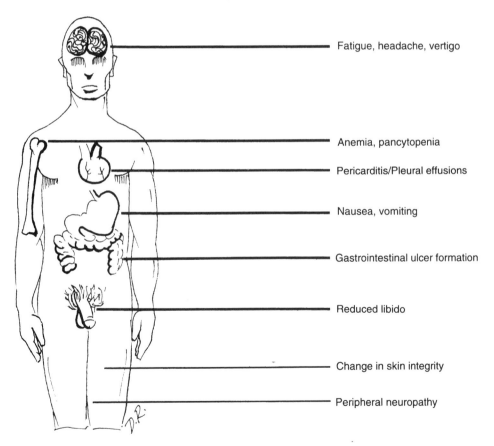

FIGURE 14-2.
Uremic syndrome. Uremic syndrome causes symptoms in every body system.

    c.   Ulceration in the gastrointestinal tract from the mouth all the way to the anus

    d.   Nausea and vomiting

    e.   Hypertension (due to accelerated renin secretion)

    f.   Pruritus and altered skin color (due to retained urochrome pigments)

    g.   Calcium and phosphorus imbalances leading to calcium phosphate precipitation (calcium deposits)

    h.   Acid–base and fluid and electrolyte imbalances

    i.   Poor blood clotting (due to inability of thrombocytes to move well and function in acid plasma)

    j.   Immunosuppression (due to hindered phagocytosis)

    k.   Pericarditis, which may lead to effusion and tamponade

  5. Symptoms are reversible when dialytic therapies are instituted.

D. **Overview of nursing interventions**

  1. Prepare the patient for hemodialysis or peritoneal dialysis to replace kidney functioning.

  2. Restrict the patient to a low-protein diet.

  3. Institute measures to manage symptoms.

  4. **While treating the patient, remember that symptoms are present in every body system and are minimized by reducing levels of uremic toxins. However minimizing symptoms requires a therapy so strict it is almost impossible to adhere to.**

IX. Diabetic nephropathy (diabetic glomerulosclerosis)

A. **Description: kidney failure due to diabetes mellitus**

B. **Etiology**

  1. Diabetic nephropathy is caused by lesions of the arterioles and glomeruli.

  2. It is associated with resulting pyelonephritis and necrosis of the renal papillae.

  3. A significant complication of diabetes mellitus, it has an adult onset.

C. **Pathophysiologic processes and manifestations**

  1. The glomeruli are affected by diffuse sclerosis and thickening of the basement membrane and mesangium.

  2. Both afferent and efferent arterioles are affected by thickened walls and hyaline deposits.

  3. As a result, GFR decreases and azotemia occurs.

  4. Symptoms of diabetic nephropathy may not manifest for years after diabetes develops.

  5. All persons with insulin-dependent diabetes can expect to develop diabetic nephropathy. Once proteinuria occurs, renal changes invariably progress.

  6. A diabetic person may appear to have uremia at GFR levels higher than a nondiabetic person.

D. **Overview of nursing interventions**

  1. Monitor electrolyte studies, observing for any abnormal values, especially K^+ and Ca^+ levels.

  2. Assess fluid volume status by observing for tachycardia, venous jugular distention, rales, and dyspnea.

3. Monitor intake and output.
4. Ensure time for sleep and rest.
5. Develop an educational plan for a patient with end-stage renal disease.
6. Treat the same as renal failure.

X. Obstructive uropathy

A. Description
1. Obstructive uropathy occurs when urine flow is obstructed as it exits from the kidney toward the bladder.
2. As a result, urine backs up from the point of the obstruction back toward the pelvis and into the kidney.

B. Etiology
1. The most common cause of obstructive uropathy is the presence of a calculus.
2. It may also result from:
   a. Congenital kinks in the ureter
   b. Tumors

C. Pathophysiologic processes and manifestations
1. Stones are aggregates of substances such as calcium or uric acids; they are formed from metabolic causes.
2. Stones tend to be painful and may cause hematuria. Costovertebral tenderness also is noted.
3. Some stones are small enough to pass through the urinary tract; others may obstruct the flow of urine through the urinary tract.
4. As the flow of urine is obstructed, it backs up into the kidney, causing hydronephrosis.
5. The fluid causes pressure on the tubules and damages the nephrons' structures.
6. Because the obstruction is usually unilateral, the urinalysis will be normal; the glomerular filtration rate may be normal as well.
7. Initially, the kidneys increase in size, then shrink.

D. Overview of nursing interventions
1. Assist with measures to relieve the obstruction (eg, insertion of nephrotomy tube or lithotripsy).
2. Monitor the patient for dehydration and electrolyte imbalances, because massive diuresis may occur as the obstruction is relieved.

XI. Fluid and electrolyte disorders

A. Description: conditions characterized by excesses or deficits of body fluids and electrolytes; commonly occur in renal failure

B. Etiology
1. Fluid and electrolyte excesses result from excessive intake or decreased output, from any cause.
2. Fluid and electrolyte deficits result from poor intake or excessive output, from any cause.
3. Fluid and electrolyte changes also occur from shifts that occur with various health disorders.

C.   Pathophysiologic processes and manifestations

1.   Alterations in the normal balance of fluids and electrolytes result in changes in the conduction of nerve and muscle cells.

2.   Manifestations include changes in mental status and in reflex response.

3.   Neuromuscular symptoms also may be present and can include paresthesia, numbness, tingling, and tremors.

4.   In the presence of renal failure, the glomerulus and tubules lose their ability to regulate electrolytes.

5.   In general, symptoms depend upon which electrolyte is effected, and how severe the alteration.

D.   Overview of nursing interventions

1.   Institute replacement therapy for a patient with a fluid or electrolyte deficit.

2.   Administer Lasix, as prescribed, for a patient with a fluid or electrolyte excess.

3.   Treat underlying cause of the disorder.

XII.   Renal cell carcinoma

A.   Description: malignant kidney tumors

B.   Etiology

1.   Renal cell carcinoma results from unknown causes.

2.   It accounts for the majority of kidney cancers.

C.   Pathophysiologic processes and manifestations

1.   The tumor may arise anywhere in the kidney.

2.   Due to its increasing mass, the tumor may compress surrounding tissue, causing ischemia, necrosis, and hemorrhage.

3.   Tumors may invade the collecting system and branches of the renal vein, even extending into the inferior vena cava.

4.   Metastasis can occur at any stage; primary sites are the lungs, liver, lymph nodes, and bones.

5.   Renal cell carcinoma metastasizes to all visceral organs.

6.   Staging of renal cell carcinoma is as follows:

    a.   Stage I: Tumor is confined within the kidney capsule.

    b.   Stage II: Tumor invades through the renal capsule but remains within the surrounding fascia.

    c.   Stage III: The regional lymph nodes, renal vein, or vena cava are involved.

    d.   Stage IV: Distant metastases occur.

    e.   Display 14-2 describes staging for renal tumors in more detail.

D.   Overview of nursing interventions

1.   Institute interventions depending on the selected treatment modality.

2.   Prepare the patient for surgery, if indicated; afterward, provide appropriate postoperative care.

3.   Monitor closely fluid and electrolyte status, intake and output, and acid–base balance.

4.   Follow appropriate cancer care protocols.

DISPLAY 14-2
TNM Classification for Tumors of the Kidney

Primary Tumor (T)

TX   Minimum requirements cannot be met

T0   No evidence of primary tumor

T1   Small tumor, minimal renal and caliceal distortion of deformity; circumscribed neovasculature surrounded by normal parenchyma

T2   Large tumor with deformity or enlargement of kidney or collecting system

T3A Tumor involving perinephric tissues

T3B Tumor involving renal vein

T3C Tumor involving renal vein and infradiaphragmatic vena cava

Note: Under T3 tumor may extend into perinephric tissues, into renal vein, and into vena cava as shown on cavography. In these instances, the T classification may be shown as T3A, B, and C, or some appropriate combination, depending on extension (*e.g.,* T3A–B is tumor in perinephric fat and extending into renal vein).

T4A Tumor invasion of neighboring structures (e.g., muscle, bowel)

T4B Tumor involving supradiaphragmatic vena cava

Nodal Involvement (N)

The regional lymph nodes are the paraaortic and paracaval nodes. The juxtaregional lymph nodes are the pelvic nodes and the mediastinal nodes.

TX   Minimum requirements cannot be met

N0   No evidence of involvement of regional nodes

N1   Single, homolateral regional nodal involvement

N2   Involvement of multiple regional or contralateral or bilateral nodes

N3   Fixed regional nodes (assessable only at surgical exploration)

N4   Involvement of juxtaregional nodes

Note: If lymphography is course of staging, add *1* between *N* and designator number; if histologic proof is provided, + if positive, and—if negative. Thus, *N1+* indicates multiple positive nodes seen on lymphography and proved at operation by biopsy.

Distant Metastasis (M)

MX   Not assessed

M0   No (known) distant metastasis

M1   Specify

Specify sites according to the following notations: Pulmonary, PUL; osseous, OSS; hepatic, HEP; brain, BRA; lymph nodes, LYM; bone marrow, MAR; pleura, PLE; skin, SKI; eye, EYE; other, OTH.

Note: Add "+" to the abbreviated notation to indicate that the pathology (p) is proved

(*Source:* DeVita, V. T., Hellman, S., and Rosenberg, S. A. *Cancer Principles and Practice of Oncology* (4th ed.). Philadelphia: J. B. Lippincott, 1993.)

Bibliography

Boggs, R., & Wooldridge, M. (Eds.). (1993). *American Association of Critical Care Nurses.* (3rd ed.). Philadelphia: W. B. Saunders.

Brenner, B. (Ed.) (1996). *Brenner and Rector's The Kidney* (5th ed.). Philadelphia: W. B. Saunders.

Brundage, D. J. (1992). *Renal disorders.* St. Louis: Mosby-Year Book, Inc.

Bullock, B. (1996). *Pathophysiology: Adaptations and alterations in function* (4th ed.). Philadelphia: Lippincott-Raven.

Ganong, William F. (1997). *Review of medical physiology* (18th ed.). Stamford, CT: Appleton and Lange.

Guyton, Arthur C., & Hall John E. (1996). *Textbook of medical physiology* (9th ed.). Philadelphia: W. B. Saunders.

Ignatavicius, D. D., & Bayne, M. V. (1991). *Medical surgical nursing: A nursing process approach.* Philadelphia: W. B. Saunders.

Kinney, M., Packa, D., & Dunbar, S. (1993). *AACN's clinical reference for critical-care nursing* (3rd ed.). St. Louis: C.V. Mosby.

McCance, K. L., & Huether, S. E. (1994). *Pathophysiology: The biologic basis for disease in adults and children* (2nd ed.). St. Louis: Mosby-Year Book.

Porth, C. (1994). *Pathophysiology: Concepts of altered health states.* (4th ed.). Philadelphia: Lippincott-Raven.

Thelan, L. A., Davie, J. K., et al. (1994). *Critical care nursing: Diagnosis and management* (2nd ed.). St. Louis: Mosby-Year Book.

STUDY QUESTIONS

1. Hypocalcemia may develop in a patient with which of the following conditions?
  a. chronic renal failure
  b. hyperparathyroidism
  c. thiazide therapy
  d. vitamin D overdose

2. Which of the following conditions would cause prerenal failure?
  a. diabetes
  b. glomerulonephritis
  c. acute tubular necrosis
  d. hypovolemia

3. Abnormal serum laboratory findings common to patients with acute renal failure are:
  a. increased potassium, BUN; decreased creatinine
  b. increased potassium, creatinine; decreased BUN
  c. decreased potassium; increased BUN, creatinine
  d. increased potassium, BUN, creatinine

4. In the diuretic phase of acute tubular necrosis (ATN), the nurse must be alert for which of the following complications?
  a. fluid overload
  b. hypokalemia
  c. hypertension
  d. hypernatremia

5. The primary acid–base disorder associated with renal failure is:
  a. respiratory acidosis
  b. metabolic acidosis
  c. respiratory alkalosis
  d. metabolic alkalosis

6. Patients with acute renal failure (ARF) may have all of the following complications except:
  a. peaked T-waves on ECG and pericarditis
  b. sinus tachycardia and ST elevations
  c. heart failure and friction rub
  d. mitral insufficiency and Mobitz type-II heart block

7. A patient's glomerular filtration rate (GFR) can be measured by evaluating:
  a. serum creatinine
  b. blood urea nitrogen
  c. serum osmolarity
  d. creatinine clearance

8. The mechanism of obstruction or reflux leading to chronic pyelonephritis may include all of the following except:
  a. presence of stones
  b. hypovolemia
  c. hypertension
  d. streptococcal infection

9. Loss of which of the following is a major factor in the pathophysiology of nephrotic syndrome?
  a. potassium
  b. protein
  c. urea
  d. sodium

10. The renal symptoms of glomerulonephritis is caused by:
  a. streptococcal infections causing inflammation
  b. complement migration to the glomerulus and tubules
  c. elimination of protein stores through proteinuria
  d. destruction of basement membrane by anti-GMB antibodies

11. When assessing a patient for possible kidney stones, the nurse should examine for:
  a. breath sounds
  b. hypercalcemia
  c. costovertebral tenderness
  d. hypervolemia

12. Hypoalbuminemia, hyperlipidemia, edema, are signs of:
  a. pyelonephritis
  b. uremia
  c. nephrotic syndrome
  d. renal failure

ANSWER KEY

Question	Correct answer	Correct answer rationale	Incorrect answer rationales
1.	a	Hypocalcemia occurs in renal failure and is due to the inability of the diseased kidneys to excrete phosphorus. As serum phosphorus levels increase, calcium decreases.	b, c, and d. These responses do not cause calcium deficiency.
2.	d	Causes of prerenal failure include factors that interfere with renal perfusion, such as hypovolemia.	a, b, and c. These are associated with the development of renal parenchymal failure.
3.	d	Laboratory studies in acute renal failure typically include elevated BUN, creatinine, and potassium levels.	a, b and c. See above.
4.	b	Hypokalemia can result from excessive loss during diuresis.	a. Fluid depletion, not fluid overload, would result. c. Blood pressure would decrease as fluid volume decreases. d. Hyponatremia occurs with diuresis.
5.	b	Metabolic acidosis occurs with renal failure; it results from the kidneys' inability to excrete hydrogen ions and conserve bicarbonate.	a and c. Respiratory conditions are not involved. d. Metabolic alkalosis results when there is an excess of bicarbonate.
6.	d	Mitral insufficiency and Mobitz type II heart block are not associated with ARF.	a, b, and c. These are potential complications of ARF.
7.	d	Creatinine clearance provides an evaluation of GFR; the creatinine clearance increases as renal function diminishes.	a, b, and c. These are indicators of renal function but not GFR.
8.	a	The presence of stones may result in chronic pyelonephritis.	b, c, and d. Hypovolemia, hypertension, and streptococcal infection are not etiologies associated with the development of pyelonephritis.
9.	b	Loss of protein facilitates third-spacing of fluids, hypoalbuminemia, hyperlipidemia, and vitamin D deficiency.	a, c, and d. These are not factors in the pathophysiology of nephrotic syndrome.
10.	d	In response to the group A beta-hemolytic streptococcus antigen/antibody complex, the anti-GBM antibody is formed.	a. This initial infection does not cause the actual damage to the kidneys. b. The complement system is activated by the anti-GBM antibodies.

Question	Correct answer	Correct answer rationale	Incorrect answer rationales
			c. Proteinuria is a symptom, not cause of the disease.
11.	c	Costovertebral tenderness is often a finding when stones are present.	a. Breath sounds will not reveal any information regarding stones. b. Hypercalcemia cannot be revealed during an examination c. Hypervolemia may be present in renal failure, but that is not the situation described.
12.	c	These symptoms are consistent with nephrotic syndrome.	a, b, and d. Other symptoms are more pronounced in these conditions.

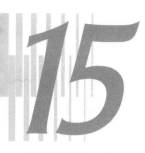

Genitourinary Disorders

I. Overview of pathophysiologic processes

A. Restrictive diseases

1. Restrictive diseases are those disorders that result in inadequate bladder emptying; micturition reflex is activated by the stretch receptors of the bladder. Bladder contraction and internal sphincter relaxation cause bladder emptying.

2. Normally, urinary volume in the bladder (approximately 250 mL) stimulates the urge to void; voiding empties the bladder and prevents overstretching of its walls.

3. Restrictive diseases can result from interstitial urinary tract disease and from obstructive causes, including:
    a. Congenital malformations
    b. Strictures
    c. Benign prostatic hypertrophy
    d. Tumors
    e. Calculi

4. **Restriction also can occur as a result of pregnancy, decreased muscle tone secondary to aging, abdominal surgery, trauma, and administration of anticholinergic medications and antihistamines.**

5. Restrictive diseases include urinary retention and urinary reflux.

6. **Persons at risk for restrictive diseases include:**
    a. **Postoperative patients who are unable to void due to the effects of anesthesia**
    b. **Middle-aged males with benign prostatic hypertrophy, which can impinge on bladder emptying and stretch the bladder**
    c. **Persons with chronic urinary tract infections, which can cause edema and prevent complete bladder emptying.**

B. Obstructive diseases

1. **Obstructive diseases include any disorders that prevent urinary flow and elimination as a result of mechanical obstruction:**
    a. **Sudden obstruction secondary to nephrolithiasis can result in acute illness.**
    b. **Chronic obstruction can be caused by increased cellular growth (benign tumors) and renal and bladder cancer.**

2. Alterations in urinary pH can increase the risk for urinary precipitates.
    a. Alkaline urine increases calcium and phosphate stone formation.
    b. Acidic urine precipitates uric acid and cystine stones.

3. Chronic urinary tract infections (caused by *Proteus* organisms) produce urea-splitting bacteria which alter urinary pH and cause stone formation.
4. Metabolic disorders, such as gout, increase uric acid formation, which can precipitate into stones.
5. Urolithiasis (renal calculi) is classified as an obstructive disease.
6. **Factors that increase the risk for stone formation include:**
    a. **Dietary intake of excessive protein, calcium, and oxalate**
    b. **Warm temperatures due to seasonal changes, which increase urinary concentration**
    c. **Family history of nephrolithiasis and gout**

C. Urinary incontinence
1. Urinary incontinence results in involuntary release of urine and the inability to retain urine.
2. Conditions that contribute to urinary incontinence include:
    a. Renal parenchymal conditions that decrease bladder capacity
    b. Relaxed pelvic muscles associated with obesity
    c. Neurologic impairments

D. Urinary tract infection (UTI)
1. UTIs include infections of the urethra, bladder, and kidney.
2. UTIs are classified as:
    a. Upper (involving the kidney)
    b. Lower (involving the bladder and urethra)
3. Common UTIs include pyelonephritis (kidney), cystitis (bladder), and urethritis (urethra).
4. **Risk factors for UTIs include:**
    a. **Stasis**
    b. **Strictures**
    c. **Structural abnormalities**
    d. **Obstructive conditions**
    e. **Metabolic diseases (eg, diabetes mellitus, gout, and renal disease)**

E. Neurologically related urinary disease
1. **Neurologically related urinary disease refers to a bladder dysfunction that results from neurologic damage.**
2. Spinal cord lesions above S-2 (upper motor neuron damage) destroy the cortical control to inhibit the voiding reflex, resulting in hypertonicity and incontinence.
3. Lower motor neuron damage to the cauda equina or sacral segments of the spinal cord result in flaccid bladder, urinary retention, and urinary incontinence secondary to overflow.
4. Neurogenic bladder is a neurologically related urinary disease.
5. **Risk factors for neurogenic bladder include:**
    a. **Spinal cord disease or injury**
    b. **CNS disorders**

F. Urinary tract cancer
1. Urinary tract cancer includes tumors and malignancies of the bladder and kidneys.

2. It may occur without significant damage or symptoms; advanced malignancies can lead to hematuria, pain, anemia, and obstruction.

3. **Risk factors for urinary tract cancer include:**
   a. **History of cigarette smoking**
   b. **Exposure to carcinogens**
   c. **Genetic predisposition**

II. Physiologic responses to urinary dysfunction

A. **Alterations in urinary pattern: urinary symptoms of frequency, hesitancy, or changes in urinary stream or urgency (with or without incontinence)**

B. **Alterations in urinary consistency**
   1. Urine color can indicate hydration status.
      a. Clear dilute urine often indicates a state of good hydration, with particles diluted in the urine.
      b. Dark amber urine indicates a dehydrated state in which the body conserves water, allowing only small amounts to be eliminated in the form of urine; dark urine may also result from metabolic conditions (eg, liver or bile duct disease).
   2. Hematuria (blood in the urine) can result from irritation due to bacteria (infection), causing tissue edema and injury.
   3. Pyuria (pus in urine) can indicate infection.

C. **Alterations in urine output**
   1. Urinary volume reflects the body's ability to eliminate volume and wastes.
   2. Urinary output decreases in obstructive and restrictive disorders; residual urine after voiding indicates retention.

D. **Pain**
   1. Dysuria (pain associated with voiding) can occur secondary to infection, obstruction, and retention.
   2. Costovertebral angle (CVA) tenderness or flank pain is indicative of kidney inflammation and edema related to upper UTI; it can be elicited by fist percussion to the posterior CVA margin.

E. **General symptoms**
   1. Changes in body weight and hypertension secondary to fluid retention can indicate obstruction.
   2. Symptoms of acute renal failure can indicate kidney damage secondary to restrictive, obstructive, and infectious urinary conditions (see Chapter 14, Renal Disorders, for more information).

III. Urinary retention

A. **Description: retention of urine in the bladder, with the inability to eliminate urinary volume**

B. **Etiology**
   1. Urinary retention can result from mechanical or functional obstruction.
   2. Mechanical obstruction exists when urine flow is blocked.
      a. Urethral strictures and spinal cord and urinary tract malformations can structurally impede urinary flow and elimination.

        b.   Calculi, tumors, inflammation, pregnancy, and trauma can cause secondary mechanical urinary retention.

    3.   Functional obstruction exists when there is a decrease in muscular control and release of urine.

        a.   Neurogenic bladder, detrusor muscle bladder atrophy, and decreased peristaltic activity contribute to structural urinary retention.

        b.   Anxiety and medications such as anesthetics, narcotics, sedatives, and antihistamines can contribute to impaired sphincter relaxation and retention.

C.   **Pathophysiologic processes and manifestations**

    1.   As the bladder becomes distended with urine, it becomes palpable; percussion of a distended bladder will produce a "kettledrum" sound.

    2.   Detrusor muscle nerve endings are stimulated as the bladder fills.

    3.   Symptoms of restlessness and diaphoresis can occur secondary to the patient's urgency to void but inability to eliminate urine.

    4.   Urinary retention can lead to overflow. Frequent voiding of very small amounts (25 to 50 mL) decreases the intravesicular pressure caused by bladder overdistention; however, the bladder continues to retain urine until obstruction is relieved.

D.   **Overview of nursing interventions**

    1.   Monitor for signs and symptoms of retention (eg, inability to void, bladder distention, and decreased urination).

    2.   Relieve primary obstruction by inserting a Foley or straight catheter.

    3.   Instruct patient/family on catheter insertion when indicated.

    4.   Maintain hydration.

    5.   Administer antispasmodics, as prescribed, to relieve spasms and pain.

IV. Urinary reflux

A.   **Description: a backflow of urine from the bladder into the ureter and renal pelvis**

B.   **Etiology**

    1.   Urinary reflux results from weakness or incompetency at the ureterovesical junction, allowing backflow of urine into the kidney.

    2.   Ureterovesical junction incompetence can occur secondary to structural malformation, infection, neurologic impairment, or urinary obstruction.

C.   **Pathophysiologic processes and manifestations**

    1.   Urinary stasis and reflux of bacteria into the kidney can lead to infection.

    2.   Bladder distention with residual urine can increase urgency and micturition; as a result, bladder total volume increases as does the threshold triggering the voiding reflex.

    3.   Renal failure symptoms can occur secondary to chronic reflux and subsequent kidney damage.

D.   **Overview of nursing interventions**

    1.   Relieve bladder distention by intermittent or continuous urinary catheterization.

    2.   Monitor for signs and symptoms of urinary tract infection (see Section VIII, C).

3. Hydrate the patient to promote urinary flow.
4. Prepare the patient for surgical reimplantation of ureter, if indicated; after surgery, provide appropriate postoperative care.
5. Teach the patient hygiene measures to prevent infection (eg, wiping from front to back and wearing cotton undergarments).

V. Urolithiasis (renal calculi)

A. **Description:** formation of stones in the urinary tract secondary to precipitates caused by calcium, urinary stasis, altered purine metabolism, or genetic predisposition

B. **Etiology**
1. Urinary pH influences stone formation.
   a. Low urinary pH precipitates calcium and phosphate stone formation.
   b. High urinary pH precipitates uric acid and cystine formation.
2. Other factors that influence stone formation include:
   a. Diet high in calcium and protein
   b. Urinary stasis
   c. Dehydration (which increases urinary concentration)

C. **Pathophysiologic processes and manifestations**
1. Manifestations of urolithiasis can include:
   a. Costovertebral angle tenderness due to inflammation and edema.
   b. Infection and fever due to urinary stasis and retention.
   c. Decreased urinary output with complaints of urgency, burning, and frequency
   d. Bladder distention due to obstruction of urinary flow.
2. If the obstruction causes kidney damage, impaired renal function secondary to hydronephrosis (backflow of urine from the point of obstruction into the ureters and kidneys) may occur.

D. **Overview of nursing interventions**
1. Increase fluid intake 1 to 3 L daily to dilute urine.
2. Strain urine to isolate the type of stone.
3. Encourage the patient to ambulate, unless contraindicated, to promote passage of the stone.
4. **Administer narcotic analgesics, as prescribed, because the pain of kidney stones can be horrific.**
5. Provide dietary counseling to prevent recurrent stone formation.
   a. Encourage an acid ash diet for calcium or phosphate stones.
   b. Encourage an alkaline ash diet for uric acid or cystine stones.
   c. Encourage a low-purine diet for uric acid stones.
6. Prepare the patient for surgery to remove stone, if indicated, including nephrolithotomy (kidney stone), pyelolithotomy (renal pelvis stone), ureterolithotomy (ureter stone), and cystostomy (bladder calculi); after surgery, provide appropriate postoperative care, including increasing the patient's activity to promote mobility and prevent urinary stasis.
7. Prepare the patient for lithotripsy (ultrasonic shock wave therapy to disintegrate stones), if indicated; afterward, administer antibiotics to prevent infection, as ordered.

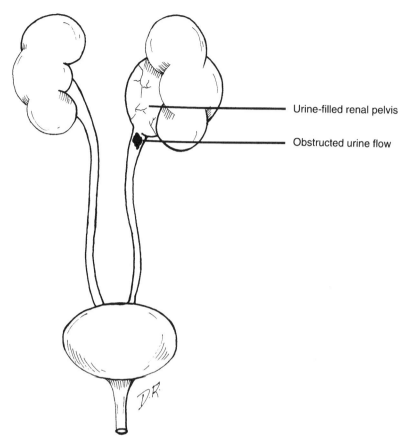

Urine-filled renal pelvis

Obstructed urine flow

FIGURE 15-1.
Urolithiasis. Obstructed urine flow backs up into the kidney causing hydrone-phrosis.

VI.　**Urinary incontinence**

A.　**Description**
　　1.　Urinary incontinence is the involuntary expulsion of urine; it may be temporary or permanent.
　　2.　It has both physiologic and psychological effects.
　　3.　Types of urinary incontinence include:
　　　　a.　*Stress incontinence:* involuntary voiding of small amounts of urine
　　　　b.　*Urge incontinence:* involuntary urination that occurs soon after the urgency to void is present
　　　　c.　*Reflex incontinence:* involuntary control of urination at intervals once a certain bladder volume is reached
　　　　d.　*Functional incontinence:* involuntary urination related to cerebral confusion and inability to recognize the urge to void.
　　　　e.　*Overflow incontinence:* continuous loss of urine

B. Etiology

1. *Stress incontinence* results from weak pelvic muscles, obesity, or incompetence of the bladder sphincters.

2. *Urge incontinence* is associated with decreased bladder capacity, bladder retention, increased fluid intake and infection.

3. *Reflex incontinence* is associated with spinal cord injuries and neurologic disorders.

4. *Functional incontinence* is related to cerebral confusion and ignorance of the urge to void.

5. *Overflow incontinence* results from abnormal bladder emptying; usually this occurs due to neurologic disorders (such as spinal cord lesions) or obstructions (such as urethral strictures or enlarged prostate). Send patient for appropriate consultation.

C. Pathophysiologic processes and manifestations

1. In *stress incontinence,* sudden increases in intraabdominal pressure (due to coughing, lifting, or straining) force urine out through the sphincter.

2. In *urge incontinence,* the patient feels the urge to void and is unable to hold the urine in the bladder.

    a. In cases of neurologic impairment, the bladder may contract uncontrollably, causing incontinence.

    b. When the bladder is irritated from infection or tumor formation, involuntary bladder contraction may occur, resulting in incontinence.

3. In *reflex incontinence,* the nervous system mechanism responsible for sphincter relaxation and bladder contraction is damaged, causing the sphincter to open.

4. In *functional incontinence,* the lower urinary tract may be intact, but other factors result in incontinence. These factors include:

    a. Inability to identify the need to void (as seen with Alzheimer's patients)

    b. Inability to reach the toilet (as seen with elderly patients placed on bedrest)

5. In *overflow incontinence,* the urine stream is steady, but the bladder never completely empties. This results in overdistention with urine leaking out constantly.

D. Overview of nursing interventions

1. Help the patient maintain urinary control.

    a. Instruct the patient to heed the urgency to void.

    b. Establish a urinary elimination pattern.

2. Institute bladder training.

3. Encourage increased fluid intake (3 L daily), unless contraindicated, to stimulate voiding reflex.

4. Limit caffeine intake.

5. Allow the patient to express feelings of embarrassment and provide emotional support.

6. Assure the patient that you will assist with achieving continence, when possible.

VII. Urinary tract infection (UTI)

A. Description

1. UTIs include infections of the kidney (pyelonephritis), bladder (cystitis), and urethra (urethritis).
2. UTIs can be classified as upper (kidney) or lower (bladder, urethra).

B. Etiology and incidence

1. UTIs are caused by bacteria, usually *E. coli.*
2. Pyelonephritis results from the spread of bacteria into the bloodstream, urinary reflux, obstruction, or ascending UTI.
3. Cystitis has been associated with obstructive urinary conditions such as benign prostatic hypertrophy. It occurs more commonly in women because of their shorter urethra, which allows contamination from the rectum and bladder secretions to travel upward.
4. Urethritis is associated with bacterial and viral infections.
5. Other factors that contribute to UTIs include:
   a. Stasis
   b. Urinary retention and bladder distention
   c. Instrumentation of the urinary tract (eg, cystoscopy, catheterization)
   d. Poor hygiene
   e. Fecal incontinence
   f. Sexual transmission of bacteria

C. Pathophysiologic processes and manifestations

1. Bacterial and viral transmission can occur through the lower urinary tract; if not adequately treated, infection can spread to the upper urinary tract. Infection begins with urethral invasion with bacteria that rapidly ascends to the bladder.
2. **Manifestations of *pyelonephritis* can include:**
   a. **Symptoms of infection such as chills, fever, dysuria, and urinary frequency**
   b. **CVA tenderness as the result of edema and inflammation of the kidney**
   c. **Cloudy, foul-smelling urine; antibody-coated bacteria can be isolated in the urine specimen**
3. Manifestations of *cystitis* and *urethritis* are similar and can include:
   a. Urinary frequency, urgency, and dysuria resulting from bacterial irritation of mucosa
   b. Suprapubic pain resulting from inflammation and edema
   c. Hematuria and pyuria resulting from irritation and elimination of bacteria (may be present)
4. Cystitis and urethritis may be asymptomatic; diagnosis results from urine specimen analysis.

D. Overview of nursing interventions

1. Administer appropriate antimicrobial agent, as prescribed.
2. Maintain hydration to dilute urine bacterial count and flush metabolites from the antimicrobials.

3. Avoid catheterization of the urinary tract if possible, because this is often a source of infections.
4. Repeat urine culture after treatment to prevent recurrence.
5. In a female patient, instruct to wipe (after going to the bathroom) from front to back.
6. Instruct patient on the importance of good hygiene practices.

VIII.   Neurogenic bladder

A. **Description: bladder dysfunction resulting from central or peripheral nervous system lesions, which affect sphincter control and bladder capacity**

B. **Etiology**
1. Upper motor neuron disease causes spastic neurogenic bladder; frequent uncontrollable urge incontinence results from damage above S-2, S-3, or S-4 segments.
2. Lower motor neuron disease causes flaccid neurogenic bladder; a lack of sensation or desire to void results from damage at S-2, S-3, or S-4 segments. As a result, bladder overdistention with overflow incontinence results in urinary retention.
3. Mixed motor disease resulting from cortical brain damage causes decreased perception and inability to control urgency to void.
4. Other causes include neurologic disorders such as cerebral vascular accident, multiple sclerosis, and congenital anomalies.

C. **Pathophysiologic processes and manifestations**
1. Manifestations of *spastic neurogenic bladder* include:
   a. Reduced bladder capacity secondary to increased detrusor tone and increased sensitivity to small amounts of urine
   b. Uncontrolled reflex voiding of less than 150 mL of urine (which can result in urge incontinence)
2. Manifestations of *flaccid neurogenic bladder* include:
   a. Increased bladder capacity (leading to hypotonia)
   b. Urinary retention with overflow resulting from bladder overdistention
3. Manifestations of mixed neurogenic bladder include those for both spastic and flaccid dysfunction.

D. **Overview of nursing interventions**
1. Maintain hydration to prevent stone formation and adequate urine flow.
2. Encourage the patient to eat a low-calcium diet to prevent stone formation.
3. Use appropriate urinary drainage methods (eg, reflex training, indwelling or intermittent catheterization, urinary surgical diversion, Credé's technique [application of gentle downward pressure over the lower abdomen and bladder]).
4. Assess for residual urine.
5. Teach the patient and family members how to manage chronic urinary care.

IX. **Bladder cancer**

A. Description
1. Bladder cancer refers to malignant papillomatous growths within the posterior and lateral walls of the bladder and the trigone; early signs and symptoms rarely are present.
2. Metastasis to the lungs, liver, and bones can occur.

B. Etiology
1. Bladder cancer results from unknown causes.
2. **Factors associated with the development of bladder cancer include:**
   a. **Cigarette smoking**
   b. **Exposure to certain dyes**
   c. **Chronic bladder infections**

C. Pathophysiologic processes and manifestations
1. Manifestations of bladder cancer include:
   a. Gross hematuria occurs secondary to bladder wall irritation and malignant cell wall invasion.
   b. Anemia may be present if hematuria is persistent.
   c. Palpable mass in bladder.
   d. Lower abdominal pain (secondary to pressure caused by malignant growth).
2. Complaints of dysuria, frequent urination, and intermittent bleeding may indicate obstruction secondary to malignancy.

D. Overview of nursing interventions
1. Monitor for signs and symptoms of urinary obstruction.
2. Administer narcotic analgesics for pain, as prescribed.
3. Maintain hydration.
4. Prepare the patient for surgical interventions (cystoscopic resection, total cystectomy with urinary diversion), if indicated; after surgery
   a. Provide appropriate postoperative care.
   b. Monitor for bleeding and elimination.
   c. Provide appropriate patient teaching if urinary diversion is used.
   d. Help the patient manage feelings of grief and loss.
5. Prepare the patient for other treatment modalities, include radiation and chemotherapy.

 X. **Kidney cancer**

A. Description
1. Kidney cancer involves malignant renal tumors, primarily adenocarcinomas.
2. Symptoms commonly are vague, making early diagnosis and treatment difficult.

B. Etiology and incidence
1. **The cause of kidney cancer is unknown; factors contributing to it include:**
   a. **Cigarette smoking**
   b. **Family history**

    2. Incidence is higher in middle-aged and older men.

C. **Pathophysiologic processes and manifestations**

    1. Vague symptoms including persistent anemia, fatigue, and weight loss indicate early stages of the disease.

     2. **Manifestations secondary to pathologic malignant growth usually occur late in the disease; these include:**

        a. **Gross hematuria**

        b. **Flank pain**

        c. **Palpable kidney mass**

        d. **Compression of internal organs**

    3. Symptoms of urinary dysfunction (eg, altered urinary patterns or abnormal constituents in the urine) and hematuria result from malignant growth and bladder wall erosion.

D. **Overview of nursing interventions**

    1. Maintain hydration.

    2. Monitor for signs of anemia secondary to hematuria.

    3. Prepare the patient for surgery (nephrectomy), if indicated; after surgery, provide appropriate postoperative care.

    4. Prepare the patient for other treatment modalities, including radiation therapy.

    5. Provide patient teaching covering:

        a. Importance of follow-up care

        b. Avoidance of UTIs

    6. Determine the patient's prognosis by noting the stage of the tumor.

Bibliography

Bullock, B. (1996). *Pathophysiology: Adaptations and alterations in function* (4th ed.). Philadelphia: Lippincott-Raven.

Carrieri-Kahlmon, V., Lindsey, A., & West, C. (1993). *Pathophysiological phenomena in nursing* (2nd ed.). Philadelphia: W. B. Saunders.

Colley, W. (1997). Know how: Female catheterization. *Nursing Times 93*(27): 34–5.

Ganong, William F. (1997). *Review of medical physiology* (18th ed.). Stamford, CT: Appleton and Lange.

Guyton, Arthur C., & Hall, John E. (1996). *Textbook of medical physiology* (9th ed.). Philadelphia: W. B. Saunders.

Haslam, J. (1997). Promoting continence and treating incontinence *Health Visit 70*(6): 237–8.

Kinney, M., Packa, D., & Dunbar, S. (1993). *AACN's clinical reference for critical-care nursing* (3rd ed.). St. Louis: C.V. Mosby.

Mastering Advanced Assessment. (1993). Springhouse advanced skills series. Springhouse, PA: Springhouse Corporation.

McCance, K., & Huether, S. (1994). *Pathophysiology. The biologic basis for disease in adults & children* (2nd ed.). St. Louis: C.V. Mosby.

Porth, C. (1994). *Pathophysiology: Concepts of altered health states.* (4th ed.). Philadelphia: Lippincott-Raven.

Price, S., & Wilson, L. (1992). *Pathophysiology: Clinical concepts of disease processes* (4th ed.). St. Louis: C.V. Mosby.

Providing Expert Care for the Acutely Ill. (1994). Springhouse Advanced Skills Series. Springhouse, PA: Springhouse Corporation.

Sampselle C. M. et al. (1997). Continence for women: Evidence-based practice. *JOGNN* 26(4): 375–85.

——. (1995). The Foley patrol: CQI team tackles UTI's. *Home Care Quality Management* 1(3): 48–52.

Wilson J. (1997). Infection control: control and prevention of infection in catheter care. *Community Nurse.* 3(5): 39–40.

STUDY QUESTIONS

1. Which of the following is a risk factors for restrictive genitourinary diseases:
   a. chronic urinary tract infections
   b. antiadrenergic medications
   c. diuretic medications
   d. prostatic cancer

2. A patient asks the nurse why he develops kidney stones only in summer months. Which of the following statements would be the most appropriate response?
   a. "There is no seasonal risk factor."
   b. "Kidney stones are related to high-calcium diet."
   c. "Warm temperatures can increase urinary concentration and increase the risk for precipitates."
   d. "The increased incidence is related to sun exposure."

3. Which of the following is a manifestation of urinary retention?
   a. urinary reflux
   b. bladder distention
   c. inability to stop voiding
   d. kidney failure

4. The pathophysiologic process of flaccid neurogenic bladder involves:
   a. spinal cord damage of CNS nerve transmission
   b. increased detrusor tone
   c. increased sensitivity to small amounts of urine
   d. reflex voiding of less than 150 mL of urine

5. All of the following are manifestations of urinary tract infections *except:*
   a. dysuria
   b. anuria
   c. frequency
   d. urgency

6. When providing patient teaching on prevention of urinary tract infections, the nurse should instruct the patient to:
   a. take diuretics to increase output
   b. use self-catheterization to avoid contact with skin

c. decrease fluid intake
d. use hygienic measures to prevent contamination

7. Nursing management of incontinence includes:
   a. dehydrating to reduce the amount of urine
   b. increasing stimulants such as caffeine
   c. hydrating to stimulate voiding reflex
   d. administering anti-incontinent drugs

8. When providing dietary instructions for a patient with cystine stones, the nurse should recommend:
   a. alkaline ash diet
   b. acid ash diet
   c. low-purine diet
   d. high-purine diet

9. Which of the following surgical interventions is commonly performed for a patient with bladder cancer?
   a. total cystectomy
   b. total cystectomy with ileal conduit
   c. total nephrectomy
   d. total nephrectomy with urinary diversion

10. Which of the following nursing interventions is appropriate for a patient with urolithiasis?
    a. bedrest
    b. fluid restrictions
    c. diuretic therapy
    d. ambulation

11. Early diagnosis of kidney cancer is difficult because symptoms are:
    a. the same as prostate cancer
    b. the same as benign prostatic hypertrophy
    c. not consistent with the disease
    d. vague in their appearance

12. Which type of neurogenic bladder results in frequent uncontrollable urge incontinence?:
    a. spastic

b. flaccid

c. mixed motor disease

d. none of the above

13. Which is most important intervention in the treatment of urinary tract infections:

a. frequent catheterization

b. obtaining urine culture and sensitivity

c. providing liberal hydration

d. obtaining white blood count

ANSWER KEY

Question	Correct answer	Correct answer rationale	Incorrect answer rationales
1.	a	Chronic urinary tract infections is a risk factor for the development of a restrictive urinary tract disease.	b. This choice is incorrect because it is anticholnergics drugs that can cause restriction. c and d. These choices are incorrect because neither diuretics or prostatic cancer contribute to the development of restrictive urinary disease.
2.	c	Warm temperatures can increase urine concentration and lead to precipitate development—a risk factor for calculi development.	a and d. These are incorrect. b. This is not related to the patient's expressed concern.
3.	b	Urinary retention will result in bladder distention as the bladder fills with urine.	a. Urinary relux may be a cause of urinary tract infection, not a manifestation. c. The person with retention cannot begin to void, stopping the stream is not the problem. d. Urinary retention refers to urine being retained in the bladder. If the patient has renal failure, urine is not produced.
4.	a	Flaccid neurogenic bladder involves spinal cord damage of afferent, efferent, or CNS nerve transmission, which interferes with the sensation or desire to void.	b, c, and d. These are pathophysiologic processes and manifestations of a spastic neurogenic bladder.
5.	b	Anuria is a manifestation of kidney failure or dehydration.	a, c, and d. These are manifestations of urinary tract infections.
6.	d	Hygienic measures to prevent contamination (eg, wiping from front to back, handwashing) are appropriate preventive measures.	a. This intervention is not related to UTIs. b. Self-catheterization is contraindicated and might cause an infection. c. The patient should increase fluid intake.
7.	c	Hydrating the patient will stimulate the urge to void and facilitate bladder-training.	a. Hydration, not dehydration, is indicated as described above. Dehydration can harm a person, so it is not wise to dehydrate an individual. b. Increasing stimulants is not a treatment for incontinence.

Question	Correct answer	Correct answer rationale	Incorrect answer rationales
			d. There are no anti-incontinent agents available.
8.	a	An alkaline ash diet is recommended for the patient with cystine stones.	b. An acid ash diet is recommended for the patient with calcium and phosphate stones. c. Lowpurine diet is recommended for the patient with uric acid stones. d. This is not a recommended diet.
9.	b	The cancerous bladder is removed and an alternative collection site for urine is created using part of the ileum.	a. If the bladder is removed, some means of collecting urine needs to be established. c and d. These surgical interventions are not indicated for bladder cancer.
10.	d	The patient should ambulate to promote passage of the stone.	a, b, and c. These interventions are contraindicated for the patient with urolithiasis.
11.	d	Symptoms of kidney cancer are often vague, making it difficult to diagnose kidney cancer early.	a, b, and c. The symptoms of kidney cancer are not consistent with either prostatic disease. The symptoms are consistent with the disease but usually appear in later stages.
12.	a	A spastic neurogenic bladder results in frequent uncontrollable urge incontinence.	b and c. These disorders are not associated with these symptoms.
13.	c	The provision of liberal amounts of fluid is the best intervention listed. The fluid will dilute the bacteria and flush the system.	a. Catheterization is contraindicated during urinary tract infections. b and d. These diagnostic tests are not helpful in treating the infection. They are valuable in monitoring progress.

16

Female Reproductive Disorders

I.   **Overview of pathophysiologic processes**

A.   Hormonal imbalances

1.   Hormonal imbalances are disorders in which the normal balance of hormones governing the female reproductive system is altered.

2.   Hormonal imbalances may be caused by stress or by drug interactions with the body's own hormones.

 3.   Some hormonal imbalances, such as dysmenorrhea and premenstrual syndrome (PMS), may be part of a woman's normal cycle.

4.   Extreme imbalances include amenorrhea (absent menses) or abnormal uterine bleeding.

5.   The sole risk factor for hormonal imbalances is age.

B.   Inflammatory and infectious conditions

1.   Inflammatory and infectious conditions are disorders that result from exogenous infections or from the proliferation of endogenous microbes.

2.   Exogenous pathogens are most often sexually transmitted (see Chapter 18 for a complete discussion).

3.   Endogenous pathogens overproliferate when bacteria that help maintain the normal balance are destroyed, usually by antibiotics.

4.   Vaginitis, cervicitis, bartholinitis, toxic shock syndrome, and pelvic inflammatory disease (PID) are inflammatory and infectious conditions.

 5.   Risk factors for inflammatory and infectious conditions include poor hygiene, instrumentation, and compromised immune system.

C.   Structural abnormalities

1.   Structural abnormalities are disorders in which a weakened pelvic support system causes abnormalities in both the structure and possibly function of the female reproductive system.

2.   Structural abnormalities may be congenital or acquired; acquired conditions usually result from a stretching of supportive ligaments, commonly due to childbearing and aging.

3.   Cystocele, rectocele, and uterine prolapse are common structural abnormalities.

D.   Gynecologic tumors

1.   Tumors of the reproductive system may occur in the cervix, ovaries, and uterus.

2.   Tumors may be benign or malignant.

a.   Benign tumors include ovarian cysts, leiomyomas, and endometriosis.

 b.   Malignant disorders include cervical and ovarian cancers.

3.   Breast tumors, fibrocystic disease, and breast cancer may also be classified as tumors of the female reproductive system.

4.   Risk factors for tumors include:

a.   Cigarette smoking

b.   High-fat diet

c.   Family history

E.   Breast tumors
  1.   Benign breast tumors are often found as palpable lumps that are felt in the breast; their presence changes with the phases of the menstrual cycle.
  2.   *Fibrocystic disease* is the term used to describe benign breast lesions.

  3.   Malignant breast lesions most often arise from ductal epithelium and spread through the lymph vessels and nodes.
    a.   Cancers of the mammary ducts include papillary, intraductal, and infiltrating.
    b.   Cancers of the mammary lobules include lobular *in situ*, infiltrating, Paget's disease, inflammatory, sarcoma, fibrosarcoma, and cystosarcoma phyllodes.

II.   Physiologic responses to female reproductive dysfunction

  A.   Abnormal vaginal discharge
  1.   Abnormal vaginal discharge refers to a purulent, white, curdlike, or grayish white discharge that can come from the vagina, urethra, or Bartholin's glands.
  2.   It can result from:
    a.   Alterations in vaginal pH
    b.   Increased number of invading organisms
    c.   Decreased resistance (due to aging, malnutrition, stress, drug use, or disease)
    d.   Allergens or irritants
    e.   Foreign objects
  B.   Pruritus: severe itching resulting from menopausal changes in the epithelium, vitamin A deficiency, glucosuria, scabies, allergies, or simple vaginitis.
  C.   Inflammation: tissue response to injury or irritation; may include erythema and edema
  D.   Dysuria: difficult or painful urination resulting from local irritation of the urinary tract
  E.   Pain: pelvic pain may be present and may be referred to the rectum
  F.   Infection: signs and symptoms depend on the specific causative organism but can include fever, erythema, discharge, itching, malaise, pain and swelling

III.   Dysmenorrhea

  A.   Description: painful menstruation; may be primary or secondary
  B.   Etiology
  1.   Primary dysmenorrhea is not associated with pelvic disease. It usually begins with the onset of ovulation or within the first year after menarche and commonly disappears or declines after pregnancy or by age 23 to 26.
  2.   Secondary dysmenorrhea is caused by organic diseases such as PID, en-

dometriosis, or cervical stenosis; occasionally, it results from a retrograde uterus.

C. **Pathophysiologic processes and manifestations**

1. The chief symptom of dysmenorrhea is pelvic pain associated with the onset of menses.

2. Although the exact cause of the pain is unknown, it probably results from excessive synthesis of prostaglandin.

3. **Prostaglandin causes the myometrium to contract, constricting blood vessels causing ischemia, endometrial bleeding, and pain. Often, the pain radiates into the groin; it may be accompanied by backache.**

4. Secondary manifestations include breast tenderness, abdominal distention, headache, diarrhea, vomiting, anorexia, and syncope.

5. Symptoms may last from a few hours to 2 days.

D. **Overview of nursing interventions**

1. **Advise the patient to keep a record of her menstrual cycle, flow, and occurrence of pain and other symptoms.**

2. Encourage adequate rest, moderate exercise, proper nutrition, and good bowel habits.

3. Apply local heat to promote vasodilation, which results in increased blood flow and relief of ischemia, increased elimination of menstrual flow, and decreased muscle hypertonus.

4. Administer analgesics such as aspirin, a prostaglandin antagonist, as ordered.

5. Administer prostaglandin inhibitors (eg, ibuprofen, naproxen), as ordered:
   a. Give these medications with milk or food.
   b. Note that these medications are contraindicated in women with aspirin intolerance or duodenal ulcer.

6. Explain the use oral contraceptives (if used) to suppress ovulation and achieve symptomatic relief.

7. Institute other relief measures, including systematic relaxation, massage, breathing techniques, muscle toning, and biofeedback.

IV. Amenorrhea

A. **Description**

1. Amenorrhea is a lack of menstruation.

2. It may be primary or secondary:
   a. Primary amenorrhea is the failure to menstruate that persists after age 16; usually, secondary sex characteristics fail to develop.
   b. Secondary amenorrhea occurs in women who have previously menstruated but who have menstruated only three times (or less) in a year.

B. **Etiology**

1. Primary amenorrhea may be caused by:
   a. Decreased or absent secretion of gonadotropin-releasing hormone (Gn-RH), follicle-stimulating hormone (FSH), or luteinizing hormone (LH)
   b. Ovarian resistance to FSH or LH

      c.   Anatomic defects (eg, absence of vagina or uterus)

      d.   Genetic disorders (Turner's syndrome)

      e.   Congenital CNS defects (hydrocephalus) or acquired CNS lesions (trauma, infection, and tumors)

   2.   Secondary amenorrhea is associated with anovulation; it may develop if the uterus is removed or if regulatory hormone levels are altered to inhibit ovulation. It also may be caused by dramatic weight loss or by nutritional disorders such as anorexia nervosa or obesity.

   3.   Secondary amenorrhea is normal during early adolescence, pregnancy, lactation, and when approaching menopause.

C.   **Pathophysiologic processes and manifestations**

   1.   The major manifestation is the absence of menses.

   2.   In primary amenorrhea

      a.   The hypothalamic pituitary ovarian axis is dysfunctional; the hypothalamus does not synthesize Gn-RH, so the pituitary does not secrete LH and FSH.

      b.   Because the ovaries do not receive the hormones necessary to initiate the ovarian and endometrial changes of the menstrual cycle, anovulation and lack of menstruation result.

      c.   Lack of ovarian hormones also results in the absence of secondary sex characteristics.

   3.   In secondary amenorrhea, anovulation may be due to:

      a.   Increased levels of prolactin.

      b.   Decreased levels or irregular secretion of gonadotropin.

      c.   Abnormally low levels of CNS neurotransmitter

D.   **Overview of nursing interventions.**

   1.   Explain hormonal replacement therapy to the patient.

   2.   Prepare the patient for surgery, if indicated; afterward, provide appropriate postoperative care.

   3.   Provide support and counseling to help the patient deal with feelings about infertility.

V.   Abnormal uterine bleeding

A.   **Description**

   1.   Abnormal uterine bleeding refers to heavy or irregular bleeding caused by a disturbance of the menstrual cycle.

   2.   Types include:

      a.   *Menorrhagia* (prolonged, profuse menstrual flow during regular menstrual period)

      b.   ***Metrorrhagia* (bleeding between menstrual periods)**

      c.   *Oligomenorrhea* (menstrual periods more than 35 days apart)

      d.   *Dysfunctional uterine bleeding* (excessive bleeding with no cyclic pattern)

B.   **Etiology**

   1.   Menorrhagia in adolescents may be caused by a blood dyscrasia or endocrine disturbance; in adult women, it may be a symptom of an ovarian tumor, uterine myoma, or PID.

    2. Metrorrhagia may be due to endometrial polyps, endometrial or cervical cancer, or exogenous estrogen administration.

    3. Oligomenorrhea may be due to pregnancy, menopause, estrogen secreting tumors, or excessive weight loss.

    4. Dysfunctional uterine bleeding has no organic cause.

C. **Pathophysiologic processes and manifestations**

    1. The major manifestation is irregular or heavy bleeding, or both, which may be associated with either ovulatory or anovulatory menses.

    2. Anovulatory menses

        a. Occurs in women over age 40

        b. Results either from low estrogen and progesterone levels, causing the endometrium to become hypoplastic (thin and underdeveloped) and to bleed, or from high estrogen levels and low progesterone levels, causing the endometrium to become hyperplastic (overproliferative)

        c. Causes tissue breakdown, sloughing, and bleeding that occurs at different sites and at different times

    3. Ovulatory menses

        a. Occurs in women over age 30 who have had two or more children

        b. Results from luteal phase defects in which the corpus luteum degenerates prematurely (if the corpus luteum degeneration is prolonged, irregular bleeding occurs)

        c. Causes normal menstrual flow that occurs too often

D. **Overview of nursing interventions**

    1. Prepare the patient for and assist with diagnostic procedures such as endometrial biopsy or dilation and curettage (D & C).

    2. Instruct the patient about the use of drug therapy (eg, oral contraceptives, antifibrolytic agents, prostaglandin synthetase inhibitors, or ovulation stimulators) and potential side effects.

    3. Prepare patient for surgery (hysterectomy), if indicated; afterward, provide appropriate postoperative care.

VI. Premenstrual syndrome (PMS)

A. **Description: the cyclic recurrence of physical, psychological, or behavioral changes that interfere with activities of daily living**

B. **Etiology**

    1. The etiology of PMS is unknown.

    2. It may result from a variety of factors including:

        a. Estrogen-progesterone imbalance

        b. Hypoglycemia

        c. Excess aldosterone or prostaglandin

        d. Excess levels of prolactin in the blood

        e. Psychogenic factors

        f. Low progesterone levels

        g. High (or falling) estrogen levels

        h. Increased renin-angiotensin or adrenal activity

        i. Endogenous endorphin withdrawal

       j.   Central changes in catecholamines

       k.   Vitamin deficiencies

C.   **Pathophysiologic processes and manifestations**

    1.   The pathophysiology of PMS is unclear.

    2.   Manifestations are categorized according to four patterns based on time of onset and duration.

    3.   Symptoms vary among women, but a health history should reveal identical symptoms that occur during the last 7 to 10 days of each cycle for three consecutive cycles to confirm a diagnosis of PMS.

    4.   Symptoms of PMS may include:

       a.   Behavioral changes (tension, irritability, mood swings, anxiety, crying, depression, insomnia)

       b.   Fatigue

       c.   Water and sodium retention (edema, weight gain, breast enlargement and tenderness, abnormal bloating)

       d.   Acne

       e.   Palpitations

       f.   Increased appetite

       g.   Migraine-like headache

       h.   Joint pain

       i.   Backache

D.   **Overview of nursing interventions**

    1.   Provide symptomatic relief.

    2.   Teach the patient about the nature of PMS and stress reduction techniques.

    3.   Encourage a diet high in complex carbohydrates, moderate in protein, and low in refined sugar and sodium.

    4.   Advise the patient to reduce or eliminate consumption of caffeine, chocolate, and alcohol, and to avoid smoking.

    5.   Encourage regular 30-minute exercise periods three to four times per week.

VII.   Nonspecific vaginitis

A.   **Description: inflammation of the lower genital tract**

B.   **Etiology**

    1.   Nonspecific vaginitis may be caused by bacterial vaginosis or unidentified organisms.

       a.   Bacterial vaginosis (formerly referred to as *Coryne-bacterium vaginale, Haemophilus vaginalis,* and *Gardnerella vaginalis*) is a general term reflecting the fact that several organisms cause the infection.

       b.   Unidentified organisms are most often introduced from outside sources (eg, clothing, hands, douche nozzle) or during sexual intercourse.

    2.   In sexually active women, reinfection occurs unless sexual partners are also treated.

C.   **Pathophysiologic processes and manifestations**

    1.   Normally, the vagina is protected by its pH and the presence of Döderlein's bacilli.

2. If the pH is altered or resistance is lowered, tissue inflammation, abnormal discharge, and itching occur.
3. During menopause, decreased estrogen causes a thin vaginal mucosa; pyogenic bacterial invasion of this mucosa results in burning, pruritus, and leukorrhea.

D. Overview of nursing interventions

1. Relieve itching with wet compresses, sitz baths, and warm vinegar-and-water douches (15 mL vinegar to 1 L water).
2. Instruct the patient in the proper administration of oral or vaginal estrogenic preparations, if prescribed.
3. Provide patient teaching including:
    a. Preventive measures (eg, washing hands, wearing cotton underwear, ensuring proper perineal care, avoiding tight clothing and feminine hygiene sprays, and avoiding sex with an infected partner and during period of treatment)
    b. Proper administration of medications and potential side effects

VIII. Cervicitis

A. Description

1. Cervicitis, a common gynecologic disorder, is an inflammation of the cervix.
2. It may be classified as mucopurulent or chronic (persistent infection and inflammation).

B. Etiology

1. Mucopurulent cervicitis (formerly referred to as acute cervicitis) usually is caused by the sexual transmission of a pathogen or fungus, such as *Candida albicans* or *Chlamydia*.
2. Chronic cervicitis can follow childbirth, abortion, or erosion.

C. Pathophysiologic processes and manifestations

1. Mucopurulent cervicitis may be asymptomatic; manifestations, if present, may include:
    a. Mucopurulent cervical discharge
    b. Gross erythema and edema of the cervix
    c. Hypertrophic ectopy of mucosa around external os (which may appear everted)
2. Manifestations of chronic cervicitis may include:
    a. Laceration or eversion of the cervix
    b. Purulent cervical discharge
    c. Erythema and hypertrophy of cervix
    d. Hyperemia (which may cause intermenstrual or postcoital spotting)
    e. Thick, viscous cervical mucus (which may interrupt sperm transport, causing infertility)
    f. Lower abdominal pain or dyspareunia (caused by pelvic congestion)
    g. Vulvar burning
3. Chronic cervicitis also may result in scarring or metaplasia.

D. Overview of nursing interventions

1. For mucopurulent cervicitis, teach the patient about appropriate drug therapy and potential side effects when medication is prescribed.

2. For chronic cervicitis, prepare the patient for cervical cauterization (silver nitrate, electrical) or cryotherapy; after treatment, instruct the patient to:
   a. Leave the tampon or packing in place (usually for about 8 to 24 hours).
   b. Avoid douching or sexual relations until after the next visit to the physician.
   c. Expect an unpleasant discharge to be present for 4 to 5 days.
   d. Seek medical assistance if bleeding is excessive (more than the amount of normal menses).

IX. Bartholinitis (Bartholin's cyst)

A. Description: inflammation of the duct system leading from the opening of the vagina to Bartholin's glands; may be acute or chronic

B. Etiology
1. Causative organisms include streptococci, staphylococci, *Escherichia coli,* sexually transmitted microorganisms, and other pathogens that typically infect the lower genital tract.
2. Acute bartholinitis typically occurs after an infection (eg, vaginitis, cervicitis, urethritis).

C. Pathophysiologic processes and manifestations
1. Inflammation due to infection or trauma occludes the duct, blocking the normal flow of secretions from the gland and resulting in cyst formation (Fig. 16-1).
2. Cysts may be asymptomatic; symptomatic cysts may be red, painful, and have a purulent discharge.
3. Other symptoms may include infection and fever.

D. Overview of nursing interventions
1. Provide pain relief by administering analgesics, as ordered, and encouraging sitz baths.
2. Instruct the patient about the use of drug therapy and potential side effects when antibiotics are prescribed.
3. Prepare the patient for incision and drainage of the cyst, if indicated.

X. Toxic shock syndrome (TSS)

A. Description: a severe, acute disorder associated with strains of *staphylococci*

B. Etiology and incidence
1. Toxic shock syndrome is caused by toxins secreted by strains of *Staphylococcus aureus.*
2. Incidence is higher during menstruation.
3. Risk factors associated with TSS include:
   a. Use of tampons (especially superabsorbent ones)
   b. Use of fingers rather than applicators to insert tampons
   c. Chronic vaginal infections (herpes)
   d. Puerperal endometriosis
   e. Use of barrier contraceptives (eg, sponge, diaphragm)

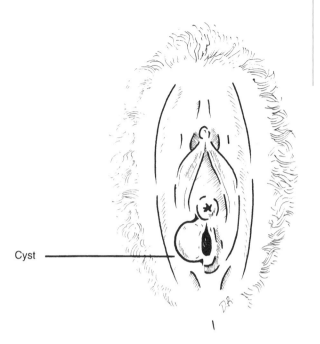

FIGURE 16-1.
Bartholinitis. Bartholin's gland with
cyst formation.

C. **Pathophysiologic processes and manifestations**

1. The organism gains entry to the circulation through vaginal lesions produced by the use of tampons.

2. Superabsorbent tampons maintain an environment favorable to bacterial growth, because they contain a large amount of menstrual blood and may be left in place for several hours.

3. The three major manifestations of TSS are:
   a. Fever of sudden onset over 102°F (38.9°C)
   b. Hypotension (systolic pressure < 90 mm Hg), orthostatic dizziness, and disorientation.
   c. **Erythematous macular desquamating rash, most prominent on the palms and soles**

4. Multisystem dysfunction—including symptoms such as vomiting or diarrhea; impaired renal, hepatic, or cardiopulmonary function; and altered levels of consciousness—may occur.

5. The acute phase lasts about 4 to 5 days; the convalescent phase lasts about 1 to 2 weeks.

6. Mortality is associated with adult respiratory distress syndrome (ARDS), uncontrollable hypotension, and disseminated intravascular coagulation (DIC).

D. **Overview of nursing interventions**

1. Teach the patient about preventive measures, including proper cleaning of the perineum, aseptic handling of tampons, use of sanitary napkins, and avoidance of superabsorbent tampons and douching.

2. Inform women who are carriers of *S. aureus* about potential risks.

3. Educate women about the signs and symptoms of TSS; instruct them to seek immediate medical treatment.
4. Monitor a patient with septic shock and provide symptomatic treatment.

XI. Pelvic inflammatory disease (PID)

A. Description

1. PID is an acute inflammatory process that may involve any organ of the upper reproductive tract, including the uterus (endometritis), fallopian tubes (salpingitis), or ovaries (oophoritis); in its most severe form, it may involve the entire peritoneal cavity.
2. PID may be acute or chronic.

B. Etiology and incidence

1. PID is caused by organisms such as *Neisseria gonorrhea, Chlamydia, Haemophilus, Streptococcus,* mycoplasmas, and anaerobic organisms.
2. PID occurs five times more often in women using intrauterine devices (IUDs).
3. PID also may result from secondary infections due to appendix rupture or pelvic peritonitis.
4. Chronic PID results from undiagnosed or inadequately treated acute PID.

C. Pathophysiologic processes and manifestations

1. Pathogenic organisms ascend through the cervical canal into the uterus during sexual intercourse, abortion procedures, childbirth, or the postpartum period.
2. Organisms pass through thrombosed uterine veins into the pelvis by way of the fallopian tubes.
3. Many of the pathogens lodge in the fallopian tubes; as a result, purulent material collects, adhesions form, and strictures and sterility may occur.
4. The clinical manifestations of PID vary from sudden, severe abdominal pain with fever to no symptoms at all.
5. Symptoms of acute PID can include
   a. Severe abdominal pain (pressure or fullness)
   b. Lower abdominal cramps
   c. Intermenstrual spotting
   d. Dyspareunia
   e. Fever and chills
   f. Malaise
   g. Nausea and vomiting
   h. Foul-smelling, purulent vaginal discharge
6. Symptoms of chronic PID can include
   a. Chronic, dull, aching lower abdominal pain
   b. Backache
   c. Constipation
   d. Malaise
   e. Low-grade fever
   f. Disturbances in menstruation

D. Overview of nursing interventions

1. Administer IV fluids, antibiotics, and analgesics, as prescribed.
2. Provide pain relief measures, as needed.

3.   Teach the patient about preventing infections of the vulva, vagina, and cervix and about recognizing the signs and symptoms of PID. Teach patient about safe sex.

4.   Identify women at risk for PID; encourage sexually active women to have a routine cervical smear or culture for sexually transmitted diseases (STDs).

5.   Provide treatment for the sexual partners of women with PID.

XII.   Cystocele

A.   **Description: prolapse or descent of the bladder into the vagina due to laceration, stretching, or weakening of supporting fascial tissue; also known as dropped bladder**

B.   Etiology: causes include prolonged labor, multiple births, birth of a large baby, repeated close pregnancies, or pelvic surgery

C.   **Pathophysiologic processes and manifestations**

1.   Muscular and fascial tissues lose tone and strength with aging and may fail to maintain pelvic organs in the proper position.

2.   Pelvic relaxation is progressive, and cystocele may occur many years after the initial injury.

3.   Progressive relaxation of the pelvic support structures may cause uterine displacement.

4.   Common manifestations include
   a.   Urinary frequency, urgency, and occasional incontinence
   b.   Difficulty in emptying the bladder completely
   c.   Low backache that worsens with standing or walking

D.   **Overview of nursing interventions**

1.   Encourage the patient to perform isometric exercise to strengthen the pubococcygeal muscles.

2.   Instruct the patient in the use of oral or topical estrogen therapy, which may be prescribed to improve fascial support tone and vascularity, and potential side effects.

3.   Prepare the patient for surgery (anterior colporrhaphy); after surgery:
   a.   Prevent pressure on the vaginal suture line
   b.   Leave indwelling catheter in place for about 4 days to avoid full bladder
   c.   Prevent constipation
   d.   Teach the patient to avoid Valsalva's maneuver, jarring activities, heavy lifting, and sexual intercourse for 6 weeks postoperatively.

XIII.   Rectocele

A.   **Description: herniation or bulging of the rectum into the vagina**

B.   **Etiology: trauma to the fascia and levator muscles, usually caused by childbirth**

C.   **Pathophysiologic processes and manifestations**

1.   Pathophysiology is the same as that for cystocele.

2. Manifestations include:
   a. Constipation or feeling of rectal fullness
   b. Difficult defecation
   c. Pressure and sensation of fullness in the vagina

D. Overview of nursing interventions

1. Encourage the patient to perform isometric exercise to strengthen the pubococcygeal muscles.
2. Instruct the patient in the use of oral or topical estrogen therapy, which may be prescribed to improve fascial support tone and vascularity, and potential side effects.
3. Prepare the patient for surgery (posterior colporrhaphy) by administering cathartic and enemas to empty bowel; after surgery:
   a. Prevent increased intraabdominal pressure or strain on the wound by placing the patient in low Fowler's or supine position.
   b. Provide a liquid diet (for approximately 5 days) and paregoric to inhibit bowel function.
   c. Institute measures to prevent constipation and straining.
   d. Avoid administration of enemas to relieve flatus or cleanse bowel for at least 1 week.

XIV. Uterine prolapse

A. Description

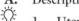

1. **Uterine prolapse is the displacement of part or all of the uterus into the vagina.**
2. It may be classified as follows:
   a. *First-degree prolapse:* The cervix descends but is still within the vagina.
   b. *Second-degree prolapse:* The cervix protrudes from the vagina.
   c. *Third-degree prolapse:* The entire uterus protrudes from the vagina.

B. Etiology: weakened supporting ligaments allow the uterus to drop

C. Pathophysiologic processes and manifestations

1. Pathophysiology is the same as that for cystocele and rectocele.
2. Typical manifestations include
   a. Chronic backache
   b. Pelvic pressure
   c. Dysmenorrhea
   d. Leukorrhea

D. Overview of nursing interventions

1. Teach the patient how to apply and care for a pessary (removable mechanical device that holds the uterus in place), if indicated.
2. Prepare patient for surgery (hysterectomy), if indicated; afterward, provide appropriate postoperative care.

XV. Ovarian cysts

A. Description

1. **These are benign cysts that can occur at any time in life, but are most common between puberty and menopause.**

2. The two most common types are follicular cysts and corpus luteum cysts.

B. Etiology

1. Follicular cysts develop from mature ovarian follicles that do not release their ova.
2. Corpus luteum cysts develop from a corpus luteum that persists abnormally and continues to secrete progesterone.

C. Pathophysiologic processes and manifestations

1. Follicular cysts are thin walled and translucent, arising during the evolution or involution of the graafian follicle. Most are asymptomatic, require no treatment, and either regress or rupture spontaneously within 60 days.

2. **A large follicular cyst may cause low back pain, dyspareunia, chronic lower abdominal pain, and menstrual irregularities; a mass may be palpated during pelvic examination.**
3. Corpus luteum cysts consist of blood or fluid that accumulates in the cavity of the corpus luteum. These are less common than follicular cysts, but cause more symptoms, especially if they rupture.
4. Manifestations of corpus luteum cysts include dull pelvic pain and amenorrhea or delayed menstruation, followed by irregular or heavier than normal bleeding. These cysts usually regress spontaneously within 2 months.
5. A ruptured corpus luteum cyst may cause massive bleeding and require immediate surgery.

D. Overview of nursing interventions

1. Prepare the patient for surgery (oophorectomy), if indicated.
2. Provide postoperative pain medication, as ordered.
3. Institute measures to control infection.

XVI. Leiomyomas (uterine fibroids)

A. Description

1. Leiomyomas, the most common benign uterine tumors, develop from smooth muscle cells in the myometrium.
2. They may be classified as:
   a. Subserosal: growth affects the serous layer of uterine tissue; this is the most superficial type
   b. Submucosal: growth is in the nest endometrial layer, the mucus layer
   c. Intramural: the deepest of fibroids, it enters the uterine muscle

B. Etiology and incidence

1. Leiomyomas result from unknown causes, but they appear to be related to hormonal fluctuations.
2. They are not seen before menarche.
3. Leiomyomas will usually shrink after menopause; they will not develop after menopause.
4. Leiomyomas occur more often in black and Asian women than in whites.

C. Pathophysiologic processes and manifestations

1. Leiomyomas usually are firm and surrounded by a pseudocapsule composed of compressed myometrium.

2. They may occur in multiples in the fundus of the uterus or singly and throughout the uterus.
3. Major manifestations include
    a. Abnormal uterine bleeding
    b. Pain
    c. Symptoms related to pressure on nearby structures (eg, backache, constipation, urinary retention or urgency)
    d. Irregular, nontender nodularity of uterus (revealed by bimanual examination)
4. Large leiomyomas may cause sterility, spontaneous abortion, or difficult delivery.

D. **Overview of nursing interventions**
1. Note that treatment depends on the symptoms, the patient's age, whether more children are desired, and how near the patient is to menopause.
2. Prepare the patient for surgery (myomectomy or hysterectomy, if severe bleeding or obstruction occurs), as indicated; afterward, provide appropriate postoperative care.

XVII.   Endometriosis

A. **Description**
1. Endometriosis is a condition characterized by the presence of endometrial cells at sites outside the uterus.
2. The most common sites of endometrial implantation are:
    a. Ovaries
    b. Uterine ligaments
    c. Rectovaginal septum
    d. Pelvic peritoneum
3. Other sites include the sigmoid colon, small intestine, rectum, appendix, bladder, uterus, vulva, vagina, cervix, lymph nodes, extremities, pleural cavity, lungs, laparotomy scars, and hernial sacs.

B. **Etiology**
1. The cause of endometriosis is unknown.
2. Theories suggest it may be caused by:
    a. Congenital presence of endometrial cells at sites outside of their normal location
    b. Transfer of endometrial cells by means of blood vessels or the lymphatic system
    c. Reflux of menstrual fluid containing endometrial cells up the fallopian tubes and into the pelvic cavity

C. **Pathophysiologic processes and manifestations**
1. Cyclic changes depend on the blood supply of the endometrial implants.
2. The ectopic endometrium proliferates, breaks down, and bleeds in conjunction with the normal menstrual cycle.
3. The bleeding causes inflammation and pain in surrounding tissues; the inflammation may lead to fibrosis, scarring, and adhesions.
4. Other manifestations include:
    a. Abnormal vaginal bleeding

   b. Dysmenorrhea
   c. Infertility
   d. Dyspareunia
   e. Constipation
   f. Dyschezia (pain on defecation)
   g. Tender, palpable masses
   h. Fixed retroverted uterus

D. **Overview of nursing interventions**

  1. If symptoms are minimal, relieve pain with mild analgesics, as prescribed.

  2. Advise the patient to have regular pelvic exams (every 6 months) to monitor the disease's progress.

  3. Encourage young patients who desire children to conceive early.

  4. For more severe symptoms, instruct the patient about the use of drug therapy (oral contraceptives, danazol) and possible side effects.

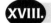

XVIII. **Cervical cancer**

A. Description

  1. **Cervical cancer is an invasive carcinoma, composed of connective tissue enclosing epithelial cells; it is the third most common cancer in women.**

  2. There are two types of cervical carcinomas:
   a. *Squamous cell carcinomas* involve the epidermal layer of the cervix.
   b. *Adenocarcinomas* involve the cervical mucus-producing gland cells.

B. Etiology and incidence

  1. Risk factors associated with cervical cancer include:
   a. First coitus before age 18 (the most important predictor)
   b. Multiple sexual partners
   c. Low socioeconomic status
   d. Exposure to herpes virus type 2
   e. Infection with STDs
   f. Intercourse with men whose previous partners have had cervical cancer
   g. Cigarette smoking or exposure to secondhand smoke
   h. Prolonged use of oral contraceptives (7 to 10 years)

  2. The death rate from cervical cancer has declined as a result of an increased use of Pap smears for mass screening and more frequent and thorough gynecologic examinations.

C. Pathophysiologic processes and manifestations

  1. Precursor lesions of cervical squamous cell carcinoma have been identified as dysplasia.

  2. The cervical intraepithelial neoplasia (CIN) system grades the three stages of dysplasia:
   a. CIN I: mild to moderate dysplasia
   b. CIN II: moderate to severe dysplasia
   c. CIN III: severe dysplasia to carcinoma *in situ*

  3. Women with the earlier stages of CIN may experience one of three courses: regression, persistence, or progression to carcinoma *in situ* or invasive carcinoma.

4. Adenocarcinoma is not preceded by a well-recognized, prolonged precursor state; it may be present for a considerable time before it can be clinically detected.
5. Stages of cervical cancer are as follows:
   a. Stage 0: Cancer is confined within the epithelium of the cervix.
   b. Stage I: Cancer is completely confined to the cervix.
   c. Stage II: Cancer extends outside the cervix but does not involve the pelvic wall or the lower third of the vagina.
   d. Stage III: Cancer involves the pelvic wall and lower third of the vagina.
   e. Stage IV: Cancer extends beyond stage III and involves the bladder, rectum, or metastatic spread.
6. In the early stages, the disease is asymptomatic; it is often detected by an abnormal Pap smear.
7. As the disease progresses, manifestations may include:
   a. Slight watery discharge
   b. Occasional bloody spotting after intercourse or between periods
   c. Abnormally long menstrual periods
   d. Dull lower backache preceding menstrual periods
8. Manifestations of advanced disease may include:
   a. Vaginal bleeding
   b. Yellow vaginal discharge
   c. Pain extending from lower back through the hip and into the thigh
   d. Weight loss
   e. Anemia
   f. Urinary symptoms

D. Overview of nursing interventions

1. Educate the patient about and assist with diagnostic procedures (eg, cervical biopsy, endocervical curettage).
2. Educate the patient about and assist with tests used to stage the disease (eg, chest x-ray, colposcopy, proctosigmoidoscopy, intravenous pyelography [IVP], and barium studies of lower colon and rectum).
3. Prepare the patient with carcinoma *in situ* for cryosurgery or excisional conization of the cervix, if indicated.
4. Prepare the patient with invasive carcinoma for surgery (radical hysterectomy with pelvic lymph node dissection) or radiotherapy.
5. Provide appropriate postoperative care to prevent complications, especially abdominal distention and thrombophlebitis.
6. Explain to premenopausal women who have pelvic irradiation that they will lose their ovarian function; offer counseling regarding the use of hormones, vaginal lubricants, and other methods to prevent or alleviate menopausal symptoms.
7. Monitor the patient for symptoms of radiation sickness (eg, nausea, vomiting, diarrhea, malaise, and fever).
8. Follow safety precautions for appropriate time and distance restrictions and discarding of linens when caring for a patient with a radiation implant.
9. Provide patient teaching including:
   a. Disease process
   b. Diet and exercise recommendations

    c.   Bladder functioning after surgery

    d.   Impact of surgery on sexuality

    e.   Need for follow-up care

XIX. Ovarian cancer

A. Description

    1.   Ovarian cancer affects the functional ovaries rather than the structural uterus.

    2.   Two major types are:

        a.   Germ cell neoplasms

        b.   Epithelial neoplasms

    3.   Germ cell neoplasms may be benign (cystic teratoma) or malignant (tending to be highly aggressive and rapidly growing, with poor prognosis).

    4.   Epithelial tumors are more common, but they also have a poor prognosis.

B. Etiology and incidence

    1.   The cause of ovarian cancer is unknown.

    2.   Risk factors for developing ovarian cancer include:

        a.   Never having borne children

        b.   Never having been pregnant

        c.   Undergoing estrogen replacement therapy after menopause

        d.   Cigarette smoking or exposure to smoke

        e.   Exposure to asbestos and talc

    3.   Incidence is highest in industrialized countries.

C. Pathophysiologic processes and manifestations

    1.   The intrapelvic location of the ovaries and the range of tumor activity (from slow to rapid growth) results in diverse signs and symptoms.

    2.   Ovarian cancer generally is considered a silent disease because by the time the woman experiences symptoms, the disease has spread beyond the primary site.

    3.   The most obvious manifestations are:

        a.   Pain and abdominal swelling from the primary ovarian mass, plaques, or ascites

        b.   Vomiting and altered bowel habits resulting from mechanical obstruction by the tumor

        c.   Abnormal vaginal bleeding

    4.   Staging of the disease, which is done during surgery, is as follows:

        a.   Stage I: limited to ovaries

        b.   Stage II: involves one or both ovaries with pelvic extension

        c.   Stage III: involves one or both ovaries with intraperitoneal metastasis outside pelvis or positive lymph nodes

        d.   Stage IV: involves one or both ovaries with distant metastasis (eg, liver or lungs)

D. Overview of nursing interventions

    1.   Educate the patient about and assist with diagnostic tests (eg, ultrasound, computed tomography [CT] scan, magnetic resonance imaging [MRI]), and exploratory surgery).

2. Prepare the patient for surgery (total abdominal hysterectomy, bilateral salpingoophorectomy), if indicated; afterward, provide appropriate postoperative care.
3. Prepare the patient for additional or adjuvant therapy, depending on the disease stage:
   a. Stage I: chemotherapy with an alkylating agent such as melphalan or intraperitoneal installation of radioactive phosphorus (^{32}P)
   b. Stage II: installation of ^{32}P, external abdominal and pelvic irradiation, or systemic combined chemotherapy
   c. Stages III and IV: combined chemotherapy, whole abdominal irradiation (stage III)
4. Provide patient teaching including:
   a. Disease process
   b. Diet and exercise recommendations during and after therapy
   c. Personal impact of the disease and changes in sexuality
   d. Need for follow-up care

Fibrocystic disease

A. Description
1. *Fibrocystic disease* is a catch-all term describing benign breast lesions of epithelial origin.
2. Benign breast lesions are classified as:
   a. Nonproliferative: lesions with no proliferative activity (includes mild hyperplasia, microcyst, epithelium-related calcification, and fibroadenomas)
   b. Proliferative: lesions without atypia (includes moderate to florid hyperplasia, papillomas, ductal involvement with atypical lobular hyperplasia, and sclerosing adenosis)
   c. Atypical hyperplasia: includes the so-called borderline lesion (a lesion with some of the morphologic characteristics of carcinoma *in situ*)
3. Many of these lesions are risk factors for breast cancer; most appear to represent breast tissue response to estrogen stimulation.

B. Etiology and incidence
1. The cause of fibrocystic disease is unknown.
2. It occurs mainly in women between age 30 and menopause.

C. Pathophysiologic processes and manifestations
1. Histologic changes may result from inappropriate responses of breast tissue to hormones rather than inappropriate hormone levels.
2. The most common manifestations include:
   a. Pain (mastodynia) or tenderness of the breast; discomfort increases as menstruation approaches
   b. Palpable masses (most commonly found in the upper outer quadrant of the breast); masses are soft, well demarcated, and freely movable
   c. Clear, milky, straw-colored, or green nipple discharge may also be present.

D. Overview of nursing interventions
1. Prepare the patient for and assist with diagnostic measures (eg, breast biopsy or aspiration).

2. Teach the patient to minimize discomfort by wearing a supportive bra, using analgesics, and applying warm compresses.
3. Encourage the patient to reduce or eliminate caffeine intake.
4. Teach the patient how to perform breast self-examination; encourage her to perform it regularly and obtain periodic mammography.

XXI. Breast cancer

A. Description

 1. **Malignant neoplasms of the breast are the most common form of cancer in women and the second leading cause of cancer deaths in women age 15 to 55.**
2. The mammary ducts or mammary lobules, or both, may be involved.
3. A danger exists if metastases occur to the lymph system.

B. Etiology and incidence
1. The cause of breast cancer is unknown; however, several factors may contribute to its development.
2. Risk factors can be classified as:

   a. **Reproductive (early menarche, late menopause, nulliparous, birth of first child after age 34)**
   b. **Hormonal (oral contraceptive use, estrogen replacement therapy)**
   c. **Environmental (radiation exposure, high-fat diet, alcohol consumption, upper socioeconomic status, Caucasian race)**
   d. **Familial (history of breast cancer in mother or sister, especially with premenopausal and bilateral condition)**
   e. **Personal (age over 40, benign breast disease, primary breast cancer, lowered immunologic defenses, other organ cancers, especially ovarian, uterine, or endometrial)**
3. Breast cancer occurs in premenopausal and postmenopausal women.

C. Pathophysiologic processes and manifestations
1. Most breast cancers arise from the ductal epithelium.
2. Infiltrating ductal type tumors do not grow to a large size, but metastasize early. This type accounts for 70% of breast cancers.
3. Metastatic spread occurs through the lymph vessels and nodes.
4. There are three major pathways of lymphatic drainage:
   a. Axillary (usual route of metastatic spread)
   b. Internal mammary
   c. Transpectoral
5. Metastasis to the axillary nodes takes place by embolization.
   a. A small mass of cells breaks off from the tumor and enters the lymphatic system.
   b. When the mass reaches a lymph node, it may remain and enlarge the node or travel to a nearby or distant node.
   c. About 60% of breast carcinomas occur in the upper outer quadrant because most of the glandular tissue is there.
6. Lymphatic spread to the opposite breast, to lymph nodes in the base of the neck, and to the abdominal cavity is caused by:

       a. Obstruction of normal lymphatic pathways
       b. Destruction of lymphatic vessels by surgery or radiotherapy
   7. Metastasis from the vertebral veins can involve the vertebrae, pelvic bones, ribs, and skull.
   8. Other sites of metastasis include the lungs, kidneys, liver, ovaries, and adrenal and pituitary glands.
   9. **The first manifestation is usually a small, painless lump in the upper outer quadrant of the breast (see Display 16-1 for additional manifestations).**

D. Overview of nursing interventions
   1. Assist in preventing the disease by:
       a. Educating women about proper breast selfexamination techniques
       b. Encouraging a healthy lifestyle and elimination of controllable risk factors
       c. Recommending periodic physical examinations
   2. Provide the patient with support and information during diagnostic testing (eg, mammography, CT scan, MRI, and biopsy).
   3. Note that therapy depends on various factors including:
       a. Tissue involvement and aggressiveness
       b. Hormonal milieu (pre- or postmenopausal patient, estrogen- or progesterone-dependent tumor)
       c. Location and size of tumor
       d. Local or regional metastasis (staging of tumor incorporates the tumor, node, metastasis [TNM] classification)
       e. Patient's lifestyle
   4. Explain the various treatment modalities (surgery, radiation, chemotherapy) to the patient.

DISPLAY 16-1
Manifestations of Breast Cancer

- Local pain (caused by obstruction)
- Skin dimpling (with dermal lymphatic invasion or pectoralis fascia involvement)
- Nipple retraction (caused by shortening of the mammary ducts)
- Skin retraction (with suspensory ligament involvement)
- Edema (caused by local inflammation or lymhatic obstruction)
- Nipple or areolar eczema (caused by Paget's disease)
- Skin pitting, similar to the surface of an orange (caused by subcutaneous lymphatic obstruction)
- Reddened skin, local tenderness, and warmth (due to inflammation)
- Dilated blood vessels (due to a fast-growing tumor obstruction of venous return)
- Nipple discharge in nonlcatating woman (caused by tumor obstruction)
- Ulceration (due to tumor necrosis)
- Hemorrhage (due to blood vessel erosion)
- Edema of the arm (due to obstruction of lymphatic drainage in the axilla)
- Chest pain (associated with lung metastasis)

    5. If surgery is performed, provide postoperative care, including:

        a. Assisting the patient in working through the loss of her breast and its significance

        b. Providing wound care and elevating the arm to promote drainage and increase comfort

        c. Teaching the patient postmastectomy or postlumpectomy exercises

        d. Providing referrals, as indicated, to self-help groups such as "Reach for Recovery."

        e. Providing information about a prosthesis, appropriate clothing styles, and reconstruction options, if appropriate.

    6. If radiation therapy is used:

        a. Teach the patient about the usual course of treatment (external beam therapy for 6 weeks, then interstitial therapy).

        b. Explain potential side effects (reduced energy, nausea, and sometimes heartburn).

        c. Educate the patient about arm exercises and precautions for lymphedema.

        d. Offer counseling to help the patient work through feelings of grief and loss.

        e. Maintain radiation safety.

    7. If chemotherapy is used:

        a. Teach the patient about the usual course of therapy and commonly used cytotoxic agents (cyclophosphamide, methotrexate, 5-fluorouracil, vincristine, prednisone, and doxorubicin).

        b. Explain the side effects (nausea, temporary hair loss, bone marrow depression, anemia, loss of appetite, fatigue, and neurotoxicity) and offer techniques for managing them.

Bibliography

ACOG. (1996). *Guidelines for women's healthcare.* Washington, D.C.

Allen, K., and Phillips, J. (1997). *Women's health across the lifespan.* Philadelphia: Lippincott-Raven.

AWHONN. (1997). *Standards and guidelines for professional nursing practice in the care of women and newborns* (5th ed.). Washington, D.C.

Carlson, K., Eisenstat, S., Frigoletto, F., and Schiff, I. (1995). *Primary care of women.* St. Louis: Mosby.

Cokingtin, P. S., et al. (1992). *Lippincott's review series: Medical-surgical nursing.* Philadelphia: J. B. Lippincott.

Edge, V., and Miller, M. (1994). *Women's health care.* St. Louis: Mosby.

Lemcke, D., Pattison, J., Marshall, L., and Cowley, D. (1995). *Primary care of women.* Norwalk, CT: Appleton and Lange.

Leppert, P., and Howard, F. (1997). *Primary care for women.* Philadelphia, PA: Lippincott-Raven.

Ramsom, S., and Mcneely, G. (1997). *Gynecology for the primary care provider.* Philadelphia, PA: W.B. Saunders.

STUDY QUESTIONS

1. In primary amenorrhea, imbalances may be found in all of the following hormones *except:*
   a. gonadotropin-releasing hormone (Gn-RH)
   b. luteinizing hormone (LH)
   c. prolactin hormone
   d. follicle-stimulating hormone (FSH)

2. Prolonged, profuse menstrual flow during regular periods is called:
   a. menorrhagia
   b. metrorrhagia
   c. oligomenorrhea
   d. dysfunctional uterine bleeding

3. A potential etiology of premenstrual syndrome is:
   a. hyperglycemia
   b. progesterone imbalance
   c. decreased renin-angiotensin activity
   d. decreased prostaglandins

4. Nursing interventions for the patient with PMS include encouraging a diet with:
   a. moderate sodium
   b. low protein
   c. moderate caffeine
   d. increased complex carbohydrates

5. All of the following are associated with vaginitis in the menopausal female *except:*
   a. decreased estrogen
   b. thicker vaginal mucosa
   c. pyrogenic bacterial invasion
   d. leukorrhea

6. All of the following infections are precursors to acute bartholinitis *except:*
   a. cervicitis
   b. cystitis
   c. vaginitis
   d. urethritis

7. Incidence of toxic shock syndrome (TSS) is greater in women:
   a. during ovulation
   b. who use tampons
   c. who insert tampons with applicators
   d. who use contraceptive pills

8. The descent of the cervix or entire uterus into the vaginal canal is called:
   a. cystocele
   b. rectocele
   c. uterine prolapse
   d. endometriosis

9. Risk factors associated with cervical cancer include all of the following *except:*
   a. multiple sex partners
   b. infection with STDs
   c. cigarette smoking
   d. first coitus at later age

10. Which one of the following manifestations is characteristic of cervical cancer?
    a. white purulent discharge
    b. amenorrhea
    c. lack of any pain
    d. occasional spotting following intercourse

11. Nursing interventions for the woman patient presenting with the following symptoms of pelvic pain radiating to the groin and associated with the onset of menses one day ago, breast tenderness, abdominal distension, and backache include:
    a. rest, moderate exercise, proper nutrition and application of local heat
    b. administer ibuprofen or naproxen on an empty stomach
    c. prepare patient for endometrial biopsy, D&C, or hysterectomy, as indicated
    d. administer IV fluids, antibiotics and analgesics; treat sexual partner(s) with antibiotics

12. A 36-year-old *Caucasian* nulliparous patient in a monogamous relationship presents with the following: T98, abnormal vaginal bleeding and dysmenorrhea, inability to conceive a pregnancy,

dysparenunia, tender abdomen, constipation and pain on defecation. The nurse recognizes these characteristics as:

a. endometriosis
b. uterine fibroids
c. ovarian cysts
d. pelvic inflammatory disease

13. Breast cancer risk factors include all of the following *except:*

a. nulliparity
b. alcohol intake and high-fat diet
c. familial history; particularly in mother or sister
d. early menopause, late menarche

14. After an initial episode of pelvic inflammatory disease, a women is more likely to experience:

a. infertility and sterility
b. reinfection
c. ectopic pregnancy
d. all of the above

15. A 30-year-old patient is diagnosed with fibrocystic breast changes. All of the following may be included in her treatment plan *except:*

a. yearly mammograms beginning *immediately*
b. low-salt diet
c. limit caffeine intake
d. Tylenol, support bra, warm compresses

ANSWER KEY

Question	Correct answer	Correct answer rationale	Incorrect answer rationales
1.	c	Abnormal levels of prolactin are associated with secondary amenorrhea.	a, b, and d. Imbalances of Gn-RH, LH, and FSH can be associated with primary amenorrhea.
2.	a	Menorrhagia is prolonged, excessive bleeding during regular periods.	b. Metrorrhagia is bleeding between periods. c. Oligomenorrhea refers to menstrual periods that are more than 35 days apart. d. Dysfunctional uterine bleeding refers to abnormal bleeding without organic cause.
3.	b	Progesterone imbalances are attributed to PMS.	a. Hypoglycemia, not hyperglycemia, is associated with PMS. c and d. Increased renin–angiotensin activity and increased prostaglandins are also associated with PMS.
4.	d	Dietary guidelines for the patient with PMS recommend increased complex carbohydrates.	a. A reduced-sodium diet is recommended. b. Moderate protein intake is recommended. c. A diet with low or eliminated caffeine intake is recommended.
5.	b	Decreased estrogen results in a thinner, not thicker, vaginal mucosa.	a, c, and d. Decreased estrogen, pyrogenic bacterial invasion, and leukorrhea are all associated with vaginitis in the menopausal female.
6.	b.	Cystitis is not typically a precursor to acute bartholinitis.	a, c, and d. All of these may precede the development of acute bartholinitis.
7.	b	The use of superabsorbent tampons is associated with TSS.	a. Incidence of TSS is higher during menstruation. c and d. Risk factors associated with TSS include use of fingers to insert tampons and use of barrier contraceptives (eg, diaphragm or sponges).
8.	c	a. Cystocele refers to the descent of the bladder and anterior vaginal wall into the vaginal canal.	b. Rectocele refers to the bulging of the rectum and posterior vaginal wall into the vaginal canal. d. Endometriosis is the presence of endometrial cells at sites outside the uterus.

Question	Correct answer	Correct answer rationale	Incorrect answer rationales
9.	d	First coitus at an early age is the most important predictor.	a, b, and c. These are risk factors for cervical cancer.
10.	d	Manifestations of cervical cancer include occasional bloody spotting after intercourse or between periods.	a. Early manifestations can include a thin watery discharge, followed by a yellow discharge. b. Abnormally long menses is a symptom of cervical cancer. c. A dull lower backache or pain extending from the lower back through the hip is often seen in cervical cancer.
11.	a.	Primary dysmenorrhea is painful menstruation not associated with pelvic disease. Application of local heat promotes vasodilation resulting in increased blood flow, relief of ischemia, and increased menstrual flow.	b. Prostaglandin inhibitors must be given with milk or food to prevent gastric irritation.
12.	a.	All are manifestations of endometriosis.	b. Uterine fibroids more often occur in black and Asian women with symptoms of abnormal uterine bleeding, pain and pelvic pressure. c. Ovarian cysts are mostly asymptomatic; cysts either regress or rupture spontaneously. d. PID manifests with sudden, severe abdominal pain with fever, or may be asymptomatic.
13.	d.	Reproductive risks indicate *early* menarche, *late* menopause, nulliparous, birth of first child after age 34.	a, b, and c. These answers are true.
14.	d.	The inflammatory process of PID may involve fallopian tubes and ovaries causing infertility and sterility.	b. Reinfection occurs from undiagnosed or inadequately treated acute PID. c. Ectopic pregnancy may result from blocked fallopian tubes (salpingitis), adhesions, and strictures.
15.	a.	Yearly mammograms beginning immediately are not the standard of care in a 30 years old. Patient teaching in proper technique of regular breast self-exam along with periodic mammograms are indicated in her plan of care.	b, c, and d. Low-salt diet, limited caffeine use, Tylenol, bra, and warm compresses are interventions to assist the patient in minimizing discomfort.

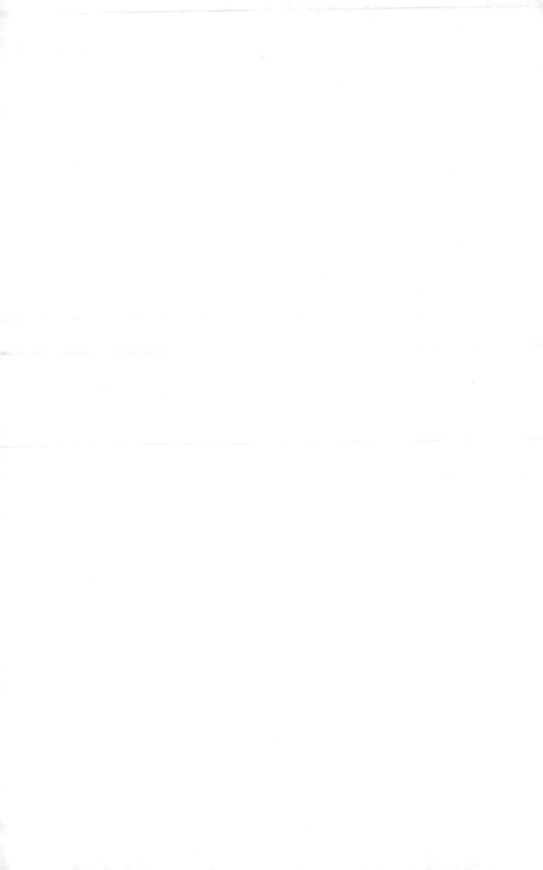

17

Male Reproductive Disorders

I. **Overview of pathophysiologic processes**

A. Congenital disorders
1. Congenital disorders are structural malformations of the penis or testicles that occur *in utero*.
2. Congenital disorders may affect either reproduction or urinary functions in adults.

3. Hypospadias and epispadias and cryptorchidism are congenital disorders; urethral stricture may be congenital or acquired.

4. There are no specific risk factors for these disorders.

B. **Acquired and inflammatory disorders**

1. Acquired or inflammatory disorders include disorders of the penis or testicles, or both, that result during the life-cycle from infection, illness, or injury.

 2. **Trauma and infection are the most common causes of these disorders (see Chapter 18 for a discussion of certain infections).**

3. These disorders may affect sexual function and reproduction.

4. Risk factors include:
   a. Trauma
   b. Poor hygiene
   c. Exposure to microorganisms

C. **Prostatic disorders**

1. Prostatic disorders affect the gland responsible for the secretion of seminal fluid.

2. Prostatic disorders result from an infection or benign enlargement.

3. Risk factors include age and exposure to pathogens.

D. **Male reproductive cancers**

1. Cancers of the male reproductive tract involve the testicles, penis, or prostate gland.

2. Incidence of these cancers depends on the person's age. Testicular cancer is common in younger men; prostate cancer, in older men; penile cancer is rare.

3. The earlier these cancers are detected, the better the prognosis; testicular self-examination is a screening test that can aid early detection.

4. There are no specific risk factors for male reproductive cancers.

II. Physiologic responses to male reproductive dysfunction

A. Urinary hesitancy: delay in initiation of urinary stream

B. Nocturia: excessive urination occurring at night

C. Dysuria: difficult and painful urination

D. Impotence: inability to achieve erection

E. Genital and lymph node swelling

III. Hypospadias and epispadias

A. Description

1. Hypospadias and epispadias are congenital deformities.

 2. In *hypospadias,* the urethral meatus opens on the ventral surface of the penis, proximal to the tip of the glans penis (Fig. 17-1); it can be classified according to location:
   a. Coronal (opening at the coronal sulcus)
   b. Glandular (opening on the proximal glans penis)

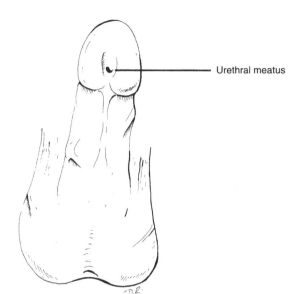

FIGURE 17-1.
Hypospadias. Urethral meatus opens on the ventral surface of the penis.

     c.   **Penile shaft**

     d.   **Penoscrotal**

     e.   **Perineal area**

  3.   Most cases of hypospadias are coronal or open on the distal penis.

   4.   **In *epispadias*, the urethra is displaced dorsally (Fig. 17-2); types include:**

     a.   **Glandular**

     b.   **Penile**

     c.   **Penopubic**

B.   **Etiology and incidence**

  1.   *Hypospadias*

     a.   Results when fusion of the urethral folds is incomplete; no specific genetic traits have been established to date, although a familial pattern has been noted.

     b.   Occurs in about 1 in 300 male children. Hormones (eg, estrogen and progestin) given during pregnancy are believed to increase the incidence.

  2.   *Epispadias*

     a.   Is a mild form of bladder exstrophy

     b.   Is less common then hypospadias, occurring in 1 in 120,000 males

C.   **Pathophysiologic processes and manifestations**

  1.   Sexual differentiation and urethral development occur between week 8 and 15 in utero.

  2.   In *hypospadias*

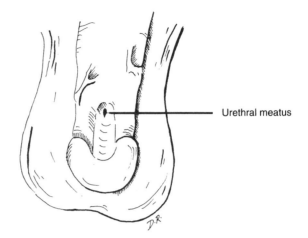

Urethral meatus

FIGURE 17-2.
Epispadias. Urethral meatus opens
on the dorsal surface of the penis.

    a. Curvature of the penis (chordee) causes ventral bending and bowing of the penile shaft, which may prevent sexual intercourse.

    b. The penis appears hooded as result of deficient or absent ventral foreskin.

    c. Older children complain of difficulty directing the urinary stream and spraying.

3. Perineal and penoscrotal hypospadias necessitate voiding in the sitting position.

4. Proximal forms of hypospadias in adults may cause infertility.

5. Hypospadias is associated with an increased incidence of undescended testicles in children.

6. In *glandular epispadias,* the urethra opens on the dorsal surface of the glans, which is broad and flattened.

7. In *penile epispadias,* the urethral meatus, which is broad and gaping, is located between the pubic symphysis and the coronal sulcus.

8. A distal groove extends from the meatus through the glans.

9. In *penopubic epispadias,* the urethral opening is at the penopubic junction (where the penis meets the pubic bone) and a distal dorsal groove extends through the glans.

10. Urinary incontinence is a common problem in penopubic and penile epispadias due to the maldevelopment of the urinary sphincters.

11. Dorsal curvature of the penis is also evident.

D. Overview of nursing interventions

1. Educate the child's parents to recognize problems early and seek medical attention.

2. Prepare the patient for surgery, if indicated; educate the parents about surgical interventions, which may include:

    a. For hypospadias: Free skin grafts to allow voiding in the standing position and ejaculation of semen into the vagina.

b.   For epispadias: Surgery to correct incontinence, remove the chordee to straighten the penis, and extend the urethra out onto the glans penis; if incontinence is not corrected, bladder augmentation with an artificial sphincter may be considered.

IV.   Cryptorchidism

A.   Description

1.   Cryptorchidism refers to failure of one or two testicles to descend from the abdomen into the scrotum during fetal development.

2.   **Testicles are most commonly located in the superficial inguinal area.**

B.   Etiology

1.   Although cryptorchidism results from unknown causes, it has been associated with the following factors:

a.   Shortened gubernaculum

b.   Testosterone deficiencies

c.   Narrow inguinal canal

d.   Adhesions of the inguinal pathway

2.   It may also result from:

a.   Congenital gonadal defect that renders the testicles insensitive to gonadotropins

b.   Deficient gonadotropic hormonal stimulation

C.   Pathophysiologic processes and manifestations

1.   Assessment findings include absence of one or both testes from the scrotum.

2.   An inguinal hernia often presents on the affected side.

3.   Pain from trauma to the testes and scrotum on the affected side may be present.

4.   Spermatogenesis will decrease.

5.   Even with surgery, 20% of males will remain infertile.

6.   A direct relationship exists between cryptorchidism and testicular cancer.

D.   Overview of nursing interventions

1.   Educate the child's parents regarding symptom recognition and treatment options.

2.   Administer hormone therapy (human chorionic gonadotropin [HCG] and luteinizing hormone releasing hormone [LHRH]), as ordered.

3.   Prepare the patient for surgery (orchiopexy), which must be done to prevent testicular atrophy; afterward, provide appropriate postoperative care.

V.   Urethral stricture

A.   Description: fibrotic stricture of dense collagen and fibroblasts resulting in a narrowed urethra and limiting urine flow

B.   Etiology: may be congenital (uncommon) or caused by infection resulting from use of indwelling catheters, trauma, or pelvic fractures

C.   Pathophysiologic processes and manifestations

1. The fossa navicularis and membranous urethra are the two most common sites of congenital urethral stricture.
2. Severe strictures cause:
    a. Bladder damage
    b. Hydronephrosis
    c. Urinary frequency and urgency
    d. Infection
3. Other symptoms can include:
    a. Decrease in urine stream
    b. Chronic urethral discharge
    c. Acute cystitis
    d. Mild dysuria
    e. Postvoiding dribbling
4. Complications can include chronic prostatitis, cystitis, chronic urinary infection, diverticula, urethrocutaneous fistulas, periurethral abscesses, and urethral carcinoma.

D.   Overview of nursing interventions
1. Educate the patient about related symptoms that indicate a stricture.
2. Prepare the patient for dilation, urethrotomy or surgical reconstruction depending on size.
3. Advise the patient to seek follow-up care to assess the stability of the stricture.

VI.   Phimosis and paraphimosis

A.   Description
1. *Phimosis* is a condition in which the tightened foreskin is unable to retract over the glans (Fig. 17-3); it may be congenital or acquired.
2. Most often phimosis is seen in uncircumcised males; however, excessive skin left after a circumcision can become stenotic and cause this disorder.
3. *Paraphimosis* is a condition in which the foreskin can be retracted but not returned to its normal position.

B.   Etiology
1. *Congenital phimosis* occurs when the foreskin does not grow along with the penis, making it too small to either retract or reduce; *acquired phimosis* usually results from chronic infection from poor local hygiene.
2. *Paraphimosis* results from chronic inflammation under the foreskin, which leads to contracture of the preputial opening and formation of a tight ring of skin when the foreskin is retracted behind the glans (Fig. 17-4). This leads to venous congestion, edema, and enlargement of the glans.

C.   Pathophysiologic processes and manifestations
1. At birth, most male infants do not have a fully retractable foreskin. As the child grows, a space usually develops between the glans and foreskin so that by age 3, most uncircumcised males have a fully retractable foreskin.

2. **In phimosis and paraphimosis, the foreskin is not retractable but is tightened.**

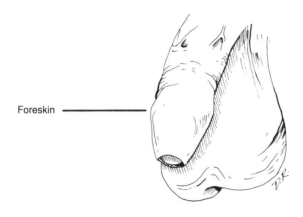

Foreskin ——————

FIGURE 17-3.
Phimosis. Tightened foreskin is
unable to retract over the glans.

3. Tightened foreskin leads to excess oil gland secretion and smegma accumulation with subsequent inflammation and infection.
4. Other manifestations include edema, erythema, and tenderness.

D. Overview of nursing interventions

1. Educate parents who opt not to circumcise their male children about the potential for these disorders to occur and how to recognize the symptoms.
2. Encourage parents to seek treatment if symptoms appear; treatment options may include:
    a. For phimosis: Administration of broad-spectrum antibiotics, slitting of the dorsal foreskin for drainage, and circumcision after the infection is controlled
    b. For paraphimosis: Firm squeezing of the glans for 5 minutes to reduce the edema and size of the glans. If this is unsuccessful, then the

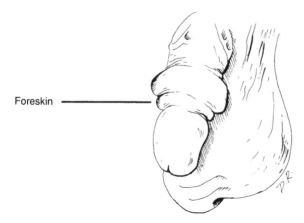

Foreskin ——————

FIGURE 17-4.
Paraphimosis. Retracted foreskin
cannot be returned to its normal
position.

constricting may need to be incised and antibiotics prescribed. Circumcision is done after inflammation is reduced.

VII. Balanitis

A. Description

    1. Balanitis is a condition in which the foreskin becomes inflamed, loses pigmentation, and undergoes atrophic sclerotic changes; it affects uncircumcised males.

    2. It is also called leukoplakia of the penis.

B. Etiology: viral (papovirus)

C. Pathophysiologic processes and manifestations

    1. The skin atrophies, and the poor cohesion between the epidermis and the underlying connective tissue develops.

    2. Manifestations include redness, swelling, pain, purulent drainage, and development of a white plaque involving the meatus, prepuce, or glans.

    3. Hemorrhagic changes may result from even the mildest trauma.

D. Overview of nursing interventions

    1. Instruct the child and parents in cleansing of the prepuce.

    2. Educate the child and parents regarding circumcision.

    3. Administer antibiotics, if indicated.

    4. If meatal stenosis occurs, prepare the patient for emergency meatomy.

    5. Assist with circumcision.

VIII. Peyronie's disease

A. Description: fibrous plaque formation on the dorsal side of the penis in the sheath of the corpus cavernosum

B. Etiology and incidence: idiopathic; usually occurs in middle-aged or elderly men

C. Pathophysiologic processes and manifestations

    1. Inflammatory cells infiltrate the perivascular region of the tunica albuginea.

    2. A fibrous plaque containing excessive collagen forms.

    3. In time, the plaque may become bony as it calcifies. The hardening of the penile tissue prevents elongation, making erection painful and sexual intercourse difficult or impossible.

D. Overview of nursing interventions

    1. Teach the patient how to assess for Peyronie's disease; note that spontaneous remission occurs in about 50% of the cases.

    2. Prepare the patient for treatment, if indicated; treatment options may include:

        a. Inject hydrocortisone, vitamin E, or parathyroid hormone into the plaque

        b. Radiation therapy

        c. Administer fibrinolytics

        d. Surgical removal of the plaque and replacement with dermal graft

IX. **Priapism**

A. Description

1. Priapism is a vascular instability in the penile corpora cavernosa that causes sustained painful nonsexual erection; it may be primary or secondary.
2. Types include:
    a. Stasis priapism: blood becomes stagnant in the corpora cavernosa
    b. High-flow priapism: blood flow is maintained or increased

B. Etiology

1. Primary priapism is idiopathic.
2. Secondary priapism results from other disorders (eg, spinal cord or penile trauma, pelvic infections, leukemia, sickle cell disease) or occurs secondary to administration of certain medications (eg, coumadin, heparin, steroids, and testosterone).

C. Pathophysiologic processes and manifestations

1. **Instability of the blood flow into and out of the corpora cavernosa leads to sustained erection, because blood pressure inside the corpora is always increased.**
2. Increased blood pressure in the corpora leads to decreased oxygen tension.

3. **This damaging pathology can lead to fibrosis and erectile failure; impotence and gangrene are the worst sequelae.**
4. When the duration of blood stasis is long and severe, the possibility of erectile failure exists.

D. Overview of nursing interventions

1. Educate the patient about the disorder.
2. Administer analgesics for pain, as ordered.
3. Administer ice cold saline enemas.
4. Prepare the patient for shunt insertion, if indicated.
5. Encourage bedrest.

X. **Epididymitis**

A. Description: inflammation of the epididymis; usually accompanied by infection

B. Etiology

1. Infectious agents in parts of the reproductive tract (urethra, bladder, prostate) spread to the epididymis.

2. **Causative organisms commonly are sexually transmitted organisms or enteric bacteria (eg, *Chlamydia*, *Neisseria gonorrhea*, *Enterobacter*, or *Pseudomonas*).**

C. Pathophysiologic processes and manifestations

1. The infection moves upward through the urethra and the ejaculatory duct, then along the vas deferens to the epididymis.
2. Symptoms include:
    a. Pain

      b.   Fever and chills

      c.   Malaise

      d.   Scrotal swelling

      e.   Testicular congestion

3. In advanced epididymitis, testicular necrosis, fibrosis, and infertility can occur.

4. Urethral discharge and overlying reddened skin are also present; these symptoms follow severe physical strain or sexual excitement.

D. **Overview of nursing interventions**

   1. Instruct the patient to avoid straining, lifting, and sexual excitement until the infection is controlled.

   2. Teach the patient the potential relationship between sexually transmitted urethritis and epididymitis.

   3. Educate the patient about safe sexual behavior.

   4. Administer antibiotics to both partners and nonsteroidal antiinflammatory drugs (NSAIDs), as ordered.

   5. Administer lidocaine to relieve pain and swelling.

   6. Apply ice packs to reduce inflammation.

   7. Encourage use of an athletic supporter.

XI. Testicular torsion

A. **Description: rotation or twisting of the testis within the tunica vaginalis; twisting of spermatic cord also occurs**

B. **Etiology: may occur spontaneously after exercise or trauma**

C. **Pathophysiologic processes and manifestations**

   1. The twisting of cords produces severe pain and leads to the following symptoms:

      a.   Nausea

      b.   Vomiting

      c.   Lower abdominal pain

      d.   Tachycardia

      e.   Urinary urgency

      f.   Diurnal frequency

      g.   Dysuria

      h.   Nocturia

   2. The affected testicle is enlarged and tender, and the skin is reddened; pain may radiate to the inguinal area.

   3. **Extensive cremasteric muscle reaction causes thickening of the spermatic cord; extravasation of blood into the scrotal sac may occur if vessels rupture.**

   4. Blood supply to the testicle is reduced.

D. **Overview of nursing interventions**

   1. Educate the patient about the importance of seeking medical attention early.

   2. Prepare the patient for manual detorsion or emergency surgery (orchiopexy), if indicated; afterward, provide appropriate postoperative care.

XII. **Orchitis**

A. Description: unilateral or bilateral inflammation of the testes

B. Etiology

1. Orchitis may result from ascending infection of the genitals or lymphatic spread, or it may occur as a complication of mumps (due to urinary excretion of the virus).

2. Common causative agents are *Staphylococcus, Streptococcus, Escherichia coli, Streptococcus pneumoniae,* and *Pseudomonas.*

C. Pathophysiologic processes and manifestations

1. Symptoms include:
   a. Pain
   b. Testicular swelling (testes may appear bluish in color)
   c. Tender and red scrotum
2. Complications include hydrocele and abscess.
3. Sequelae may include impotence, sterility, or marked atrophy.

D. Overview of nursing interventions

1. Administer antibiotics, as ordered, to treat infection.
2. Administer steroids, as ordered, to reduce inflammation.
3. Administer analgesics and antipyretics, as prescribed, to relieve pain and reduce fever.
4. Apply ice packs.

XIII. **Hydrocele**

A. Description: accumulation of clear or straw-colored fluid within the tunica or processus vaginalis sac

B. Etiology

1. Hydrocele results from unknown causes; it may occur after epididymitis, orchitis, injury, or neoplasm.
2. Late closure of the tunica vaginalis during fetal life results in infant hydrocele.

C. Pathophysiologic processes and manifestations

1. Manifestations include:
   a. Scrotal changes (small and soft in the morning and large and tense at night); this usually is painless unless accompanied by epididymal infection
   b. Possible scrotal tension
2. Transillumination is positive and helps distinguish hydrocele from a tumor or hernia.

D. Overview of nursing interventions

1. Instruct the patient to use an athletic supporter for comfort and support.
2. Prepare the patient for surgery, if indicated; afterward, provide appropriate postoperative care.

XIV. Varicocele

A. Description: abnormal dilation of pampiniform plexus above the testes, usually occurring on the left side

B. Etiology

   1. Varicocele results from unknown causes.
   2. It commonly occurs in males between the ages of 15 and 25.

C. Pathophysiologic processes and manifestations

   1. Symptoms include pain, tenderness, and discomfort in the inguinal area.
   2. On palpation, the mass feels like a bag of worms.

D. Overview of nursing interventions

   1. Prepare the patient for surgery, if fertility is a concern.
   2. Apply an ice bag to the area to reduce edema after surgery.
   3. Instruct the patient to wear a scrotal support.

XV. Spermatocele

A. Description: painless, cystic mass containing sperm; located above and posterior to the testis

B. Etiology

   1. Spermatocele results from unknown causes.
   2. It may arise from the tubules that connect the rete testis to the head of the epididymis or from cystic structures on the upper pole of the testis or epididymis.

C. Pathophysiologic processes and manifestations

   1. Spermatocele is usually small and is discovered on routine examination.
   2. It is a freely movable mass with dead sperm inside its fluid center.

D. Overview of nursing interventions

   1. Apply scrotal support.
   2. Apply ice packs.
   3. Prepare the patient for surgery (excision), if necessary; afterward, provide appropriate postoperative care.

XVI. Pyoderma

A. Description and etiology

   1. Pyoderma is an infection in the genital area; types of lesions include:
      a. Follicular pustule (folliculitis)
      b. Superficial blister impetigo
   2. *Staphylococcus aureus* is the most common causative organism.

B. Pathophysiologic processes and manifestations

   1. Folliculitis presents as a superficial infection of a follicle; it usually is acute but can become chronic.

2. Recurrent folliculitis is commonly seen in patients with acquired immuno-deficiency syndrome (AIDS).

3. Impetigo is a superficial blister that breaks quickly, leaving a crusted, weeping erosion.

C. Overview of nursing interventions

1. Teach the patient about personal hygiene habits to avoid recurrences.

2. Instruct the patient to wash with antibacterial soap.

 3. **Administer penicillinase-resistant penicillin, as ordered, because topical treatment alone is inadequate.**

XVII. Prostatitis

A. Description: inflammation of the prostate gland; may be bacterial (acute or chronic) or nonbacterial (most common form)

B. Etiology

1. Bacterial prostatitis can be caused by Gram-negative or Gram-positive organisms.

2. Bacterial prostatitis is associated with cystitis and urinary retention.

3. Chronic bacterial prostatitis may result after acute prostatitis.

4. Nonbacterial prostatitis results from unknown causes; it may be related to excessive consumption of alcohol, caffeine, or spicy foods.

C. Pathophysiologic processes and manifestations

1. In bacterial prostatitis, microbes may ascend from the urethra or may descend from the bladder or kidneys.

2. Hematogenous spread (from the skin or the respiratory system) or lymphogenous spread (from rectal bacteria) may also occur.

3. In *acute bacterial prostatitis*
   a. Manifestations include fever, dysuria, urinary frequency, urinary urgency, and hematuria.
   b. Palpation reveals large, tender, and warm prostate.
   c. Seminal vesicles may be palpable.
   d. Hematuria or pyuria may be present.

4. In *chronic bacterial prostatitis*
   a. No symptoms may be present; diagnosis may occur in routine urinalysis.
   b. Manifestations include low-grade fever, perineal and back pain, nocturia, and dysuria.

5. In *nonbacterial prostatitis*
   a. Manifestations include low back pain, urinary frequency, urinary urgency, rectal or perineal discomfort.
   b. The prostate is nontender.
   c. This is the most common form of prostatitis.

D. Overview of nursing interventions

1. For acute bacterial prostatitis:
   a. Administer antimicrobial therapy (Bactrim), as prescribed.

b. **Avoid catheterization because it may spread the infection into the urinary tract.**

2. For chronic bacterial prostatitis:
   a. Administer antimicrobial therapy for at least 12 weeks, as prescribed.
   b. Prepare the patient for transurethral prostatectomy if medical therapy fails.
   c. Encourage hot sitz baths.
   d. Administer NSAIDs to relieve symptoms, as ordered.
3. For nonbacterial prostatitis:
   a. Administer antimicrobial therapy, as prescribed.
   b. Administer NSAIDs, as ordered.
   c. Encourage hot sitz baths.
4. Instruct patient to avoid sexual arousal and intercourse during periods of acute inflammation.
5. Tell the patient to avoid sitting for prolonged periods.
6. Encourage the patient to have a 1-year medical follow-up.
7. Administer antibiotics and analgesics as ordered.

XVIII. Benign prostatic hypertrophy

A. **Description: benign enlargement of the prostate**
B. **Etiology**
   1. Possible causes of benign prostatic hypertrophy include:
      a. Hormonal factors
      b. Histologic and age-related changes
   2. It usually affects men over age 50.
C. **Pathophysiologic processes and manifestations**
   1. Hyperplasia produces the following symptoms:
      a. Large discrete nodules in the median and lateral lobes
      b. Urethral compression, which causes signs of urinary obstruction

 2. **Symptoms can be initiated as a result of alcohol intake, low temperature, ingestion of certain medications (eg, anticholinergics, psychotropics, and adrenergic agents), and ignoring the first desire to void.**
   3. Other symptoms may include:
      a. Decrease in force and caliber of the urinary stream due to ureteral compression
      b. Urinary urgency, hesitancy, intermittency, and dribbling
      c. Nocturia
      d. Dysuria
      e. Enlarged prostate (palpated on rectal examination)
D. **Overview of nursing interventions**
   1. Prepare the patient for transurethral dilation of the prostate, if indicated; afterward, provide appropriate postoperative care.
   2. Instruct the patient in perineal exercises after surgery to regain urinary control.
   3. Administer medications such as antiandrogens.

XIX.   Prostate cancer

A.   Description and etiology

1. Carcinoma of the prostate gland is the most commonly occurring male cancer; it generally affects men over age 50.

2. Adenocarcinoma is the typical type of cancer; it usually occurs in the posterior lobe.

3. Although the exact etiology is unknown, factors associated with prostate cancer include:

    a. Age
    b. Race (more common in African Americans)
    c. Genetic predisposition
    d. Hormonal factors
    e. History of sexually transmitted diseases
    f. Exposure to chemical carcinogens
    g. High-fat diet

B.   Pathophysiologic processes and manifestations

1. **Manifestations include hard, fixed nodules palpated on rectal examination.**

2. Acid-phosphatase and serum prostatic specific antigen may be elevated.

3. The most common sites of metastases are bones, lungs, lymph nodes, and liver.

4. If signs of urinary obstruction are present, the tumor is large enough to cause metastasis.

5. Staging of prostatic cancer involves digital examination followed by computed tomography (CT) or magnetic resonance imaging (MRI). Transrectal ultrasonography with a biopsy can stage extracapsular extension.

6. Bone scintigraphy and serum acid phosphatase are also used to rule out metastasis.

C.   Overview of nursing interventions

1. Advise men over age 40 to have digital rectal examinations annually to aid early detection of prostate cancer.

2. Prepare the patient for treatment, which may include

    a. Radical nerve-sparing prostatectomy (low-stage disease)
    b. Radiation therapy
    c. Hormonal therapies (metastatic cancer)

XX.   Testicular cancer

A.   Description and etiology

1. Cancer of the testes occurs in young men between ages 20 and 40 (Fig. 17-5).

2. Types include germinal cell tumors and nongerminal cell tumors.

    a. Germinal cell tumor types include seminoma and nonseminoma.
    b. Seminomas are the most common type, occurring in men ages 30 to 40.

3. As with most cancers, the etiology is unknown.

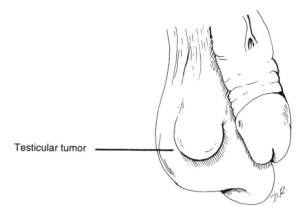

FIGURE 17-5.
Testicular cancer. Visible tumor in
scrotal sac.

    4. Risk factors associated with testicular cancer include:
        a. History of cryptorchidism
        b. Trauma
        c. Exogenous estrogen administration to the mother during pregnancy

B. **Pathophysiologic processes and manifestations**
    1. Germinal cell tumors arise from spermatozoa and their derivations.
    2. Seminoma germinal cell tumors arise from seminiferous epithelium of the testes.
    3. Nonseminoma germinal cell tumors include three types:
        a. Embryonal carcinoma: more aggressive; may begin *in utero*
        b. Teratoma: can occur at any age as a benign mass
        c. Choriocarcinoma: highly malignant
    4. Nongerminal cell tumors arise from other cellular components of the testes (eg, Leydig's cells, Sertoli's cells, and gonadoblastoma).
    5. Symptoms can include:
        a. Painless enlargement of the testes
        b. Dull ache in the testes
        c. Back pain
        d. Cough
        e. Dyspnea
        f. Bone pain
        g. Lower extremity swelling
    6. A mass does not transilluminate (when a flashlight is pressed against the mass, transillumination occurs when the light shines through); possible lymphadenopathy.
    7. If the tumor secretes HCG or estrogen, gynecomastia may be seen.

C. **Overview of nursing interventions**

    1. **Teach male patients how to perform a testicular self-examination monthly and when to recognize the need for medical attention.**
    2. Stress importance of follow-up examinations when a tumor of the testes has been treated.

3. Prepare patient for orchiectomy, radiation, or chemotherapy depending on the stage and histology of the tumor.

XXI.   Penile cancer

A. Description

1. Penile cancer (squamous cell carcinoma) is a rare type of malignant lesion.
2. Three types of tumors have been identified:
   a. Precancerous dermatologic lesions
   b. Carcinoma in situ (Bowen's disease, erythroplasia of Queyrat)
   c. Invasive carcinoma (comprises most penile cancers)

B. Etiology and incidence

1. Causes of penile cancer include poor hygiene and smegma accumulation under the phimotic foreskin, which results in chronic inflammation.
2. Penile cancer accounts for a small percentage of male cancers in the United States.
3. Typically, it occurs in the sixth decade of life.

C. Pathophysiologic processes and manifestations

1. Precancerous dermatologic lesions manifest as leukoplakia on the meatus, prepuce, or glans.
2. Carcinoma *in situ* involves the penile shaft; it appears as a red plaque with encrustation. Erythroplasia of Queyrat is a velvety, red lesion with ulcerations involving the glans.
3. Invasive carcinoma appears on the glans, prepuce, or shaft as papillary or ulcerative lesions.
4. It is inoperable when the lymph nodes are involved or distant metastases occur.
5. Manifestations include:
   a. Pain
   b. Discharge
   c. Irritating voiding symptoms (such as dysuria)
   d. Bleeding

D. Overview of nursing interventions

1. Prepare the patient for biopsy.
2. Prepare the patient for chemotherapy or surgery, the extent of which is indicated by the pathology of the lesion.
3. Refer the patient for psychological counseling.
4. Manage the patient's pain.

Bibliography

Bullock, B. (1996). *Pathophysiology: Adaptations and alterations in function* (4th ed.). Philadelphia: Lippincott-Raven.

Droller, M. M. A. (1992). *Surgical management of urologic diseases: An anatomic approach.* St. Louis: Mosby-Year Book.

Ganong, William F. (1997). *Review of medical physiology* (18th ed.). Stamford, CT: Appleton and Lange.

Gillenwater, J., Grayback, J., et al. (1991). *Adult and pediatric urology, Vols. 1 & 2* (2nd ed.). St. Louis: Mosby-Year Book.

Gray, M. (1992). *Genitourinary disorders.* St. Louis: Mosby-Year Book.

Guyton, Arthur C., & Hall John E. (1996). *Textbook of medical physiology* (9th ed.). Philadelphia: W. B. Saunders.

Hanno, P., & Wein, A. (1994). *Clinical manual of urology* (2nd ed.). New York: McGraw-Hill.

Kinney, M., Packa, D., & Dunbar, S. (1993). *AACN's clinical reference for critical-care nursing* (3rd ed.). St. Louis: C.V. Mosby.

McCance, K. L., & Huether, S. E. (1994). *Pathophysiology: The biologic basis for disease in adults and children* (2nd ed.). St. Louis: Mosby-Year Book.

Porth, C. (1994). *Pathophysiology: Concepts of altered health states* (4th ed.). Philadelphia: Lippincott-Raven.

Tanagho, E., & McAninch, J. (1992). *Smith's general urology* (13th ed.). Norwalk, CT: Appleton & Lange.

STUDY QUESTIONS

1. Which of the following are risk factors for acquired disorders of the male reproduction system:
   a. influenza
   b. good hygiene
   c. exposure to organisms
   d. congenital defects

2. Hesitancy can be defined as:
   a. urination that occurs at night
   b. delay in initiation of urinary stream
   c. painful urination
   d. inability to urinate

3. Hormones administered to the mother during pregnancy may increase the incidence of:
   a. hypospadias
   b. varicocele
   c. phimosis
   d. balanitis

4. When educating new parents about the possible consequences of not circumcising their son, the nurse would explain that which of the following conditions might occur?
   a. hypospadias
   b. phimosis
   c. varicocele
   d. spermatocele

5. Manifestations of epididymitis may include:
   a. pain
   b. testicular necrosis
   c. pale skin locally
   d. infertility

6. Nursing interventions for a patient with epididymitis can include:
   a. application of warmth
   b. encouragement of sexual activity
   c. avoidance of athletic supporters
   d. lidocaine injections into spinal cord

7. Patient education for the patient with epididymitis should focus on:
   a. surgical treatment
   b. safe sexual behavior
   c. heat application
   d. hormonal therapy

8. A cardinal symptom of prostate cancer is:
   a. soft movable mass
   b. hard fixed nodules palpated on rectal examination
   c. velvety red ulcerative lesion
   d. painless enlargement of testes

9. Risk factors for testicular cancer may include:
   a. cryptorchidism
   b. priapism
   c. testosterone administration
   d. balanitis

10. Patient education regarding the prevention of penile carcinoma should focus on the importance of:
    a. using condoms
    b. self-examination of the testicles
    c. treatment of inflammation
    d. yearly rectal digital examinations

ANSWER KEY

Question	Correct answer	Correct answer rationale	Incorrect answer rationales
1.	c		a, b, and d. Influenza does not influence the development of male cancers. Good hygiene helps prevent the development of male cancers. Congenital defects are related to congenital disorders.
2.	b	Hesitancy is defined as a delay in initiation of urinary stream.	a. Nocturia is urination that occurs at night. c. Dysuria is painful urination. d. This response is incorrect.
3.	a	Administration of estrogen or progesterone to a pregnant woman increases the risk of hypospadias.	b, c, and d. These are not associated with hormone administration.
4.	b	Phimosis is a condition in which the tightened foreskin is unable to retract over the glans. Most often it is seen in uncircumcised males.	a, c, and d. These conditions are not related to circumcision.
5.	c	In epididymitis, the skin appears reddened, not pale.	a, b, and d. Manifestations of epididymitis may include pain, testicular necrosis, and infertility.
6.	d	Nursing interventions can include lidocaine injections into the spinal cord to relieve pain and swelling.	a. Apply ice, not warmth. b. Instruct the patient to avoid sexual activity, lifting, and straining until the inflammation has abated. c. Encourage the patient to use an athletic supporter.
7.	b	The nurse should focus patient education on safe sexual practices, including the relationship between sexually transmitted urethritis and epididymitis.	a. Surgery is not a treatment. c. Ice packs, not heat applications, are encouraged. d. This response is incorrect.
8.	b	Assessment includes hard, fixed nodules palpated during a rectal examination.	a. This response is incorrect. c. A velvety red ulcerative lesion is seen in penile carcinoma. d. Painless enlargement of testes is a sign of testicular cancer.
9.	a	Cryptorchidism, exogenous administration of estrogen to the mother during pregnancy, and trauma are all considered risk factors for testicular cancer.	b, c, and d. Priapism, phimosis, and balanitis are not associated with an increased risk of testicular cancer.

Question	Correct answer	Correct answer rationale	Incorrect answer rationales
10.	c	Patient education should focus on the importance of hygiene, self-examination of the penis, and treatment of inflammation.	a, b, and d. Condoms, testicular examination, and digital rectal examinations are not used to diagnose penile carcinoma.

18 Sexually Transmitted Diseases

I.   Overview of pathophysiologic processes

A.   Description

1.   Sexually transmitted diseases (STDs) are acute infections of the genitals and reproductive system that are acquired through sexual practices including, but not limited to, vaginal intercourse, anal–genital intercourse, anal–oral contact, anal–digital activity, and close direct contact with infected persons.

2.   STDs are most likely to occur in sexually active adolescents and young adults; incidence is highest in persons ages 18 to 19 years. Incidence of all STDs is increasing.

3.   The severity of STDs is greatest in women and in homosexual males. A person may be infected with more than one STD at a time.

B.   Bacterial STDs

1.   Bacterial STDs are caused by:
    a.   *Neisseria gonorrhoeae,* a Gram-negative organism
    b.   *Chlamydia trachomatis,* an intracellular parasite
    c.   *Treponema pallidum,* a spirochete

2.   Gonorrhea, chlamydia, and syphilis are bacterial STDs and are caused by the above organisms respectively.

C.   Viral STDs

1.   Viral STDs are caused by:
    a.   Herpes virus type 2
    b.   Human papillomavirus (HPV)
    c.   Hepatitis B virus

2.   Genital herpes, condylomata acuminata (genital warts), and viral hepatitis B are viral STDs, caused by the above organisms respectively.

II.   Physiologic responses to STDs

A.   Responses in women

1.   Cervicitis: inflammation of the cervical tissue

2.   Bartholinitis: inflammation of Bartholin's gland, which may result in abscess formation

3.   Systemic symptoms, including pharyngitis, joint pain, fever, and conjunctivitis

4.   Alterations in the mucous membrane and skin, including skin lesions and vaginal discharge

B.   Responses in men

1.   Prostatitis: inflammation of the prostate

2.   Epididymitis: inflammation of the epididymis that occurs as organisms move up the urethra and invade testicular structures

3.   Penile lymphangitis (rare): inflammation of the lymph vessels in the penis, which results in pain and tenderness, and penile discharge

4.   Systemic symptoms, including pharyngitis, joint pain, fever, and conjunctivitis

III. **Gonorrhea**

A. **Description**

1. The most commonly reported communicable disease in the United States, gonorrhea is an acute infection typically affecting the mucous membranes of the genitals.

2. It can also affect the mouth, throat, and anus.

B. **Etiology and incidence**

1. Gonorrhea is caused by *N. gonorrhoeae,* a Gram-negative organism.

2. It is transmitted sexually by way of direct contact with epithelial surfaces.

3. It also can be transmitted from an infected mother to a fetus across amniotic membranes or during passage through the birth canal.

4. The risk of acquiring gonorrhea rises with increased exposure. The risk of male-to-female or male-to-male transmission is greater than female-to-male or female-to-female transmission.

C. **Pathophysiologic processes and manifestations**

1. *N. gonorrhoeae* attaches itself to the walls of epithelial cells, which are located in mucous membranes. As the organism invades the cells, it damages the mucosa.

2. Damage to the mucosal cells stimulates the intrinsic inflammatory response, which causes a variety of symptoms associated with infection.

3. Although there is an incubation period, symptoms generally begin 10 days after infection.

4. Clinical gonorrhea is manifested by a broad spectrum of symptoms including:

   a. Symptomatic local infections (eg, urethritis, cervicitis, proctitis, pharyngitis, bartholinitis, conjunctivitis)

   b. Asymptomatic local infections (common sites include urethra, endocervix, rectum, and pharynx)

   c. Local complications (eg, salpingitis, epididymitis, Bartholin's abscess, lymphangitis, penile edema, periurethral abscess, prostatitis)

   d. Systemic dissemination

5. *In men*

   a. The incubation period is about 2 to 5 days but may be as long as 3 weeks.

   b. Common manifestations include dysuria, a mucopurulent discharge at the urethra meatus, and edema and erythema of the urethral meatus.

   c. Severity of symptoms varies with the infecting strain of *N. gonorrhoeae;* some patients will develop only a scant exudate, whereas a minority of patients will not develop any overt symptoms.

   d. Without treatment, gonococcal urethritis will self-resolve within several weeks; more than 95% of untreated patients will be asymptomatic within 6 months.

6. *In women*

   a. The infection usually starts in the inner part of the cervix; it may affect the Skene or Bartholin glands.

   b. Hormonal and cervical mucus changes associated with menstruation lower the normal bacterial protection in the uterus and fallopian tubes and foster ascension of organisms. This may cause an extensive infection called pelvic inflammatory disease (PID).

    c.   Symptoms of gonorrhea are the same as those of most lower genital tract infections and include increased vaginal discharge, dysuria, intermenstrual uterine bleeding, and menorrhagia.

    d.   Physical examination may reveal purulent exudate from the urethra or Bartholin's duct as well as cervical abnormalities.

    e.   Common complications include salpingitis, PID, infertility, ectopic pregnancy, and Bartholin's gland abscess.

    f.   During pregnancy, manifestations may include spontaneous abortion, premature rupture of fetal membranes, premature delivery, and acute chorioamnionitis.

    7.   *In neonates,* manifestations include:

        a.   Ophthalmia neonatorum

        b.   Pharyngeal infections

D.   **Overview of nursing interventions**

    1.   Obtain cultures, sensitivity tests, and Gram stains of affected sites, as ordered.

    2.   Institute serologic testing for *N. gonorrhoeae* antibodies.

    3.   Administer antimicrobials as prescribed. Injectable penicillin and oral Probenecid (a drug that delays excretion of penicillin) have been the accepted treatment. Ceftriaxone and doxycyline are the most often used combination because they destroy the bacteria and protect against penicillin-resistant strains.

    4.   Administer Tetracycline to patients who are allergic to penicillin.

    5.   Provide patient teaching covering use of condoms, diaphragm, cervical cap, and topical spermicidal and bactericidal agents.

    6.   Inform the patient that the disease is reportable.

    7.   Provide written information for the patient and his or her sexual partners.

    8.   Provide appropriate referrals for diagnosis and treatment to the patient's sexual partners.

    9.   Conduct examinations, obtain cultures, and provide presumptive treatment for all persons exposed within 30 days.

    10.   Prevent ophthalmia neonatorum by instilling a prophylactic agent into the eyes of all newborns.

IV.   **Chlamydia**

A.   **Description**

    1.   *Chlamydia* causes acute infections of the reproductive tract.

    2.   Chlamydial organisms are classified as bacteria, although they share properties of both bacteria and viruses. They have cell walls similar to Gram-negative organisms. But like viruses, they are obligate intracellular parasites and can only reproduce within host cells.

    3.   The species of *Chlamydia* organism transmitted in humans is *C. trachomatis.*

B.   **Etiology and incidence**

    1.   All *Chlamydia* infections are acquired either through sexual contact or perinatally.

2. Maternal-fetal transmission is associated with high fetal morbidity.
3. The incidence of *Chlamydia* in men has not been well defined because it is not a reportable disease in many countries, it is not microscopically confirmed, and it may be asymptomatic. In men, *C. trachomatis* is found in up to 60% of patients with nongonococcal urethritis and 70% of patients with postgonococcal urethritis.
4. *Chlamydia* is the most prevalent STD.

C. **Pathophysiologic processes and manifestations**

1. The incubation period for *C. trachomatis* is approximately 2 weeks after exposure. Some degree of immunity is conferred with repeated infections; however, the immunity usually is not strong enough to guard against repeat infections, which are common.
2. *C. trachomatis* has a twopart reproductive cycle, accounting for its virulence.
3. It begins with a small, inactive component, called an elementary body, that can survive outside of host cells. This is the infectious particle that enters uninfected cells.
4. The elementary body attaches to a host cell and enters. Once inside the cell, the organism reorganizes into the reticulate body which is the metabolically active form of the organism and is capable of reproducing.
5. Cell rupture releases all the elementary bodies that have been produced. The chlamydial growth cycle is illustrated in Figure 18-1

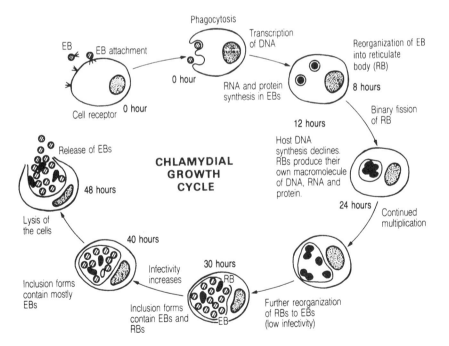

FIGURE 18-1.
Chlamydial growth cycle. [*Source:* EB, elementary body; RB, reticulate body. Thompson, S. E., & Washington, A. E. 1983]. Epidemiology of sexually transmitted *Chlamydia trachomatis* infections. *Epidemiologic Reviews, 5,* 96–123]

6. Chlamydial infections cause permanent tissue scarring.
7. Many chlamydial infections (especially those in women) are difficult to diagnose because there are few or no symptoms; any symptoms that may exist are nonspecific.
8. Clinical manifestations of genital infections caused by *Chlamydia* closely parallel infections caused by *N. gonorrhoeae*.
9. *In men,* manifestations can include:
   a. Epididymitis
   b. Conjunctivitis
   c. Prostatitis
   d. Reiter's syndrome (urethritis, conjunctivitis, arthritis, and mucocutaneous lesions); this has been found in up to 80% of men with preceding or concurrent *C. trachomatis* infection
10. *In women,* chlamydial infections typically are asymptomatic. The most common findings are mucopurulent discharge and hypertrophic ectopy (an area of the cervix that is congested, edematous, and bleeds easily).
11. Hypertrophic ectopy is normally present in 80% of sexually active adolescents; incidence declines around age 40.
    a. Ectopy may predispose women to chlamydial infections by exposing a greater number of cervical cells, making infection more likely on exposure.
    b. Ectopy may also increase shedding of *C. trachomatis* from the cervix, making transmission to sexual partners easier.
    c. The use of oral contraceptives promotes ectopy, which may explain the high prevalence of chlamydial infections in adolescent females (28%) who use oral contraceptives.
12. Other manifestations can include acute urethral syndrome, bartholinitis, cervicitis, salpingitis, conjunctivitis, perihepatitis (occurring after or with salpingitis), and reactive arthritis.
13. Severe complications may include pneumonitis in immunocompromised adults, endocarditis, and meningoencephalitis.
14. With maternal–fetal transmission, the neonate may be born prematurely or may suffer from pneumonia or newborn conjunctivitis.

D. Overview of nursing interventions

1. Administer antimicrobials (doxycycline, tetracycline) as prescribed.

2. Instruct the patient receiving tetracycline to:
   a. Avoid sunlight or ultraviolet light (due to photosensitivity)
   b. Be aware of potential side effects (gastrointestinal [GI] problems, *Candida* overgrowth in genital area, skin rashes, blood disorders)
   c. Avoid antacids and dairy products
3. Instruct the patient to avoid intercourse or to use condoms until treatment is complete.
4. Evaluate and provide treatment for the patient's sexual partners.

V.   Syphilis

A. Description: a chronic STD characterized by four different stages: primary, secondary, latency, and tertiary

B. Etiology: caused by *Treponema pallidum,* a spirochete. Due to the nature of its cell wall and its response to antibiotic therapy, *T. pallidum* is considered a bacterium.

C. Pathophysiologic processes and manifestations

1. *T. pallidum* is contained in the mucosal secretions of an infected person; it is thought to enter the subcutaneous tissue by way of microabrasions that occur during sexual contact.

2. A person is usually able to transmit syphilis sexually only during the first few years of infection. In contrast, *in utero* transmission may occur for up to 8 years after the initial infection.

3. The clinical course of syphilis is long and variable; it becomes a systemic disease shortly after infection.

 4. If left untreated, syphilis progresses through several stages: primary, secondary, latency, and tertiary.

5. *Primary syphilis*

   a. The primary chancre (the typical lesion), appears 5 to 10 days after infection. The incubation period ranges from 12 days to 12 weeks.

   b. The chancre, which commonly appears at the infection site, is usually painless and may be accompanied by inguinal lymphadenopathy.

   c. Typically, the chancre is a dull red macule that develops into a papule; it may also appear as a round or oval lesion with a clearly defined border that is firm on palpation.

   d. Extragenital lesions may appear on the fingers, anus, mouth, lips, tonsils, breasts, and axillae. Lesions in nongenital areas may have an atypical appearance.

   e. If left untreated, the lesion will heal spontaneously in 2 to 8 weeks.

6. *Secondary syphilis*

   a. Approximately 6 weeks after the initial infection, a systemic illness develops.

   b. Symptoms are similar to those of other infections and include low-grade fever, general malaise, headache, adenopathy, anorexia, and joint pain.

   c. A flat, white, moist, elevated papule known as condylomata lata may appear on the labial folds, groin, thighs, and anus.

   d. A rash, ranging from macular to pustular, may appear on the palms of the hands and soles of the feet as well as over the whole body.

   e. Mucous membrane lesions are common, especially in the mouth.

   f. Patchy alopecia may appear on the eyebrows and beard.

   g. Symptoms of secondary syphilis often resolve without treatment within 2 to 10 weeks.

   h. Relapses of secondary syphilis may occur for up to 2 years.

7. *Latent syphilis*

   a. There are usually no clinical or serologic manifestations associated with latent syphilis, although relapses of secondary syphilis may occur, especially in the first year.

   b. Early latency (defined as 1 year from onset of infection by the U.S. Public Health Service) is a potentially infectious period.

   c. Latency is described as the period until manifestations of tertiary syphilis occur. This latent stage may be as short as 1 year, or the individual may remain in this stage permanently.

8. *Tertiary syphilis*

   a. The principal cause of morbidity and mortality of syphilis in adults is related to complications of tertiary syphilis.
   b. Manifestations are present in the skin, central nervous system (CNS), bones, and viscera, particularly the heart and great vessels.
   c. Manifestations of tertiary syphilis can occur as early as 1 year or as late as 40 years after initial infection.
   d. Gumma, lesions that destroy bone or soft tissue, appear but are usually treatable.
   e. Neurosyphilis is a manifestation of tertiary syphilis. It may be asymptomatic, with abnormalities found in the cerebral spinal fluid (CSF). It also may manifest as acute syphilitic meningitis; general paresis; impaired speech, memory and concentration; and tremors. Optic atrophy and intracranial masses may also occur.
   f. When the heart is affected, aortic aneurysm or coronary artery disease may occur.

9. Manifestations of *in utero* transmission may include preterm delivery, congenital infection, and stillbirth.

D. Overview of nursing interventions

1. Prevent the transmission by counseling sexually active patients, especially adolescents, on use of condoms.
2. Conduct a serologic evaluation (VDRL), as ordered. Treatment varies depending on the stage of illness present.
3. Institute CSF testing for neurosyphilis, including cell count, protein, and VDRL, as ordered.
4. Administer antimicrobials, as prescribed.
5. Teach the patient about the nature of the disease and mode of transmission.
6. Instruct the patient to avoid intercourse until all evidence of primary or secondary syphilis is gone.
7. Explain to the patient the need to notify all sexual partners.

VI. Chancroid

A. Description

1. Chancroid is a disease affecting the genitals and lymph nodes.
2. It is differentiated from syphilis by its soft, painful chancre.

B. Etiology

1. Chancroid is caused by *Haemophilus ducreyi*, a Gram-negative bacillus.
2. It commonly occurs in heterosexual males, particularly those who are not circumcised.

C. Pathophysiologic processes and manifestations

1. *H. ducreyi* enters the body through small abrasions in the mucous membranes that occur during sexual contact.
2. As the bacteria multiply, they form a papule on the area of contact. The papule enlarges, then erodes into a soft ulcer that contains exudate.

3. Underneath the ulcer lies tissue filled with lymphocytes and plasma cells.
4. Lymph nodes may become inflamed in response to infection.
5. In females, the lesions may occur internally; there also may be no symptoms.
6. In males, the ulcer occurs on the penis, usually on the internal surface of the foreskin.

D. Overview of nursing interventions
1. Assess the patient to differentiate chancroid from syphilis.
2. Administer antibiotics—the drug of choice—as ordered.
3. Provide treatment for the patient's sexual partners.

 4. **Counsel patient on the use of condoms.**

VII. Herpes genitalis

A. Description: infectious genital lesions

B. Etiology
1. Two strains of herpesvirus are responsible for sexually transmitted herpes infections; these are herpesvirus type 1 (HSV-1) and herpesvirus type 2 (HSV-2).
2. HSV-1 is acquired by most people during the first year and a half of life.
    a. Infection occurs by way of respiratory transmission.
    b. Manifestation occurs in the oral mucosa.

 3. **HSV-2 is acquired during sexual activity; lesions occur in the genital region.**

 4. **As a result of certain sexual practices, HSV-1 may sometimes be seen in the genital region and HSV-2 may be seen in the oral region.**

 5. **HSV can be disseminated by way of the bloodstream, as evidenced by lesions over the thorax and extremities.**

6. HSV also can be transmitted to the fetus through the placenta or during passage through the birth canal (if active lesions are present in the vagina).

C. Pathophysiologic processes and manifestations
1. HSV enters the body by way of mucocutaneous tissues, then resides in the cells of the nervous system.
2. The virus can remain latent, with clinical attacks of varying frequency and duration; the incubation period is variable, ranging from 1 to 26 days.
3. Viral replication occurs at the point of contact. After vesicles form on the skin, the virus will spread to adjacent cells and move into cells of the sensory nervous system.
4. HSV is transported through nerve cells, where it remains latent in the dorsal roots. Figure 18-2 illustrates the viral occupation in the nerve cell root.
5. **Reactivation can occur at any time, causing vesicles to reappear. Reactivation may be precipitated by physical or emotional stress or hormonal changes occurring with menstruation.**
6. Symptoms can be local or systemic, and may last up to 3 weeks.
7. Systemic symptoms include fever, malaise, and myalgia.

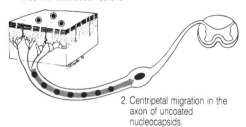

1. Penetration of virus into skin. Local replication and entry of virus into cutaneous neurons.

2. Centripetal migration in the axon of uncoated nucleocapsids.

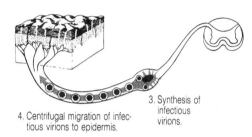

4. Centrifugal migration of infectious virions to epidermis.

3. Synthesis of infectious virions.

FIGURE 18-2.
Pathogenesis of primary mucotunaneous herpes simplex virus infection. [*Source:* Corey, L., & Spear, P. G. [1986]. Infections with herpes simplex viruses. Pt. 1. *New England Journal of Medicine, 314,* 686]

8. Local symptoms include painful lesions (which may ulcerate), itching, vaginal or urethral discharge, tender inguinal lymphadenopathy, and papules or vesicles. Viral shedding occurs up to 12 days.

9. In recurrent episodes, only local symptoms usually are present, and the disease course is shorter; viral shedding lasts up to about 4 days.

10. **Because of HSV's nerve cell pathology, meningitis and encephalitis are potential complications. Other complications can include arthritis, hepatitis, and proctitis.**

11. In immunosuppressed individuals, HSV can spread to multiple organs.

D.   Overview of nursing interventions

1. Administer acyclovir, as prescribed.
2. Teach the patient to gain symptomatic relief by:
   a. Placing warm compresses or ice packs on the affected site, two or three times a day
   b. Bathing in water that is at body temperature and using a hair dryer instead of a towel for drying
   c. Applying hydrogen peroxide or Burrow's solution to aid drying after vesicles rupture
   d. Using a topical anesthetic
   e. Wearing loose-fitting clothes and cotton underwear
   f. Using aspirin to relieve pain and systemic symptoms
3. Instruct the patient to keep the rash area clean and dry and to avoid breaking blisters.
4. Discuss with the patient preventive measures, including:
   a. Avoiding intercourse when lesions are present
   b. Avoiding oral sex if oral or genital lesions are present

c.   Using a condom when prodromal signs are present
d.   Avoiding rough handling of tissue
e.   Washing hands after contact with area

VIII.   Condylomata acuminata

A.   **Description: a viral STD characterized by warts in the genital region**

B.   **Etiology: Condylomata acuminata is caused by the human papillomavirus (HPV); persons exposed to HPV experience a high rate of infection**

C.   Pathophysiologic processes and manifestations

1.   Incubation period for condylomata acuminata is long and variable, perhaps lasting up to 3 months.
2.   As a result of trauma that occurs during sexual intercourse, HPV is able to enter the mucous membranes.
3.   HPV infects the basal cells of the epithelium and multiplies there.
4.   The epithelial cells transform, multiply, and form the soft, fleshy, and vascular warts within 2 to 3 months after infection.

5.   **In men, papular warts usually appear on the penis shaft.**

6.   **In women, manifestations include cervical, vaginal, vulvar, or clitoral lesions. Multiple lesions are likely to coalesce, forming large lesions resembling cauliflower. Lesions tend to grow during pregnancy (Fig. 18-3).**

7.   Laryngeal papillomata and airway obstruction may occur in neonates born vaginally to mothers infected with HPV.

D.   Overview of nursing interventions

1.   Prepare the patient for cryotherapy with liquid nitrogen or cryoprobe, the treatment of choice, as ordered.

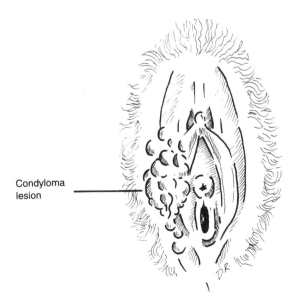

Condyloma
lesion

FIGURE 18-3.
Condylomata acuminata. Condyloma
formation on vulva.

2. Provide patient teaching covering:
    a. Possibility of recurrence (because current therapies do not eliminate HPV)
    b. Use of condoms to protect against HPV
3. Advise the patient that all sexual partners should be checked.
4. Counsel women on the need for lifetime screening for cervical cancer.

IX. Lymphogranuloma Venereum

A. Description
1. Lymphogranuloma Venereum is a venereal disease that may be acute chronic.
2. The disease is more common in men.

B. Etiology: caused by the *Chlamydia trachomatis* bacteria

C. Pathophysiologic processes and manifestations
1. The incubation period of the lesions occurs anywhere from days to weeks.
2. Small painless papules and vesicles develop and often go undetected.
3. The hallmark of the disease is the appearance of large, tender, inguinal lymph nodes known as *buboes*.
4. The buboes may be noticed from 1 to 4 weeks after infection.
5. In the early stages, the patient presents with flulike symptoms.
6. Joint pain, rash, pturia, dysuria, weight loss, splenomegaly, and proctitis follow.
7. If lymphatic obstruction occurs from scarring, elephantiasis of the testicles occurs.
8. Scarring may occur in the anal area as well.

D. Overview of nursing interventions.
1. To diagnose this disease, use the complement fixation test for *Chlamydia* group antibody. High titers will distinguish this from other chlamydial groups.
2. Administer antibiotics, as prescribed.
4. Counsel patient on use of condoms.
5. Prepare patient for surgery if scar tissue is to be surgically removed.

X. Hepatitis B

A. Description and etiology: a liver infection caused by the sexual transmission of the hepatitis B virus (HBV)

B. Pathophysiologic processes and manifestations
1. Clinical symptoms of hepatitis caused by HBV may be indistinguishable from those caused by hepatitis A virus (HAV) or hepatitis non-A, non-B (NANB) virus.
2. Early symptoms of hepatitis B can include:
    a. Skin eruptions
    b. Urticaria
    c. Arthralgia
    d. Arthritis
    e. Anorexia

        f.   Nausea

        g. Vomiting

        h. Headache

        i.   Fever

  3. Late symptoms can include:

        a. Clay-colored stool

        b. Dark urine

        c. Jaundice

  4. **Complications of HBV infection can include:**

        a. **Chronic, persistent active hepatitis**

        b. **Chronic carrier state**

        c. **Cirrhosis of liver**

        d. **Hepatocellular carcinoma**

        e. **Hepatic failure**

C. **Overview of nursing interventions**

  1. Prevent the disease by providing the series of hepatitis vaccines for persons with multiple sex partners, persons who inject drugs, homosexual and bisexual men, prostitutes, and persons seeking treatment for STDs.

  2. Provide postexposure prophylaxis by administering hepatitis B immune globulin (HBIG) followed by the series of hepatitis vaccines.

  3. Counsel all infected persons to avoid:

        a. Sexual contact involving exchange of body fluids

        b. Sharing of personal items such as razors and toothbrushes

  4. Instruct intravenous drug users to avoid sharing needles.

Bibliography

Bullock, B. (1996). *Pathophysiology: Adaptations and alterations in function* (4th ed.). Philadelphia: Lippincott-Raven.

Diebel N. D. Jr., & Williams, J. K. (1995). Chlamydia trachomatis. A trojan horse. *J Fla Md Assoc.* 82(6):411–4.

Fanaroff, A., & Martin, R. (1992). *Neonatal-perinatal medicine: Diseases of the fetus and infant.* St. Louis: C. V. Mosby.

Guyton, A. (1991). *Textbook of medical physiology* (8th ed.). Philadelphia: Saunders.

Kinney, M., Packa, D., & Dunbar, S. (1993). *AACN's clinical reference for critical care nursing* (3rd ed.). St. Louis: C.V. Mosby.

Lichtman, R., & Papera, S. (1990). *Gynecology: Well-woman care.* Norwalk, CT: Appleton-Lange.

McCance, K. L., & Huether, S. E. (1994). *Pathophysiology: The biologic basis for disease in adults and children* (2nd ed.). St. Louis: Mosby-Year Book.

Porth, C. (1994). *Pathophysiology: Concepts of altered health states* (4th ed.). Philadelphia: Lippincott-Raven.

Quinn T. C. (1994). Recent advances in diagnosis of sexually transmitted diseases. *Sexually Transmitted Disease.* 21(2):s19–27.

Soper D. E. (1994). Pelvic inflammatory disease. *Infectious disease clinics of North America.* 8(4):821–840.

STUDY QUESTIONS

1. In a male patient, which of the following symptoms would suggest a diagnosis of *Chlamydia*?
   a. extragenital lesions
   b. Reiter's syndrome
   c. a chancre
   d. papular warts

2. Ms. Penny, age 17, was treated with acyclovir for an initial HSV infection 3 weeks ago. She came to the clinic complaining of a new painful ulcerated genital lesion. This probably indicates:
   a. treatment with the incorrect antimicrobial
   b. treatment was not continued long enough
   c. reactivation of HSV infection
   d. reinfection by a new partner

3. The risk of contracting gonorrhea is higher in:
   a. female-to-male transmission
   b. female-to-female transmission
   c. male-to-female transmission
   d. maternal–fetal transmission

4. In women with gonorrhea, the pathophysiologic processes that foster the development of PID include:
   a. an autoimmune response
   b. a mutation of the bacteria
   c. suppression of normal flora protection secondary to hormonal changes
   d. suppression of the intrinsic inflammatory response

5. In women, manifestations of *Chlamydia* infections usually are:
   a. specific and easily diagnosed
   b. nonspecific with few symptoms
   c. accompanied by severe left lower quadrant pain
   d. accompanied by a yellow discharge

6. Patients who are taking tetracycline for treatment of *Chlamydia* should be instructed to:
   a. take the medication with milk
   b. take the medication with meals
   c. avoid prolonged periods of sunlight
   d. limit fluid intake

7. Gonococcal urethritis will resolve:
   a. after a prolonged course of treatment
   b. within a few weeks without treatment
   c. within 1 year without treatment
   d. only with antimicrobial treatment

8. During which of the following stages is syphilis most easily diagnosed?
   a. primary
   b. early latency
   c. tertiary
   d. secondary

9. A definitive cure for STDs caused by viruses is:
   a. treatment with antiretroviral medications
   b. acyclovir
   c. not yet known
   d. erythromycin

10. HSV-1 can be distinguished from HSV-2 because it usually involves:
    a. acquisition by age 15
    b. genital lesions
    c. acquisition during sexual activity
    d. oral mucosal lesions

11. A prostitute presents with complaints of arthralgia, anorexia, nausea, vomiting, fever, headache. The nurse suspects which of the following:
    a. gastric ulcer
    b. syphilis
    c. hepatits
    d. gastritis

12. A nurse caring for a patient with *Condylomata* infection must *first* prepare the patient for:
    a. use of antifungals
    b. cryosurgery
    c. administration of antibiotics
    d. phototherapy

13. Appearance of large, tender, inguinal

lymph nodes known as *buboes* is a hallmark of:

a. Herpes infection
b. Chancroid
c. Gonorrhea
d. Lymphogranuloma Venereum

14. The principal cause of morbidity and mortality of syphilis in adults is related to complications of:

a. tertiary syphilis
b. latent syphilis
c. secondary syphilis
d. primary syphilis

ANSWER KEY

Question	Correct answer	Correct answer rationale	Incorrect answer rationales
1.	b	In men with *Chlamydia*, Reiter's syndrome manifests as urethritis, conjunctivitis, arthritis, and mucocutaneous lesions.	a and c. These symptoms are present in syphilis. d. This is a manifestation of genital warts.
2.	c	After initial HSV infection, reactivation can occur anytime with the appearance of vesicles. Reactivation is usually precipitated by stress or hormonal changes.	a and b. Treatment of HSV requires acyclovir for 10 days; some patients take this drug to prevent reactivation. d. Based on the course of this disease, this response is incorrect.
3.	c	The risk of contracting gonorrhea by male-to-female or male-to-male transmission is highest.	a, b, and d. These are not as high as letter c.
4.	c	Suppression of normal flora protecting against infection occurs in women secondary to hormonal changes. This allows bacteria to ascend to the uterus and fallopian tubes, leading to PID.	a, b, and d. These are incorrect.
5.	b	Typically, *Chlamydia* infections—especially those in women—are difficult to diagnose because there are few, or no, symptoms. Any symptoms that may exist are nonspecific.	a, c, and d. These are incorrect.
6.	c	Patients taking tetracycline should be instructed to avoid sunlight and ultraviolet light due to photosensitivity.	a. Patients should avoid concomitant ingestion of dairy products with this drug. b. Patients should take this drug on an empty stomach. d. Patients should increase their fluid intake.
7.	b	Without treatment, gonococcal urethritis will self-resolve within several weeks. Within 6 months, 95% of untreated patients will be asymptomatic.	a, c, and d. These choices do not describe the resolution of gonococcal urethritis.
8.	a	A diagnosis of syphilis is made most easily with the presence of a chancre, which is characteristic of the primary stage.	b, c, and d. In these stages, diagnosis is made based on a positive serologic test.
9.	c	Prevention of STDs is the goal.	a, b, and d. These are treatment options, not cures.

Question	Correct answer	Correct answer rationale	Incorrect answer rationales
10.	d	HSV-1 is usually acquired during the first 1.5 years of life and involves oral mucosal lesions.	a. Age of onset is incorrect. b and c. These refer to HSV-2.
11.	c	These are symptoms consistent with hepatitis.	a and d. These gastrointestinal disorders present with different symptoms. b. This STD presents with symptoms not described here.
12.	b	Cryosurgery is used to remove the warts from the area of infection.	a, c, and d. Antifungals, antibiotics, and phototherapy are not part of the treatment for Condomata infection.
13.	d	Appearance of buboes is consistent with lymphogranuloma venereum.	a, b, and c. These STDs do not present with buboes.
14.	a	In tertiary syphilis, tissue is destroyed and the nervous system is effected, making this a dangerous condition.	b, c, and d. In these stages, extensive damage has not occurred.

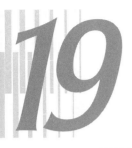

19 Oncologic and Hematologic Disorders

I. **Overview of pathophysiologic processes**

A. Description

1. Cancer is one of the leading causes of death in the United States, affecting persons in all age groups.
2. The term *cancer* describes all forms of malignant neoplasms, also known as carcinomas, which may affect nearly any body system.
3. *Neoplasia* refers to altered cell growth and replication; neoplasms may be benign or malignant.

B. Cellular disorders

1. **In cancer development, disorders of cell proliferation and differentiation exist.**
2. *Proliferation* refers to the process of cell renewal or replacement; normally, a balance exists between cell production and cell loss. In cancer, the proliferation process continues unabated as normal control mechanisms are unable to halt the process (Display 19-1).
3. *Differentiation* refers to the process by which cells diversify, acquire specific structural and functional characteristics, and mature. In cancer, cells are poorly differentiated.

C. Characteristics of cancer cells

1. Cells and tumors may be benign or malignant:
   a. *Benign cells* typically are encapsulated, noninvasive, and highly differentiated. Mitosis is rare and growth is slow. Little or no anaplasia exists, and metastasis does not occur.
   b. *Malignant cells* typically are nonencapsulated, invasive, and poorly differentiated. Mitosis is common and, therefore, cell growth is rapid. Varying degrees of anaplasia exist, and metastasis is present.
2. Other distinguishing characteristics of cancer cells include:
   a. Uncontrolled proliferation
   b. Poor differentiation: Cells contain few identified tissue characteristics; the more undifferentiated the tumor cell, the more malignant the tumor.
   c. Altered biochemical properties, such as hormone secretion
   d. Chromosomal instability: Cell mutations are caused by alterations in

DISPLAY 19-1
Proliferative Patterns

Hyperplasia: increased numbers of cells due to increased cellular reproduction

Metaplasia: differentiation of a stem cell into another cell type

Dysplasia: unusual cell growth resulting in cells that differ in arrangement, size, and shape from cells of the same tissue type

Anaplasia: growth resulting in poorly differentiated cells that are irregularly shaped and organized and lack normal cell characteristics.

Neoplasia: uncontrolled cell growth not based on physiologic demand; may be benign or malignant

DNA; genetic instability causes new mutations with unique characteristics that are increasingly resistant to therapy.

    e. **Capacity to metastasize: Metastasis is the spread of cancer cells from a primary site to distant secondary sites; a correlation exists between the degree of cell malignancy and its metastatic capacity.**

D. **Theories of carcinogenesis**
    1. Carcinogenesis is the process by which normal cells are transformed into neoplastic cells as a result of exposure to certain agents or transforming factors.
        a. A *carcinogen* is an agent that can permanently and irrevocably change the DNA of a cell, predisposing the cell to change.
        b. A *cocarcinogen* is an agent that alters genetic information of the cell, enhancing cellular transformation.
        c. A *complete carcinogen* is an agent that can induce cancer on its own (eg, radiation).
    2. Specific agents associated with the development of cancer include:
        a. *Genetic factors* (eg, familial predisposition, as in breast cancer, and genetic transmission, as in retinoblastoma)
        b. *Hormonal factors:* Hormones may make cells more sensitive to the process of carcinogenesis or may encourage the growth and spread of an established tumor; hormone-responsive tissues are considered targets for four types of cancers: prostate, brain, breast, and endometrial.
        c. *Chemical carcinogens* (eg, tobacco [chewing and smoking], secondary smoke, ether, benzene, coal tar, and asbestos)
        d. *Viruses:* Viruses infect host DNA or RNA, resulting in cell mutation (eg, adenoviruses, herpes viruses, human T-cell virus, and lymphoma leukemia viruses).
        e. *Radiation:* Ultraviolet rays from diagnostic or therapeutic x-rays, radioisotopes, sunlight, or other sources alter the structure of DNA; the effects of radiation exposure are cumulative, and cancer is usually detected long after the time of exposure.
        f. *Immune system alterations* (eg, defective or suppressed immunocompetence, as seen in patients with immunodeficiency disease, those receiving immunosuppressive therapy, and the elderly)
    3. Although the role of dietary agents is still being investigated, theories exist that high levels of fat, nitrosamines, coffee, and vitamin deficiencies may be associated with cancer development.

E. **Routes and patterns of metastasis**

    1. *Metastasis* **is the spread of cancer cells from a primary site to distant secondary sites.**
    2. It occurs by:
        a. Direct spread to adjacent tissues caused by invasion, serosal seeding, or surgical instrumentation
        b. Metastatic spread to nonadjacent tissues due to invasion through lymphatic and vascular systems
        c. A combination of both direct and metastatic spread
    3. Patterns of metastasis include:

        a.   *Tumor-specific spread* to particular organs (eg, primary breast cancer potentially spreads to lung, liver, lymph nodes, brain, and bone; primary colon cancer potentially spreads to lung, liver, and lymph nodes; primary prostate cancer potentially spreads to bone, lung, liver, and lymph nodes)

        b.   *Lymphatic spread* by way of regional lymph nodes that drain the tumor site; spread is to other areas by way of lymphatic channels

        c.   *Hematologic spread* by way of the circulatory system to organs and tissues

    4.   Metastatic tumors generally retain many of the characteristics of the primary tumors.

    5.   Cancer *in situ* is a localized, preinvasive lesion.

F.   **Tumor grading and staging**

    1.   Tumors are classified according to *grade* and *stage*.

    2.   Grading involves categorizing tumors according to cell differentiation and the relationship to the tissue of origin (Display 19-2).

    3.   Staging involves categorizing the disease progression, including the presence or absence of organ involvement (Display 19-3).

G.   **Cancer treatment modalities**

    1.   Common cancer treatment modalities include

DISPLAY 19-2
TNM Clinical Classification

Primary Tumor (T)

TX	Primary tumor cannot be assessed
T0	No evidence of primary tumor
Tis	Carcnoma *in situ*
T1, T2, T3, T4	Increasing size and/or local extent of the primary tumor

Regional Lymph Nodes (N)

NX	Regional lymph nodes cannot be assessed
N0	No regional lymph node metastasis
N1, N2, N3	Increasing involvement of regional lymph nodes

Note: Direct extension of the primary tumor into lymph nodes is classified as lymph node metastasis.

Note: Metastasis in any lymph node other than regional is classified as a distant metastasis.

A *grossly* recognizable metastatic nodule in the connective tissue of a lymph drainage area without histologic evidence of residual lymh node is classified in the N category as a regional lymph node metastasis. A *microscopic* deposit, up to 2 or 3 mm, is classified in the T category, that is, as discontinuous extension.

Distant Metastasis (M)

MX	Presence of distant metastasis cannot be assessed
M0	No distant metastasis
M1	Distant metastasis

Note: For pathologic stage grouping, M1 may be either clinical (cM1) or pathologic (pM1).

DISPLAY 19-3
Staging of Hodgkin's Disease

Stage Grouping

Stage I   Involvement of single lymph node region (I) or localized involvement of a single extralymphatic organ or site (I_E).

Stage II   Involvement of two or more lymph node regions on the same side of the diaphragm (II) or localized involvement of a single associated extralymphatic organ or site and its regional lymph node(s) with or without involvement of other lymph node regions on the same side of the diaphragm (II_E).

Note: The number of lymph node regions involved may be indicated by a subscript (e.g., II_3).

Stage III   Invovlement of lymph node regions on both sides of the diaphragm (III), which may also be accompanied by lcoalized involvement of an associated extralymphatic organ or site (III_E), by involvement of the spleen (III_S), or both $III_{(E+S)}$.

Stage IV   Disseminated (multifocal involvement of one or more extralymphatic organs, with or without associated lymh node involvement, or isolated extralymphatic organ involvement with distant (nonregional) nodal involvement.

Used with the permission of the American Joint Committee on Cancer (AJCC®), Chicago, Illinois. The original source for this material is the AJCC Manual for Staging of Cancer, 4th ed. (1992) published by Lippincott-Raven Publishers, Philadelphia.

    a.   Surgery
    b.   Radiation
    c.   Chemotherapy
    d.   Biotherapy

2. *Surgery* may be done for curative, palliative, reconstructive, or prophylactic or preventive purposes; surgical removal is usually more successful with slow-growing, encapsulated tumors than with rapidly growing, metastasizing tumors. During surgery, minimal palpation and manipulation of the tissue minimize seeding and damage.

3. *Radiation* is used for radiocurable cancers (eg, skin cancer and stage-I Hodgkin's disease), and for adjuvant therapy, prophylactic therapy, and palliative therapy (eg, relieve pain and bleeding, reduce tumor size, or control tumor growth). Cancer cell response to radiation depends on the cell type and the phase of the cell cycle.

4. *Chemotherapy* involves administering cytotoxic drugs to intervene in and interrupt the cell cycle.

5. Uses of chemotherapy include:
    a.   Adjuvant therapy: treatment in conjunction with surgery, radiation, and biotherapy
    b.   Primary therapy: localized cancer treatment; alternative treatment may be available but is less effective
    c.   Induction chemotherapy: primary treatment; no alternative treatments are available
    d.   Combination chemotherapy: use of two or more chemotherapeutic agents; each agent enhances the other or acts synergistically with it.

6. Chemotherapeutic drugs can be cell-cycle phase specific or nonspecific:

a. Cell-cycle phase specific chemotherapeutic drugs act on cells undergoing division in the cell cycle; agents include antimetabolites, vinca plant alkaloids, L-asparaginase, and decarbazine.

b. Cell-cycle phase nonspecific drugs act on cells in a dividing or resting state; agents include antitumor antibiotics, alkylating agents, hormones, and steroids.

7. *Biotherapy* involves treatment with agents derived from biologic sources or with agents that affect biologic responses; agents include interferons, interleukins, colony-stimulating factors, tumor necrosis factor, and monoclonal antibodies.

II. Physiologic responses to oncologic and hematologic disorders

A. Pain

1. Pain is experienced due to compression by the mass on the blood supply, causing ischemia, nerve compression, or invasion by the tumor.

2. It also may be due to invasion and tissue destruction by the cancer.

2. Adequate assessment of pain is vital to treatment and control.

B. Cachexia

1. Cachexia is a syndrome characterized by anorexia, weight loss, and weakness and fatigue.

2. It occurs despite normal dietary intake because of selective redistribution of carbohydrates, proteins, and fats to the growing tumor mass instead of to healthy tissue.

3. Nutritional status is also compromised by the side effects of treatment modalities.

C. Anemia (decreased hemoglobin): results from direct blood loss by erosion from the tumor mass, from nutritional deficits, or secondary to treatment modalities

D. Thrombocytopenia (abnormally reduced number of platelets): occurs as a side effect of chemotherapy or due to bone marrow involvement; results in bleeding disorders (eg, petechiae, ecchymosis, and gingival bleeding)

E. Leukopenia (decreased white cell count): may result from bone marrow suppression from treatment modalities, or invasion by carcinoma, or infection.

F. Infection: occurs commonly in cancer patients; low white blood cell count, nutritional deficits, and overall debilitation are contributing factors

G. Neurologic changes: a decrease in neurologic function (eg, confusion, impaired judgment) may be due to direct invasion of the brain, metastasis, electrolyte disturbances, or medication side effect.

H. Respiratory distress: shortness of breath, hypoxia, abscess formation, and pneumonitis result from direct invasion of the lung tissue by a tumor mass, secondary affect of radiation or infection.

I. Abdominal dysfunction: can include bowel obstruction (caused by direct tumor mass) anorexia, abdominal discomfort (due to hepatomegaly, splenomegaly, lymphadenopathy, and as a side effect of treatment modalities).

J. Paraneoplastic syndromes: include any manifestations that are systemic in nature, but that direct attention away from the primary site of the carcinoma (eg, endocrine neoplastic syndrome is manifested as Cushing's syndrome, which occurs secondary to a small cell carcinoma of the lung) and syndrome of inappropriate antidiuretic hormone (SIADH).

J. Fatigue: a key symptom and debilitating factor for cancer patients

III. Leukemias

A. Description

1. Leukemias are malignant neoplasms of white blood cells that infiltrate bone marrow, peripheral blood, and other organs (eg, kidney, skin, and the gastrointestinal [GI] tract)
2. Leukemias can be acute or chronic; they are classified according to cell type as either lymphocytic, myelocytic, and the less common promyelocytic.
3. Types of leukemias include:
   a. Acute lymphocytic leukemia (ALL)
   b. Chronic lymphocytic leukemia (CLL)
   c. Acute myelocytic leukemia (AML)
   d. Chronic myelocytic leukemia (CML)
   d. Acute promyelocytic leukemia (APL)

B. Etiology and incidence

1. Although the cause of leukemia is unknown, theories suggest it may be associated with the following factors:
   a. Exposure to radiation or known carcinogens (eg, benzene, alkylating chemotherapeutic agents)
   b. Genetic predisposition
   c. Viruses (eg, human T-cell leukemia virus I [HTLV-I])
2. ALL occurs most commonly in young children and affects males more than females; survival rates are improved, with 50% of children surviving to at least 5 years.
3. CLL affects persons over age 40 and has a higher incidence in men than in women; survival rate is approximately 7 years.
4. AML affects all age groups, with incidence increasing with age. Survival rate is 2 to 5 months if untreated and 1 year if treated; affected persons usually succumb to infection or hemorrhage.
5. CML is uncommon before age 20; incidence increases with age. Survival rate is approximately 4 years.

C. Pathophysiologic processes and manifestations

1. Normal cell differentiation is altered by an unknown carcinogen.
2. Leukemia cells are immature, poorly differentiated, and capable of an increased rate of proliferation.
3. Lymphocytic leukemia is a malignant proliferation of lymphoblasts, which interfere with normal hematopoiesis.
4. Myelocytic leukemias are malignancies of the stem cells (eg, basophils, monocytes, neutrophils).
5. Leukemia cells function abnormally, tending to crowd out normal cells; this results in altered white and red cell activity.

6. Manifestations can include:
   a. Bleeding dyscrasias (due to anemia and thrombocytopenia)
   b. Fatigue
   c. Anorexia
   d. Neurologic changes (eg, headache, visual disturbances)
   e. Abdominal discomfort (due to generalized lymphadenopathy, hepatomegaly, splenomegaly, ascites, or bleeding)
   f. Bone pain may be present from excess infiltration of leukemic cells.
   g. Fever and symptoms of infection

D. **Overview of nursing interventions**
   1. Assess for evidence of bleeding in urine, stool, gums, vaginal discharge, and heavy menses.
   2. Avoid possible trauma that could precipitate a bleeding episode.
   3. Provide oral hygiene.
   4. Monitor for manifestations of infection (eg, fever, redness, pain).
   5. Maintain reverse isolation precautions.
   6. Assess nutritional status and encourage adequate nutritional intake.
   7. Administer pain medications, as ordered.
   7. Encourage the patient to discuss concerns about diagnosis and prognosis; provide counseling as needed.
   9. Provide patient teaching covering:
      a. Recognition of bleeding
      b. Scheduled treatments
      c. Manifestations of infection
   10. Refer the patient and family members to appropriate support groups.

IV. Malignant lymphomas

A. **Description**
   1. Lymphomas are neoplasms of cells that originate in lymphoid tissue.
   2. Lymphomas affect the lymph nodes, spleen, GI tract, bone marrow, and liver; spread occurs to other tissues and structures (eg, lungs, kidneys, skin).
   3. Types of lymphomas include:
      a. Hodgkin's disease
      b. Non-Hodgkin's lymphoma
   4. *Hodgkin's disease* is a malignant disease of unknown origin; it is characterized by painless and progressive enlargement of the lymphoid system involving a single node or group of nodes. Spread to other organs (eg, spleen and liver) and to any area of the body accounts for the variety of cells manifested; the Reed-Sternberg cell is considered the pathologic hallmark and essential diagnostic criterion for this disease.
   5. *Non-Hodgkin's lymphomas* are malignancies of the lymphoid tissue other than Hodgkin's disease. These lymphomas are divided into three groups, according to the cell type involved:
      a. Lymphocytic lymphoma (lymphosarcoma)

        b.   Histiocytic lymphoma (reticulum cell sarcoma)

        c.   Mixed cell lymphoma

B. Etiology

    1.   Although the exact cause of malignant lymphomas is unknown, a viral etiology is generally suspected.

    2.   Immunosuppressive therapy and immune deficiency states may also be associated with the development of this disease.

    3.   Non-Hodgkin's lymphoma also occurs in immunosuppressed patients and is associated with B-cell abnormalities.

    4.   Incidence of lymphomas is higher in men than in women and is associated with high socioeconomic status.

C. Pathophysiologic processes and manifestations

    1.   In *Hodgkin's disease*

        a.   Chromosomal abnormalities are noted.

        b.   The characteristic cell, the Reed-Sternberg cell, is derived from monocyte-macrophages.

        c.   Transformation of the cell occurs in the lymphoid tissue and extension occurs by way of lymphatic channels.

        d.   Cell-mediated immunity is altered and is associated with T-lymphocytopenia and B-lymphocytosis.

        e.   Manifestations include painless lymphadenopathy (commonly in the neck), intermittent fever, night sweats, weight loss, and extremity involvement (may involve pain and neurovascular impingement).

        f.   Staging indicates progression of the disease and potential response to treatment modalities (see Display 19-3).

    2.   In *Non-Hodgkin's lymphoma*

        a.   Mononuclear phagocytes are affected.

        b.   Painless lymphadenopathy occurs, and the disease may progress to extranodal involvement including the nasopharynx, gastrointestinal tract, and abdomen.

        c.   Enlarged nodes or lymph tissue impinging on other structures may cause cough, chest pain, ascites, abdominal pain or fullness, jaundice, or gastrointestinal or genitourinary problems.

D. Overview of nursing interventions

    1.   Prepare the patient for radiation, chemotherapy, or a combination of both depending on the disease staging.

    2.   Institute measures to relieve nausea, abdominal fullness, pain, or other symptoms.

    3.   Monitor and assess for increased risk of infection, bleeding, and anemia.

    4.   Provide supportive care to help the patient cope with side effects related to medical management.

    5.   Monitor tissues and surrounding organs and structures for function and edema.

    6.   Monitor and intervene if there is evidence of central nervous system (CNS) involvement or neurovascular compromise.

    7.   Provide emotional support to the patient and family members; encourage them to discuss their concerns.

V.   Multiple myeloma

A.   Description
1.   Multiple myeloma is a plasma cell malignancy of osseous tissue.
2.   It is characterized by uncontrolled proliferation of abnormal plasma cells.
3.   Survival rate is generally 2 to 3 years without treatment.

B.   Etiology and incidence
1.   Although the exact cause of multiple myeloma is unknown, associated factors include:
    a.   Genetic factors
    b.   Chronic stimulation of the mononuclear phagocyte system
2.   Incidence increases in persons with a history of chronic infections (eg, tuberculosis, osteomyelitis, and pneumonitis).
3.   Incidence of multiple myeloma has doubled in the last decade, but this is believed to be due to improved detection.

C.   Pathophysiologic processes and manifestations
1.   B cells (immature plasma cells) and mature plasma cells are affected.
2.   Abnormal plasma cells are scattered throughout the skeletal system and deposit in the bone, leading to erosion.
3.   Lymph nodes, liver, spleen, and kidneys are also affected.
4.   Manifestations are related to bony infiltration and abnormal immunoglobulins and may include:
    a.   Bone pain (associated with pathologic fractures and hypercalcemia from bone reabsorption)
    b.   Weakness and fatigue
    c.   Weight loss
5.   Impaired humoral immunity results in recurrent infections.
6.   Renal failure occurs because of toxic proteinuria, which damages the tubular epithelial cells.

D.   Overview of nursing interventions
1.   Administer pain medications, as prescribed.
2.   Evaluate the patient for evidence of bony deterioration and provide protection from injury.
3.   Increase hydration to reduce risk of renal damage and decrease calcium retention.
4.   Monitor for evidence of kidney failure.
5.   Encourage mobility and hydration to prevent hypercalcemia and improve strength.
6.   Monitor for evidence of infection; if present, manage appropriately.
7.   Educate the patient and family members regarding diagnosis, prognosis, and treatment modalities.
8.   Provide counseling as needed.

VI.   Sickle cell disease

A.   Description
1.   Sickle cell disease is a hemoglobinopathy characterized by an inherited de-

fect in the shape or configuration of the hemoglobin structure; this defect leads to premature red blood cell (RBC) destruction and anemia.

2. Sickle cell disease is marked by the presence of two hemoglobin S-chains; sickle cell trait is marked by the presence of one hemoglobin S-chain and a normal hemoglobin B-chain.

B. Etiology

1. In sickle cell disease, a single amino acid is replaced in the globin chain; a valine is substituted for a glutamic acid in the sixth position of the B chain, creating a new hemoglobin structure called hemoglobin S.
2. Although the cause of this genetic alteration is unknown, epidemiologic studies have found an increased incidence of hemoglobin S in areas endemic for malaria, and in African Americans.
3. Risk factors that precipitate sickling attacks include infection, dehydration, stress, fatigue, and acidosis.

C. Pathophysiologic processes and manifestations

1. Neonates with sickle cell disease are asymptomatic on clinical examination; several months after birth, a severe hemolytic anemia manifests when fetal hemoglobin is replaced by abnormal hemoglobin.
2. In cases associated with desaturation, the cells change shape to a sickle formation and become rigid instead of compliant.
3. Cells clog up the vasculature and impair perfusion.
4. Clinical manifestations include joint pain and fever, which are indicative of vascular occlusion and ischemia.
5. Anoxia leads to thrombosis in tissues with resultant end organ damage; organs most vulnerable to damage are the brain, kidneys, and spleen.
6. Pulmonary manifestations include shortness of breath and pulmonary compromise.
7. Symptoms may be widespread and related to the areas of vascular occlusion.

D. Overview of nursing interventions

1. Administer oxygen and fluids to improve perfusion and oxygen delivery.
2. Administer pain medications, as prescribed.
3. Assess for systemic complications (eg, respiratory failure, renal disease, and CNS dysfunction); if present, manage appropriately.
4. Provide patient teaching covering:
   a. Chronic nature of the disease
   b. Recognition of complications
   c. Avoidance of precipitating risk factors

VII. Anemias

A. Description

1. Anemia is a reduction in the overall number of RBCs or the quantity of hemoglobin.
2. Anemias are classified according to morphology, shape, and hemoglobin content; types include:
   a. Normocytic, normochromic anemias (eg, aplastic or sickle cell disease)
   b. Hypochromic, microcytic anemias (eg, iron-deficiency anemia)
   c. Macrocytic, normochromic anemia (eg, pernicious anemia)

B.   Etiology
1.   Anemias result from:
a.   Frank blood loss (posthemorrhagic anemia)
b.   Deficiencies in components needed for RBC production (iron deficiency or folic acid deficiency anemias)
c.   Loss of factors necessary for absorption of dietary components (pernicious anemia)
d.   Genetic alterations (sickle cell or thalassemias)
e.   Bone marrow destruction (aplastic anemia)
2.   Anemias occur in all age groups and are considered manifestations of underlying disease, rather than diseases themselves.

C.   Pathophysiologic processes and manifestations
1.   The anemia may be of acute onset (eg, frank blood loss) or chronic (eg, dietary deficiencies). Acute anemia manifests as hemodynamic compromise; chronic anemia is typically asymptomatic in the early stages.
2.   When RBC volume is low, cardiovascular compromise with hypotension, orthostatic changes, and tachycardia may occur.
3.   Hemoglobin and hematocrit levels drop, with decreases in mean corpuscular volume (MCV), mean corpuscular hemoglobin (MCH), and mean corpuscular hemoglobin concentration (MCHC).
4.   Other common manifestations may include:
a.   Anorexia and weight loss
b.   Fatigue
c.   Shortness of breath on exertion and extreme malaise (may occur secondary to decreased oxygen delivery to the tissues)
d.   Decreased mental status and lethargy (may occur with CNS hypoperfusion)

D.   Overview of nursing interventions
1.   Assess cardiovascular status and administer fluids or blood products as indicated.
2.   Evaluate the patient for evidence of secondary hypoperfusion and end organ damage.
3.   Monitor CBC and coagulation factors.
4.   Administer oxygen to improve oxygen delivery.
5.   Evaluate the patient's ability to provide self-care in the presence of weakness and malaise; provide assistance as indicated.
6.   Provide patient teaching covering:
a.   Type of anemia
b.   Causative agents
c.   Prognosis and management

VIII.   Disseminated intravascular coagulation (DIC)

A.   Description: an acquired coagulopathy; normal homeostatic coagulation mechanisms are altered, resulting in a pathologic process
B.   Etiology
1.   No common mechanism has been identified as the single cause of DIC.

2. Preexisting conditions associated with a higher incidence of DIC development include:
   a. Shock states
   b. Trauma
   c. Infection
   d. Malignant disease
   e. Obstetric complications
   f. Cardiovascular disease

C. Pathophysiologic processes and manifestations

1. A primary event causes the normal coagulation cascade to become overstimulated and overproductive.
2. Excessive thrombin is released throughout the body, overwhelming regulatory mechanisms.
3. Activation of fibrinogen leads to the deposition of fibrin clots in the capillary bed, resulting in tissue ischemia.
4. Fibrinolysis is also accelerated, resulting in rapid breakdown of existing clots.
5. A consumptive coagulopathy is established as coagulation products are used in the microvasculature and are rapidly depleted.
6. Fibrinolysis releases fibrin degradation products into the circulation; these are natural anticoagulants and therefore contribute to further clot breakdown.
7. Microvascular clotting and systemic hemorrhage occur concomitantly.
8. Manifestations vary depending on the severity of the process and preexisting medical condition.
9. Bleeding or oozing from puncture sites, mucous membranes, and wounds occurs.
10. A major hemorrhagic episode (eg, intracranial bleeding) may result.
11. Microvascular clotting is manifested by petechia, hematoma development, and, eventually, tissue necrosis.
12. Acrocyanosis of the digits occurs, extending into gangrene.
13. Multisystem organ dysfunction is commonly associated with the development of DIC.

D. Overview of nursing interventions

1. Assess the patient to determine the primary event that precipitated DIC.
2. Administer blood products, including packed RBCs, platelets, fresh frozen plasma (FFP), and coagulation factors, as ordered.
3. Administer heparin, as ordered, to inhibit further clot formation.
4. Provide supportive care if there is evidence of major organ damage (eg, intracranial bleeding, adult respiratory distress syndrome [ARDS]).
5. Assess for occult or frank bleeding and manage potential bleeding sites.
6. Administer analgesics, as ordered, to relieve pain associated with thrombosis.
7. Provide oral care.
8. Identify potential causes of tissue damage (eg, IM injections, rectal thermometers).
9. Provide patient teaching covering prognosis and treatment protocols.

Bibliography

Bullock, B. L., & Rosendahl, P. P. (1992). *Pathophysiology: Adaptations and alterations in function* (3rd ed.). Philadelphia: J. B. Lippincott.

Clark J. McGee, R. (1997). *Core curriculum for oncology nursing.* St. Louis: W.B. Saunders.

Devine S. M., & Larson, R. A. (1994). Acute leukemia in adults. *Cancer Journal for Clinicians,* 44:326–353.

Groenwald, S. L., Frogge, M. H., Goodman, M., & Yarbo, C. H. (1994). *Cancer nursing; Principles and practice* (4th ed.). Boston: Jones and Bartlett.

Kohlman, V. C., Lindsey, A., & West, C. (1993). *Pathophysiological phenomena in nursing* (2nd ed.). Philadelphia: W. B. Saunders.

McCance, K. L., & Huether, S. E. (1994). *Pathophysiology: The biologic basis for disease in adults and children* (2nd ed.). St. Louis: Mosby-Year Book.

Porth, C. M. (1994). *Pathophysiology: Concepts of altered health states* (4th ed.). Philadelphia: J. B. Lippincott.

Yarbo, C. H. (1996). *Cancer nursing: comprehensive textbook* (2nd ed.) Philadelphia: W. B. Saunders.

STUDY QUESTIONS

1. Which one of the following characteristics does *not* describe benign cells?
   a. encapsulated
   b. noninvasive
   c. highly differentiated
   d. poorly differentiated

2. Which of the following can infect host DNA and RNA, resulting in cell mutation?
   a. radiation
   b. ultraviolet light
   c. virus
   d. asbestos

3. When assessing a patient for leukemia, the nurse would expect to see which one of the following symptoms?
   a. dysphagia
   b. swollen lymph nodes
   c. fever
   d. chest pain

4. A patient with lymphoma angrily tells the nurse, "I want my treatment started. I am tired of all these tests. Now my doctor wants to stage my disease." The nurse should respond by explaining that staging:
   a. involves cell differentiation
   b. involves categorizing the disease extension
   c. can be determined after treatment is initiated
   d. is the treatment modality

5. Manifestations of thrombocytopenia include all of the following *except:*
   a. petechiae
   b. leukopenia
   c. ecchymosis
   d. gingival bleeding

6. For the patient with thrombocytopenia, the nurse should focus patient teaching on:
   a. expected course of chemotherapy
   b. expected course of radiation therapy
   c. avoidance of infections
   d. avoidance of injury

7. Leukemia cells are:
   a. well differentiated
   b. past mature
   c. capable of increased proliferation
   d. the Reed-Sternberg cell

8. Pathophysiologic processes involved in multiple myeloma primarily affect:
   a. T cells
   b. B cells
   c. platelets
   d. RBCs

9. Which of the following interventions should the nurse undertake when caring for a patient with multiple myeloma?
   a. decrease fluids
   b. immobilize the patient
   c. manage pain
   d. administer exogenous calcium

10. The abnormal hemoglobin found in sickle cell disease is:
    a. hemoglobin B chain
    b. hemoglobin S chain
    c. hemoglobin R chain
    d. hemoglobin C chain

11. The most common type of childhood leukemia is:
    a. AML
    b. CLL
    c. ALL
    d. CML

12. The hallmark cell in Hodgkins lymphoma is:
    a. Philadelphia chromosome
    b. Lymphocytes
    c. Auer rods
    d. Reed-Sternberg cell

12. Specific agents associated with cancer development include:
    a. genetic factors
    b. hormonal factors

c.   chemical factors
d.   All of the above

12.   Tumors are classified according to:
a.   size
b.   grade and stage
c.   metastasis
d.   none of the above

15.   Chemotherapy intervenes and interrupts the:
a.   blood flow
b.   effect of radiation
c.   cell cycle
d.   all of the above

ANSWER KEY

Question	Correct answer	Correct answer rationale	Incorrect answer rationales
1.	d	Malignant cells are poorly differentiated.	a, b, and c. Benign cells are highly differentiated, noninvasive, and encapsulated.
2.	c	A virus can infect host DNA and RNA, leading to cell mutation.	a. Radiation alters DNA. b and d. Ultraviolet light and asbestos cannot infect DNA and RNA
3.	c	Fever and signs of infection are common manifestations of leukemia.	a. Anorexia, not dysphagia, may be seen with leukemia. b and d. Swollen lymph nodes and chest pain are manifestations of lymphoma.
4.	b	Staging determines how far the disease has progressed and the appropriate treatment.	a. Grading involves cell differentiation. c. Staging must be done before treatment begins. d. This response is incorrect. Staging is a process in which progress of the tumor is analyzed; it is not the treatment.
5.	b	Leukopenia is not a manifestation of thrombocytopenia (decreased platelets).	a, c, and d. Petechiae, ecchymosis, and gingival bleeding are all manifestations of thrombocytopenia, which might lead to bleeding.
6.	d	Because of an increased tendency to bleed, avoidance of injury is a major focus of patient teaching for a patient with thrombocytopenia.	a, b, and c. These may be part of the overall teaching, plan, but are not the major focus.
7.	c	Leukemia cells are capable of increased proliferation.	a and b. Leukemia cells are poorly differentiated and immature. d. The Reed-Sternberg cell is associated with lymphoma.
8.	b	B cells, plasma cells, are affected in multiple myeloma.	a. T cells are involved in immunosuppression. c and d. Platelets and RBCs are involved in anemias and bleeding disorders.
9.	c	Pain management is an important component of care for a patient with multiple myeloma.	a. Fluids should be increased. b. Encourage activity. d. This response is incorrect.
10.	b	In sickle cell disease, there are two hemoglobin S chains.	a. In sickle cell trait, there is one normal hemoglobin B chain and one hemoglobin S chain.

Question	Correct answer	Correct answer rationale	Incorrect answer rationales
			c and d. These are not present in this disorder.
11.	C	The most common type of childhood leukemia is acute lymphocytic leukemia (ALL).	a, b, and d. These leukemias are not as common as ALL
12.	D	The hallmark cell in Hodgkin's disease is the Reed-Sternberg cell.	a, b, and c. These choices are not the hallmark of Hodgkins.
13.	D	All of these factors are associated with the development of cancer.	
14.	B	Tumor classification is determined by grade and stage.	a, c, and d. Size and metastasis are not related to tumor classification.
15.	C	Chemotherapy intervenes and interrupts the cell cycle. It does not affect blood flow or radiation.	

20 Immunologic Disorders

I.   Overview of pathophysiologic processes

A.   Allergic and hypersensitivity reactions

1.   **Allergies and allergic reactions are abnormal immunologic reactions to an antigen that result in allergic diseases.**

2.   Generally, allergic diseases are mediated by immunoglobulin E (IgE) antibodies; they also can be associated with IgG and IgM.

3.   Exposure to an antigen causes IgE antibodies to be produced by selected B cells (the cells that produce immunoglobulins).

4.   The IgE then binds to the receptors on the plasma membrane of the mast cells (cells found along the walls of blood vessels and throughout body tissue).

5.   The allergen will attach itself to the IgE and the cells respond by degranulating (also known as exocytosis).

6.   On reexposure to an allergen, mast cell degranulation occurs. Mast cells contain vasoactive substances such as histamine. These agents are released into the circulation upon degranulation.

7.   Vasoactive agents act on the target organs, causing bronchial constriction, increased vascular permeability, and peripheral vasodilation.

8.   There are two types of IgE mediated allergic responses; atopic and anaphylactic (see chapter 4 for a full description of anaphylaxis)).

9.   Atopic reactions include allergic rhinitis, contact dermatitis, food allergies, and asthma.

10. Food allergies are commonly the first manifestation of a propensity for allergic disease.

11. Allergic disorders may be immediate or delayed, depending upon how much time elapses between the exposure and onset of symptoms.

12. Allergic reactions are divided into four categories. These types are described in Table 20-1, and illustrated in Figure 20-1.

13. Delayed hypersensitivity disorders are also known as cell mediated disorders.

14. This type of reaction involves T cells that serve as intermediaries in the inflammatory response. This process takes more time for the reaction to occur, therefore the allergic response occurs many hour after contact with the antigen.

B.   Autoimmune responses

1.   **Autoimmunity refers to a disruption in the body's ability to tolerate its own cells; instead, it recognizes those cells as antigens.**

2.   Autoimmune responses occur when the immune system reacts against its own cells by forming autoantibodies, which then destroy its own tissue.

3.   Once the tissue is recognized as foreign, a tissue-specific reaction, an immune complex-mediated reaction, or a cell-mediated reaction occurs.

4.   In tissue-specific reactions:

   a.   IgG and IgM are the antibodies most commonly affected.

   b.   Tissue is destroyed through the action of antibodies on the cell's plasma membrane.

   c.   Tissue destruction occurs by way of complement-mediated cell lysis,

TABLE 20-1
Classification of Hypersensitivity States

TYPE	CAUSE	RESPONSIBLE CELL OR ANTIBODY	IMMUNE MECHANISM	EXAMPLES OF DISEASE STATES
I—Immediate hypersensitivity (anaphylaxis, atopy)	Foreign protein (antigen)	IgE	IgE attaches to surface of mast cell and specific antigen, triggers release of intracellular granules from mast cells	Hay fever, allergies, hives, anaphylactic shock
II—Cytotoxic hypersensitivity	Foreign protein (antigen)	IgG or IgM	Antibody reacts with antigen, activates complement, causes cytolysis or phagocytosis	Transfusion, hemolytic drug reactions, erythroblastosis fetalis, hemolytic anemia, vascular purpura, Goodpasture's syndrome
III—Immune complex disease	Foreign protein (antigen) Endogenous antigens	IgG, IgM, IgA	Antigen–antibody complexes precipitate in tissue, activate complement, cause inflammatory reaction	Rheumatoid arthritis, systemic lupus erythematosus, serum sickness, glomerulonephritis
IV—Delayed/ cell-mediated	Foreign protein, cell, or tissue	T lymphocytes	Sensitized T cell reacts with specific antigen to induce inflammatory process by direct cell action or by activity of lymphokines	Contact dermatitis, transplant graft reaction, granulomatous diseases

macrophage phagocytosis, and antibody-dependent cell-mediated cytotoxicity.

5. In immune complex-mediated reactions:
   a. Antigen–antibody complexes form and deposit in tissue.
   b. Complement activation occurs. (Complement refers to a series of enzymatic proteins that, when activated, cause activation of other parts of the immune system.) As a result of complement activation, neutrophil digestion of immune complexes and lysosomal enzyme release occur.
   c. Tissue destruction is diffuse, affecting a number of target organs.
6. In cell-mediated reactions:
   a. Antibodies and sensitized T lymphocytes mediate this type of reaction.
   b. Cytotoxic T cells destroy the host tissue directly.
   c. Lymphokine-producing T cells have a widespread effect by attracting phagocytic cells to the tissue.

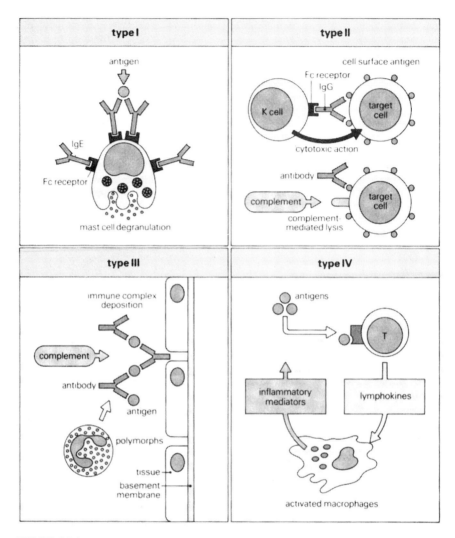

FIGURE 20-1.

Summary diagram of the four types of hypersensitivity reactions. Type 1. Mast cells bind IgE by way of their F_c receptors. On encountering antigen, the IgE becomes cross-linked, inducing degranulation and release of mediators. Type II. Antibody is directed against antigens on a person's own cells (target cell). This may lead to cytotoxic action by K (killer) cells or complement-mediated lysis. Type III. Immune complexes are deposited in the tissue. Complement is activated, and polymorphs are attracted to the site of deposition, causing local damage. Type IV. Antigen-sensitized t cells release lymphokines after a secondary contact with the same antigen. Lymphokines induce inflammatory reactions and activate and attract macrophages, which release mediators. (From Roitt, I., Brostoff, J., and Male, D., Immunology [3rd ed.] Philadelphia: J. B. Lippincott, 1989.)

7. According to several theories, autoimmunity develops:
    a. Due to the presence of a previously hidden antigen
    b. Secondary to infectious diseases
    c. As a result of alterations in suppressor T cell function
8. Systemic lupus erythematosus (SLE), rheumatoid arthritis, and scleroderma are autoimmune disorders.
9. The body's tolerance to self-antigens decreases with age, so the incidence of autoimmune diseases rises with age.
10. Autoimmunity also appears to be familial.

C. **Immunodeficiency states**

1. **Immunodeficiency states are abnormal deficits in humoral or cellular immunity, resulting in increased susceptibility to infections.**
2. Immune deficiencies can be primary (congenital) or secondary (acquired).
3. Acquired immune deficiencies can result from:
    a. Nutritional deficits
    b. Iatrogenic causes (eg, drug induced)
    c. Infectious or viral agents
4. Immunodeficiency is caused by a disruption of lymphocyte function.
5. If the disruption occurs at the level of the stem cell, normal lymphocyte production will be impaired, leading to total collapse of the immune system.
6. If the defect occurs at the level of a lymphoid organ, then maturity of the stem cells into B or T lymphocytes may not occur.
7. If the defect occurs in the final stages of maturation, then specific groups of antibodies may not be able to develop.
8. Immunodeficiency also may render the two components of the immune system unable to coordinate activities (eg, if suppressor T-cell activity increases because of a deficiency of helper T cells, the immune response will be suppressed instead of mediated).

9. **Alterations in the inflammatory process, such as macrophage or complement function, also can affect the immune response.**
10. AIDS is a commonly occurring severe secondary immunodeficiency state.

II. **Physiologic responses to immunologic dysfunction**

A. Urticaria
1. Urticaria, commonly known as hives, is a cutaneous manifestation characterized by wheals and flares.
2. It is caused by localized release of histamines.

B. **Conjunctivitis: inflammation of the membranes of the eyelids**

C. **Rhinitis: inflammation of the mucous membranes of the nasal passages**

D. **Angioedema: generalized swelling due to release of histamine and increased capillary permeability**

E. **Bronchoconstriction: swelling of the airway and constriction of bronchial smooth muscle caused by the release of vasoactive agents**

F. **Pruritus: itching associated with erythema and urticaria**

G. **Hypotension**

1. Hypotension is abnormally decreased blood pressure.
2. It commonly occurs in anaphylactic shock due to the release of vasoactive agents and the loss of intravascular volume secondary to increased capillary permeability.

H. **Leukocytopenia: abnormal decrease in both types of white blood cells or certain subcategories of cells, occurring secondary to disruption in cell development**

I. **Opportunistic infections: secondary infectious or malignant processes associated with immune system deficiencies**

III.   Allergies

A. **Description**

1. Allergies result from IgE-mediated hypersensitivity reactions and are characterized by manifestations associated with histamine release.
2. Allergies may be localized or systemic.
    a. Localized allergies include allergic rhinitis (nasal passages), contact dermatitis (skin), and food allergies (gastrointestinal [GI] tract).
    b. A systemic allergy results in anaphylaxis.

B. **Etiology**

1. Allergic rhinitis is when allergic symptoms occur in the nose. This commonly results from exposure to pollens, molds, and dust.
2. Contact dermatitis results when the skin comes in contact with a substance that triggers the allergic reaction. Common substances are poison oak, poison ivy, or metals such as nickel.
3. Food allergies result from ingesting specific foods that trigger the allergic response. Shellfish is a common allergy.

4. **Anaphylaxis is a severe life-threatening reaction that results from ingestion or exposure to an allergenic agent. An example of this reaction occurs when an allergic person is stung by a bee. Medications can cause this or any of the less severe reactions.**

C. **Pathophysiologic processes and manifestations**

1. Most allergies are mediated by IgE hypersensitivity reactions.
2. Exposure to an allergen produces antibodies. After reexposure to the offending agent, the antibodies bind to the mast cells (which are released in reaction to the allergen) and are termed *cytotropic antibodies.*
3. After further exposure, mast cell degranulation occurs, releasing the chemicals histamine, neutrophil chemotactic factor, and eosinophil chemotactic factor of anaphylaxis (Fig. 20-2).
4. Histamine's vascular effects produce increased vascular permeability, vasodilation, and angioedema.
5. The chemotactic factors cause neutrophils and eosinophils to move into the area and begin phagocytosis.
6. Manifestations vary depending on the allergen and the severity of the response.
7. Characteristic symptoms of allergic rhinitis include:

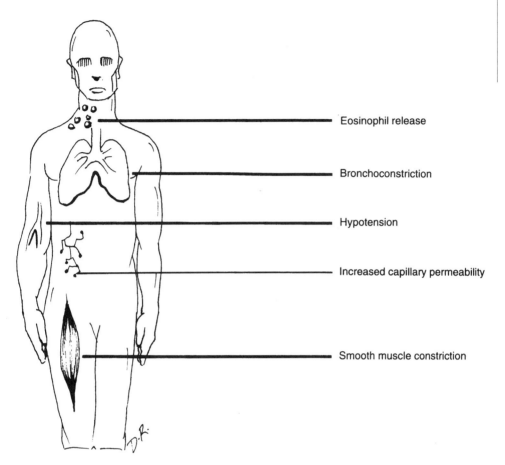

FIGURE 20-2.
Systemic effects of chemotactic factor release.

  a. Conjunctivitis
  b. Rhinitis
  c. Itching and swollen nasal passages
 8. Characteristic symptoms of contact dermatitis include:
  a. Urticaria
  b. Pruritus
 9. Characteristic symptoms of food allergies include:
  a. Vomiting
  b. Abdominal cramping and malabsorption
  c. Diarrhea
  d. Oral swelling

 10. **Some allergies may progress into anaphylactic shock, in which systemic manifestations such as hypotension, dysrhythmias, bronchoconstriction, and laryngeal edema can occur. (See Chapter 4 for more detailed information on anaphylactic shock.)**

D. Overview of nursing interventions

1. Maintain airway if edema of the respiratory tract is evident.
2. Provide supportive care of the cardiovascular system.
3. Administer antihistamines to reduce the histamine reaction.
4. In acute situations where anaphylaxis is present, administer epinephrine to reverse the symptoms.
5. Administer fluid to replace intravascular volume lost due to edema or diarrhea.
6. Monitor and evaluate possible causes of the allergic reaction.
7. Educate the patient and family members regarding avoidance of the allergen and appropriate treatment.
8. Be persistent because the identification and treatment of allergies is often frustrating.

IV. Asthma (Extrinsic)

A. Description

1. An episodic respiratory disease, asthma is associated with bronchospasm triggered by exposure to certain allergens.
2. It is related to IgE-mediated hypersensitivity reactions.

B. Etiology

1. Predisposition to asthma appears to be genetically transmitted. Most cases develop during childhood, but adult-onset asthma also occurs.
2. Allergens that can trigger asthmatic episodes include pollens, dust, animal fur, and pollutants; episodes typically occur seasonally.
3. Stress may precipitate an asthma attack.

C. Pathophysiologic processes and manifestations

1. Airways become hyperreactive due to the allergen–antibody interaction.
2. IgE-bound mast cells rupture and spill their contents, including histamine and chemotactic factors (Fig. 20-3).

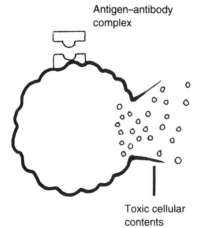

Antigen–antibody complex

Toxic cellular contents

FIGURE 20-3.
Mast cell rupture. Ruptured mast cell releases the toxins histamine and chemotactic factors into the bloodstream.

3. Increased vascular permeability and movement of inflammatory cells into the airways causes edema formation and the production of a thick tenacious exudate.

4. **The increased exudate blocks off smaller airways and causes air trapping, which contributes to ventilation–perfusion abnormalities and increased work of breathing.**

5. Airway obstruction also contributes to impaired expiration and subsequent hyperinflation.

6. Hypoxemia and respiratory acidosis also may occur.

7. **Symptoms can include:**
   a. **Wheezing on auscultation**
   b. **Dyspnea**
   c. **Increased mucus production**
   d. **Increased work of breathing**
   e. **Tachypnea**
   f. **Shortness of breath**
   g. **Nonproductive cough**
   h. **Cardiovascular manifestations, including tachycardia and mild hypertension**
   i. **Use of accessory muscles**

D. Overview of nursing interventions
   1. Assess pulmonary function, including evaluation of arterial blood gases and spirometry.
   2. Administer oxygen and bronchodilators (including sympathomimetics such as epinephrine, terbutaline, and steroids) to decrease inflammation as prescribed.
   3. Educate the patient and family members regarding the disease process and avoidance of the offending agent.
   4. Work hard to identify the offending agent and find the appropriate treatment (prevention is of primary importance).

V. Systemic lupus erythematosus (SLE)

A. **Description: an autoimmune disease, SLE is a chronic, inflammatory, multisystem disorder characterized by periods of remission and exacerbation.**

B. Etiology and incidence
   1. SLE is associated with a genetic predisposition to the disease as well as a family history of other autoimmune disorders.
   2. It occurs most commonly in women, especially among those ages 20 to 30; incidence is higher among African Americans than whites.

C. Pathophysiologic processes and manifestations
   1. SLE is characterized by the formation of antibodies (IgG and IgM) against the body's nucleic acids, phospholipids, white blood cells, red blood cells, and coagulation components.
   2. Antigen–antibody complexes against host DNA form and deposit in a variety of tissues, causing diffuse damage.

3. Neutrophils attempt to phagocytize the antigen–antibody complexes, but are ineffective.
4. Lysosomal enzymes are released, further propagating the tissue damage.

5. **The glomerular basement membrane of the kidneys is particularly susceptible to complex deposition; as a result, there is a high incidence of renal failure secondary to SLE.**
6. Deposition of complexes also occurs in the brain, heart, lung, GI tract, spleen, and skin.

7. **The most common symptoms of SLE include:**
    a. **Arthralgias and arthritis, typically affecting proximal joints**
    b. **Vasculitis (Raynaud's phenomenon) and the appearance of a facial butterflylike rash**
    c. **Renal dysfunction**
    d. **Anemia**
    e. **Cardiovascular disease (eg, pericarditis)**
8. Other symptoms can include:
    a. Photosensitivity
    b. Scaly, patchy rash
    c. Fever
    d. Myalgia
    e. Weight loss
    f. Ulceration of the mucous membranes
    g. Alopecia
9. In severe forms of SLE, neurologic dysfunction such as seizures and cranial nerve palsies may occur.

D. Overview of nursing interventions
1. Administer steroids, disease-modifying antimalarial agents, immunosuppressive agents, and nonsteroidal antiinflammatory agents as prescribed.
2. Assess the severity of the disease.
3. Provide supportive care for patients with target organ dysfunction.
4. Vary treatment according to the stage of the illness.

VI. Rheumatoid arthritis

A. Description: a chronic autoimmune disease that causes connective tissue destruction, which results in joint deformity and loss of function

B. Etiology and incidence
1. Etiology is unknown, although theories regarding its development point to bacteria, mycoplasmas, and viruses as possible causes.
2. Incidence is higher in women than in men.
3. The disease is characterized by exacerbations and remissions, and an attack may be preceded by an acute infection.

C. Pathophysiologic processes and manifestations
1. Rheumatoid arthritis is characterized by a cell-mediated tissue destruction process directed toward type-II collagen.
2. In response to an environmental stimulus, a normal antigen–antibody reaction occurs.

3. The antibodies mutate into autoantibodies called rheumatoid factors, which have been isolated in persons with rheumatoid arthritis and consist primarily of IgM and IgG.
4. Antigen–antibody complex deposition occurs.
5. Secondary destruction of tissue also occurs, initially in the synovial membrane causing synovitis.
6. Complement activation occurs, stimulating prostaglandin and kinin release and increasing vascular permeability into the synovial membrane.
7. The immune response proceeds further with the release of sensitized T lymphocytes, which are then activated and enter the inflamed area.
8. Cytotoxic T cells and lymphokine-producing T cells phagocytize tissue and release lysosomal enzymes.
9. As the inflammatory response is perpetuated, tissue destruction increases.
10. Swelling secondary to fluid and cell infiltration within the joint occurs, leading to joint hyperplasia.
11. Small veins within the area become blocked by fibrin, platelets, and other inflammatory products, decreasing perfusion to the joint.
12. Hypoxia and metabolic acidosis occur; this stimulates the release of enzymes from the synovial cells, which eventually erodes the articular cartilage, ligaments, and tendons.
13. Granulation tissue called pannus develops, leading to joint immobilization.
14. **Common symptoms include:**
    a. **Anorexia**
    b. **Fatigue**
    c. **Weakness, stiffness, and achiness**
    d. **Swollen and painful joints, including early morning stiffness**
    e. **Decreased range of motion (eventually, contractures including boutonnière and swan neck deformities of the metacarpals may develop)**
15. Secondary atrophy of muscles also may occur.
16. Cysts in the articular cartilage develop and can extend into fistulas.
17. Rheumatoid nodules composed of inflammatory cells can be found on the skin, heart, spleen, and lung, leading to dysfunction in these systems.

D. Overview of nursing interventions
1. Assess the patient's ability to carry out activities of daily living and self care.
2. Encourage the patient to rest the inflamed joint and use hot and cold packs.
3. Assist the patient with physical therapy.
4. Administer nonsteroidal anti-inflammatory and antineoplastic agents as prescribed.
5. Prepare the patient for surgery, if indicated, to correct contractures or remove synovial membrane to decrease inflammation and remove granulation tissue.

VII. Scleroderma

A. Description
1. Scleroderma literally means sclerosis of the skin.

2. It may affect the viscera as well as the skin, with symptoms occurring in one or more organs (eg, kidneys, heart, lungs, esophagus, intestine).

B. Etiology and incidence
1. Possible causes include autoimmunity and an immune reaction.
2. Incidence is higher in women than in men.

C. Pathophysiologic processes and manifestations

1. **An immune reaction causes deposits of collagen, with fibrosis in the dermis, subcutaneous tissue, and sometimes deep fascia.**
2. These deposits are accompanied by vascular changes in the capillaries in the area.
3. The collagen deposits and the fibrosis cause the skin to assume a shiny, taut appearance. The skin feels firm; when palpated, it may feel connected to the underlying tissue.
4. When visceral involvement exists, symptoms congruent with failure of the particular organ will be present (eg, kidney involvement results in renal failure).
5. The effects on the face and neck make the individual assume a masklike appearance. The hands, if involved, assume a waxy, manikin-like appearance; use of the fingers may be lost.
6. The blood vessels in the fingers may constrict (Raynaud's phenomenon), with subsequent ulcer formation on the fingers.
7. As the disease progresses and end organs become involved, death eventually results.

D. Overview of nursing interventions
1. Provide warmth for the hands.
2. Avoid trauma to the hands.
3. Treat symptoms as they appear in each organ.
4. Provide adequate nutrition.

VIII. Acquired immunodeficiency syndrome (AIDS)

A. Description
1. AIDS is a severe immunodeficiency caused by the human immunodeficiency virus (HIV).
2. It is characterized by the occurrence of opportunistic infections and direct HIV infiltration into some tissues.

B. Etiology and incidence
1. AIDS is caused by HIV, which is a retrovirus.
2. It is contracted through direct blood or body fluid contamination by way of open skin or mucous membrane lesions. It can also be transmitted *in utero*.
3. Infection was initially limited to intravenous drug abusers, homosexual men, and persons who had received blood transfusions. Now the disease is prevalent in the heterosexual community and is a common cause of death in young women as well as men.
4. Health care workers may risk contamination by way of needle sticks or excessive skin exposure to blood or body fluids.

C. Pathophysiologic processes and manifestations

1. The HIV virus carries genetic information as RNA; by attaching to a surface antigen on the cell membrane called CD4, it transmits its genetic information into the human cell.
2. The primary cells affected are the T helper cells, although direct infiltration into the central nervous system (CNS) cells has also been found.
3. Once the HIV RNA enters the cell, reverse transcriptase converts the RNA to DNA material; as DNA, the virus is able to replicate as the cell replicates.
4. After the genetic information is integrated with the host cell, rapid cell destruction and proliferation can occur. Or the virus can lie dormant for approximately 10 years.
5. Primary infection is associated with a flulike syndrome that often goes unrecognized as related to HIV infection.
6. After the primary infection, the patient will test positive for HIV but will remain asymptomatic for a span of 5 to 10 years.

7. **As the T-helper cell count drops and the immune system begins to fail, the patient will experience mild symptoms, including:**
   a. **Lymphadenopathy**
   b. **Weight loss**
   c. **Night sweats**
   d. **Diarrhea**

8. **AIDS occurs with the appearance of opportunistic infection or malignancy or evidence of CNS involvement.**

9. **Common opportunistic diseases include:**
   a. *Pneumocystis carinii* **pneumonia**
   b. **Kaposi's sarcoma**
   c. **Candidiasis**
   d. **Toxoplasmosis**
   e. **Cytomegalovirus**
   f. **Cryptococcal meningitis/pneumonia**
   g. **Tuberculosis**
10. CNS involvement is thought to be due to direct HIV infiltration into CNS tissue; called AIDS dementia, it is characterized by behavioral, cognitive, and motor deterioration. (See Chapter 7 for more detailed information.)

D. Overview of nursing interventions

1. Assess clinical manifestations.
2. Provide supportive pulmonary and cardiovascular care.
3. Assess the patient's coping skills and ability to carry out activities of daily living.
4. Protect the patient from further infection.
5. Administer antiviral, antibacterial, and antifungal medications as prescribed.
6. Ensure a safe environment.
7. Follow protocol for use of universal precautions.

Bibliography

Bullock, B., & Rosendahl, P. (1992). *Pathophysiology: Adaptations and alterations in function* (3rd ed.). Philadelphia: J. B. Lippincott.

Groer, M., & Shekleton, M. (1989). *Basic pathophysiology: A holistic approach* (3rd ed.). St. Louis: C. V. Mosby.

Guyton, A. (1992). *Human physiology and mechanisms of disease* (5th ed.). Philadelphia: W. B. Saunders.

McCance, K. L., & Huether, S. E. (1990). *Pathophysiology: A biologic basis for disease in adults and children*. St. Louis: C. V. Mosby.

Price, S. A., & Wilson, L. M. (1986). *Pathophysiology: clinical concepts of disease processes* (3rd ed.). New York: McGraw-Hill.

STUDY QUESTIONS

1. Hypersensitivity responses result in:
   a. deficiency syndromes
   b. autoimmune diseases
   c. allergic diseases
   d. degranulation

2. The release of histamine causes:
   a. increased vascular permeability
   b. complement-mediated cell lysis
   c. antigen–antibody complex binding
   d. tissue destruction

3. In immune system deficiencies in which the disruption is at the level of the stem cell, which of the following manifestations will occur?
   a. disruption of specific antibody production
   b. total collapse of the immune system
   c. alterations in the inflammatory process
   d. maturation into B or T lymphocytes

4. Urticaria is caused by:
   a. wheal and flare formation
   b. histamine
   c. pruritus
   d. mast cell degranulation

5. Allergic rhinitis is characterized by:
   a. swelling and itching of nasal passages
   b. oral edema and vomiting
   c. urticaria
   d. laryngeal edema

6. Increased expiratory effort associated with asthmatic attacks is directly related to:
   a. increased vascular permeability
   b. hyperreactive airways
   c. hypoxemia
   d. airway obstruction by exudate

7. The primary antibody affected in asthmatic patients is:
   a. IgM
   b. IgG
   c. IgE
   d. sensitized T lymphocytes

8. In SLE, the immune response primarily targets host:
   a. nucleic acids
   b. phospholipids
   c. coagulation components
   d. white blood cells

9. The diffuse manifestations of SLE are due to the fact that:
   a. antigen–antibody complex deposition is always diffuse
   b. phospholipids are found in all cell membranes
   c. lysosomal enzymes do most of the destruction
   d. molecular substances affected are widely distributed throughout the body

10. In rheumatoid arthritis, tissue destruction occurs primarily in the:
    a. synovial membrane
    b. ligaments and tendons
    c. pannus
    d. articular cartilage

11. A nurse is caring for a patient having an acute asthmatic attack. Which of the following will reverse bronchoconstriction?
    a. epinephrine
    b. atropine
    c. steroids
    d. claritin

12. An immune reaction that causes deposits of collagen, with fibrosis of the dermis, subcutaneous tissue, and sometimes deep fascia occurs in:
    a. asthma
    b. systemic lupus erythematosis
    c. scleroderma
    d. none of the above

13. Hypoxemia and respiratory acidosis are possible sequelae of:
    a. scleroderma
    b. asthma

c. arthritis

d. allergies

14. A patient presents to the nurse with lymphadenopathy, weight loss, night sweats, diarrhea. These symptoms are consistent with:

a. scleroderma

b. AIDS

c. asthma

d. rheumatoid arthritis

ANSWER KEY

Question	Correct answer	Correct answer rationale	Incorrect answer rationales
1.	c	Allergic diseases occur because of a hypersensitive response to antigens.	a. Deficiency is due to a defect in component cell production. b. Autoimmune diseases occur because of a disruption in the body's ability to tolerate self antigens. d. Mast cell degranulation occurs during allergic responses but is not the result of them.
2.	a	Histamine release results in increased vascular permeability, bronchial constriction, and peripheral vasodilation.	b. Complement-mediated cell lysis occurs in autoimmune responses, but is not due to histamine release. c and d. These are not related to histamine release.
3.	b	If the stem cell is affected, then all further generations of cells will be affected and the entire immune system will collapse.	a. Disruption of specific antibody production will occur if the defect happens in the final stages of maturation. c. Alterations in inflammation will have an effect on the immune response because of the collaborative relationship. d. B and T lymphocyte production will be altered if the defect is at the level of the lymphoid organ.
4.	b	Urticaria is caused by histamine release.	a. Wheal and flare formation characterize urticaria and not the reverse. c. Pruritus is an associated manifestation. d. Mast cell degranulation causes histamine to be released.
5.	a	Allergic rhinitis is characterized by swelling and itching of nasal passages and increased mucus production.	b. Oral edema and vomiting are associated with GI reactions. c. Urticaria is seen with contact dermatitis. d. Laryngeal edema is associated with anaphylaxis.
6.	d	Airway obstruction occurs because the presence of a thick tenacious exudate blocks off the distal alveoli, impairing expiration.	a. Increased vascular permeability leads to edema formation and exudate production but does not directly cause difficult expiration. b. Hyperreactive airways are associated with asthmatic disease but do not cause difficult expiration.

Question	Correct answer	Correct answer rationale	Incorrect answer rationales
			c. Hypoxemia may be associated with asthma but is more directly related to inspiration, not expiration.
7.	c	IgE is the antibody most frequently associated with asthmatic disease.	a, b, and d. These are not commonly associated with asthma.
8.	a	In SLE, nucleic acids are the primary target cells.	b, c, and d. All of these cells may also be affected but are secondary to nucleic acids.
9.	d	SLE affects such diffuse organ systems because the molecular substances affected (eg, nucleic acids, phospholipids, and white blood cells) are widely distributed throughout the body.	a. Antigen–antibody deposition may be diffuse, but this is not the reason. b. Phospholipids are found in cell membranes, but this is not the direct cause of systemic involvement. c. Lysosomal enzymes do destroy tissue, but this is not the reason for systemic involvement.
10.	a	In rheumatoid arthritis, the primary site of tissue destruction is the synovial membrane.	b and d. Ligaments, tendons, and the articular cartilage are eventually affected, but the process begins with inflammation of the synovial membrane. c. Pannus is the granulation tissue that forms within the joint.
11.	a	Epinephrine is given in acute asthma to reverse bronchoconstriction.	b, c, and d. These drugs will not reverse the acute bronchoconstriction of asthma.
12.	c	The physiologic changes described here are consistent with scleroderma.	a, b, and d. These disorders are not consistent with the pathology described.
13.	b	Hypoxemia and respiratory acidosis are associated with asthma.	a, c, and d. These disorders do not result in hypoxemia and respiratory acidosis.
14.	b	These symptoms are consistent with acquired immunodeficiency syndrome (AIDS) from infection with the human immunovirus.	a, c, and d. These symptoms are not consistent with the diseases listed in these choices.

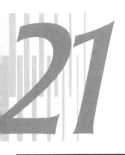

Disorders Related to Aging

I.   **Overview of the pathophysiologic processes**

A.   **Facts about aging:**

1.   ~~The aging process occurs in all living things.~~

2.   Aging causes physical, psychological, and social changes that increase as a person gets older.

3.   **How people adapt to these changes depends on their underlying physical condition, their mental health, and the amount of family support.**

4.   People age at various rates.

5.   Different societies define aging differently.

6.   Every day, 3,000 people turn 65, but only 2,000 65-year-olds die—so the geriatric population is increasing.

B.   **Theories of aging**

1.   The underlying physiologic cause of aging is not well understood, although several theories exist.

2.   According to one theory, aging occurs secondary to cellular damage through mutation of genes, accumulation of toxic substances, protein degradation, and free radical damage.

a.   Gene mutations can occur from exposure to free radicals, radiation, and other environmental toxins.

b.   Protein degradation is caused by biochemical degenerative processes and can hamper DNA's ability to repair itself.

c.   Immunologic processes that contribute to aging include a decrease in T-cell function and the production of abnormal monoclonal antibodies.

3.   Another theory states that cellular death is a normal, genetically determined process.

a.   There is evidence that stem cells have a limited proliferative capability and a finite end to their replicating ability.

b.   Evidence exists that organisms with a longer life span have more cell replication ability than organisms with a shorter life span.

c.   In progeria, a hereditary disease that causes extremely rapid aging, mitotic capability is only half of normal.

C.   **The sixth decade: normal changes**

1.   Physiologic changes in the eye result in loss of contrast capability and night vision.

2.   The ability to hear higher tones diminishes, resulting in difficulty understanding conversations.

3.   The pancreas functions less efficiently, resulting in higher glucose levels.

4.   Joints stiffen as cartilage deteriorates from wear and tear, resulting in pain on movement.

D.   **The seventh decade: normal changes**

1.   Blood pressure is 25% higher than at age 20, which can lead to hypertension.

2.   Coronary artery disease secondary to thickening of arterial walls occurs in 50% of men.

3.   Short-term memory declines, along with the ability to learn spoken material.

4.   Sweat glands decrease in number, increasing the risk of heat stroke.

E. The eighth decade: normal changes

    1. Risk of falls increases, resulting in hip fractures and permanent disability.

    2. Bone mass in the lower extremities decreases by half in many women in this age group.

    3. Heart rate decreases by 25%.

    4. Cognitive ability deteriorates and 50% of patients over age 85 show some signs of Alzheimer's disease.

II. Physiologic responses to aging

A. Common physical changes

    1. *Arcus senilis:* pale rim surrounding the cornea of the eye that has no clinical significance

    2. *Presbycus:* hearing loss

    3. *Cataracts:* opacity of the lens resulting in vision loss

    4. *Nutritional deficits:* secondary to tooth loss and alterations in smell, taste, and gastrointestinal function

B. Common syndromes

    1. Confusion states (delirium and dementia)

    2. Falls

    3. Immobility

    4. Incontinence

    5. Failure to thrive

III. Neurologic system disorders

A. Description

    1. Some neurologic changes in the central nervous system and special senses occur normally with aging.

    2. Delirium and dementia are abnormal changes.

    3. *Delirium* is the acute effect of physical illness on cerebral function.

    4. *Dementia* is a syndrome characterized by multiple cognitive deficits severe enough to cause impairment in mental function, and a decline in previous levels of cognitive functioning.

    5. *Failure to thrive* is a term used to describe a patient who makes poor progress and appears to have given up. It can exacerbate chronic medical conditions, or it can occur in a relatively healthy elderly patient.

B. Etiology

    1. Neurologic deterioration associated with aging is most profound after age 75 and results from loss of neurons, pigment accumulation within the neurons, dendritic changes, and decreased neurotransmitter activity.

    2. Changes in the special senses result from crystalline changes in the lens of the eye, reduction in the number of rods in the retina, and reduced pupillary size.

    3. Hearing loss is caused by changes in the inner ear.

    4. **Delirium can occur secondary to polypharmacy drug interactions or as the result of an underlying disease.**

5. Dementia may be chronic, as in Alzheimer's disease or hypoxic brain injury, or it may have a reversible cause.
6. Failure to thrive is usually caused by depression, but it may also be caused by metabolic disturbances, malnutrition, infectious diseases, and pharmacologic effects.

C. **Pathophysiologic processes and manifestations**
1. Normal changes
    a. Muscle strength, agility, and reaction times decrease.
    b. Muscle atrophy occurs, leading to decreased muscular strength.
    c. Reflexes and vibratory sense lessen.

    d. Position sense may decline, leading to unsteady gait and increased risk of falling.
    e. The incidence of tremors may increase.

    f. Cognitive ability does not diminish greatly, although short-term memory and the ability to rapidly retrieve information from long-term memory decreases.
    g. Contrary to popular opinion, personality does not change with age.
    h. Pupillary size may diminish, pupils may become irregular, and diminished pupillary reactivity to light and accommodation and alterations in extraocular movements may occur.

    j. Sleep deprivation may occur due to decreases in stage-IV sleep and total sleep time and increases in the time it takes to fall asleep.
    k. Brain weight decreases by 7%, and cerebral blood flow is reduced by 20%.
2. Special senses: normal changes
    a. Changes begin as early as age 40.
    b. Visual acuity decreases gradually from age 50 to 70 and more rapidly after that.
    c. Loss of eyelid muscle tone and a decrease in fat surrounding the eyes can result in a senile ptosis, ectropion, or entropion.
    d. Loss of lacrimal secretions may cause eye dryness.
    e. Thickening of the lens may eventually result in cataracts.
    f. Continuing lens growth often pushes the iris forward, leading to narrow-angle glaucoma.

    g. The ability to hear high-pitched sounds decreases, resulting in sound distortion and trouble understanding conversations.
3. Delirium and dementia
    a. Delirium is a reversible medical emergency that affects 30 to 40% of hospitalized geriatric patients.

    b. It is characterized by rapid onset of disorganized thinking with the inability to maintain attention and may cause sleep–wake cycle disturbances and altered psychomotor behavior.
    c. The patient is cognitively impaired and has a perceptual disturbance.
    d. The condition develops rapidly in hours or days and can fluctuate over the course of the day.

e. **Treatment is aimed at identifying and removing the cause.**

f. Dementia has a gradual onset that usually cannot be dated and can progress over years.

g. Disorientation occurs later in the disease, often after years of diminishing cognitive capability.

h. Patients commonly have a reversal of sleep–wake cycles (*Sundowner's presentation*).

4. Failure to thrive

   a. Signs and symptoms of failure to thrive include fatigue; functional decline; loss of interest in surrounding activities; anorexia and weight loss; medical noncompliance; personality change; resistant behaviors, such as unwillingness to eat, be fed, or participate in self-care; increased dependency on others and decreased ability to perform activities of daily living; and lack of drive and apathy in a previously active, involved person.

   b. Lack of responsiveness and motivation can eventually result in decreased capability, increased immobility, and their subsequent consequences.

   c. Chronic disease states can be exacerbated, eventually resulting in deterioration and death.

D. Overview of nursing interventions

1. Assess neurologic status on a regular basis.

2. Assess the patient's level of understanding and ability to communicate.

3. Ask about vision or hearing problems, and provide information on glasses, hearing aids, or surgical procedures to remedy these problems.

 4. **Help prevent falls in the patient with tremors or decreased motor ability by keeping bed side rails up at all times and enforcing other safety measures.**

5. Try to reduce environmental stimulae (eg, turn off the television or radio and close the door) when talking to the patient.

6. Ensure adequate sleep and encourage normal diurnal variation.

7. Orient the patient frequently to time, date, and his surroundings.

 8. **Review all the patient's medications to make sure no drug interactions are occurring. In delirium or dementia, give central nervous system depressants sparingly, as ordered.**

9. In the patient with failure to thrive:

   a. Assess for evidence of medical causes.

   b. Perform screening lab work, as ordered.

   c. Assess mental and emotional status to assist with a diagnosis of depression.

   d. Review medications to ascertain the impact of pharmacologic agents.

   e. Encourage the performance of activities of daily living and assist when needed.

   f. Maintain adequate diet and fluid balance.

   g. Stress the need for compliance with the medical regimen and the consequences of noncompliance.

   h. Administer antidepressants or other psychotropic agents, as ordered

IV.   Cardiovascular system disorders

A.   Description

1.   Hypertension and coronary artery disease are the major cardiovascular diseases of the elderly.

2.   Coronary artery disease increases rapidly with age and remains the most common cause of death in the elderly

3.   Hypertension occurs in 54% of patients aged 65 to 74.

B.   Etiology

1.   Although some changes occur with aging, much cardiovascular dysfunction is caused by disease states rather than normal aging.

2.   The cardiovascular system rarely fails except as a result of a disease state.

3.   Cardiovascular changes are due to changes in the vasculature and decreased compensatory ability of the myocardium.

C.   Pathophysiologic processes and manifestations

1.   **As blood pressure rises with age, cardiac reserve decreases from 4.6 to 3.3 times resting cardiac output, which can lead to hypertension and cardiac compromise.**

2.   As cardiac contractility decreases, risk of myocardial failure increases, especially when combined with a cardiac disease state.

3.   Left ventricular relaxation may prolong, contributing to dysrhythmias and altered cardiac output.

4.   Thickening of the bases of the valves can obstruct blood flow and cause valvular dysfunction.

5.   Atherosclerois causes the aorta and large vessels to become less flexible

6.   As peripheral vessels lengthen, they become tortuous and less resilient, leading to peripheral vascular disease.

D.   Overview of nursing interventions

1.   Evaluate the patient's blood pressure and heart rate, and check for orthostatic changes.

2.   **Review the patient's cardiovascular medications, and be aware that side effects may be exacerbated in the elderly (eg, postural hypotension from vasodilators).**

3.   Administer medications as prescribed, ensuring that vital signs are within designated parameters, if indicated.

4.   Listen to heart sounds and document clicks, murmurs, and rubs

5.   **Make sure that patients taking diuretics can get to the bathroom easily and safely without falling.**

V.   Pulmonary system disorders

A.   Description: minor alterations in pulmonary function associated with aging

B.   Etiology

1.   Most pulmonary problems are caused by disease states, rather than aging.

If deterioration in pulmonary function occurs in an elderly patient, a patho-logic cause must be ruled out.

2. Pulmonary dysfunction in the elderly is often caused by smoking, environ-mental exposures, and bacterial/viral infections.

3. The elderly have a higher incidence of pulmonary disease secondary to de-creased immune response and the long-term effects of toxic exposure.

C. **Pathophysiologic processes and manifestations**

1. Vital capacity and maximal rate of expiration decrease by age 70.

2. Skeletal changes, such as kyphosis and increased anterio-posterior diameter of the chest, can alter pulmonary function.

3. **Chest-wall compliance and elastic recoil of the lungs decreases, reduc-ing ventilatory reserve and leading to pulmonary compromise.**

4. PaO_2 and the total number of functioning alveoli decrease with age.

5. Pulmonary diseases—especially pneumonia and tuberculosis (TB)—are more common in the elderly.

   a. Pneumonia occurs in 15 to 70% of the elderly, because host-defense mechanisms become impaired with age.

   b. Reactivation accounts for 80% of active TB cases, with a high inci-dence in the elderly.

   c. Signs and symptoms of pulmonary disease in the elderly are often non-specific compared to younger adults, and might include weak-ness, poor appetite, or altered mental status.

   d. **Tachypnea and tachycardia are often the first signs of pul-monary compromise.**

D. **Overview of nursing interventions**

1. Obtain an accurate history of previous pulmonary conditions, as well as in-formation on smoking and exercise.

2. Auscultate the lungs to assess for adventitious sounds, and measure di-aphragmatic excursion.

3. Monitor arterial blood gases and chest x-rays.

4. **Observe the patient for pursed-lip breathing, use of accessory muscles, and tachypnea.**

5. Administer respiratory treatments as ordered, and assess the patient's re-sponse to treatments and medications.

6. Administer oxygen as ordered, and measure oxygen saturation regularly.

7. Obtain sputum cultures as ordered.

VI. **Gastrointestinal (GI) system disorders**

A. **Description**

1. Changes in the gastrointestinal system range from tooth loss to malabsorp-tion.

2. Poor nutritional intake is compounded by loss of taste buds and smell, so malnutrition occurs often in elderly patients.

B. **Etiology**

1. Tooth loss results from poor oral hygiene and lack of dental care.

2. Lower GI symptoms such as constipation occur from poor diet, drug effects, or disease.

C. **Pathophysiologic processes and manifestations**

1. Fifty percent of people over age 65 have lost a tooth, and many others have gum recession and other dental problems.

 2. **Diminished peristalsis results in increased absorption times, leading to constipation and alterations in drug absorption.**

3. Constipation is caused by environmental factors, such as immobility and poor hydration; psychological factors such as depression; or diseases, such as colon cancer and diverticulitis.

4. If no disease is present, treatment includes increasing fluids, fiber, and exercise.

5. Gastric acid secretion is reduced, and achlorhydria may occur.

6. Villous atrophy occurs in the small intestine, although the effect on absorption is limited.

7. The pancreas and liver shrink, but in the absence of disease, this should not effect function.

D. **Overview of nursing interventions**

1. Assess nutritional status and obtain information on eating habits, bowel habits, and any identified problems.

2. Ensure adequate hydration and fiber intake.

 3. **Review the patient's medications, and monitor for GI adverse reactions or side effects.**

4. Administer medications, such as stool softeners or histamine-2 blockers, as indicated.

5. Teach the patient about the importance of diet in controlling GI symptoms.

VII. Urinary system disorders

A. **Description**

1. Urinary system disorders affect almost all elderly people and lead to incontinence, frequent urination, and prostatic hypertrophy in men.

2. Incontinence is the inability to retain urine. It occurs in 15 to 30% of the elderly, with 20 to 30% having daily or weekly episodes.

3. In nursing facilities, the incidence of urinary incontinence rises to between 50 to 70%.

B. **Etiology**

1. Changes in the urinary tract are often a direct result of the aging process.

 2. **In hospitalized patients, urinary incontinence often occurs because patients who need help getting to the bathroom don't receive it in time.**

3. The remainder of cases are due to loss of muscle tone and diminished bladder function related to childbirth, aging, and prostatic hypertrophy.

 4. **Diuretics, hypnotics, alpha-adrenergic agents, and anticholinergics may contribute to urinary incontinence.**

C. **Pathophysiologic processes and manifestations**
1. Normal changes
   a. Peak bladder capacity is reduced, and the percentage of urine retained in the bladder at end-urination is mildly elevated.
   b. Renal blood flow decreases by 50% and the renal tubules are less able to concentrate urine. This requires the kidneys to continue working during the night to efficiently remove all substances from the blood.
   c. These factors result in urinary frequency and nocturia.
   d. Prostatic hypertrophy is seen in 100% of men, with the organ doubling in size. This can lead to urinary hesitancy, decreased urine stream, and nocturia.

 e. **Creatinine clearance decreases after age 40 at a rate of 1% per year, increasing an older adult's risk of toxicity when taking drugs excreted by the kidneys.**

2. Urinary incontinence
   a. Increased residual volume secondary to loss of bladder tone predisposes patients to urinary tract infections and incontinence.
   b. Reduction of muscle mass in the bladder wall and decreased bladder compliance results in decreased bladder capacity, urinary frequency, and nocturia.
   c. Decreased number and deterioration of sensory receptors in the bladder wall, which signal bladder fullness, don't respond as well in the elderly. So the patient may not feel the urge to void until the bladder is near capacity.
   d. Benign prostatic hypertrophy causes outlet obstruction resulting in weak stream, difficulty in starting stream, frequency, urgency, and incontinence.
   e. Sphincter weakness in women may be due to parity, giving birth to high birthweight babies, use of forceps, and vaginal tears during delivery.

 f. **Tars in cigarettes have been identified as bladder irritants that contribute to incontinence.**

D. **Overview of nursing interventions**
1. Ask the patient about nocturia, incontinence, urinary frequency, and other urinary problems.
2. Assess the patient's general state of health and perform an abdominal exam to determine bladder fullness

 3. **Make sure that the patient with nocturia has safe and easy access to the bathroom to prevent falls and secondary complications.**
4. Prevent hospital-induced urinary incontinence by putting patients on a bladder schedule.
5. Help prevent drug toxicity by monitoring the patient's medications, particularly those excreted through the kidney.

 6. **Monitor drugs taken by incontinent patients for their potential impact on urinary incontinence.**
7. Monitor intake and output and renal function, as indicated.

8. Educate patients about common urinary problems in their age group.
9. Ensure privacy.
10. Tell patients to avoid bladder irritants such as caffeine, and to limit late night fluid intake.
11. Assist the patient with practicing urge control, as indicated.

VIII.   Musculoskeletal system disorders

A.   Description:
1. Musculoskeletal changes associated with bone density, muscle mass, and joint flexibility normally occur with the aging process.
2. Immobility is complete limitation of movement (patient requires bedrest).
3. Dysmobility is partial limitation of movement secondary to a disease state.
4. A fall is an involuntary change in position not explained by syncope, trauma, or seizures.
5. Falls are markers of present disability and future morbidity:
    a. Falls occur in 25% of elderly patients
    b. Fifty percent of people who fall are repeaters.
    c. About 1 in 40 are hospitalized, with 40% becoming long-term patients.
    d. Twenty-five percent die within 6 months of injury, 25% lose functional ability and 50% have decreased mobility.
6. Forty-five percent of the elderly have mobility restrictions that affect their functional abilities.
7. Many musculoskeletal changes can be slowed down or halted by early intervention.

B.   Etiology
1. Changes in musculature are associated with microscopic lipofuscin deposition, a decrease in the number of myofibrils, and a reduction in glycolytic oxidative enzyme activity.
2. Changes in bone occur secondary to demineralization.
3. Causes of limited mobility include osteoarthritis, rheumatoid arthritis, osteoporosis, and trauma.
4. Causes of complete immobility include cerebral vascular accident, cardiovascular disease, and other chronic conditions.
5. Falls are dependent on the individual characteristics of the patient and on the environment in which he or she lives.
6. The major cause of falls is impaired postural control or dynamic balance.

C.   Pathophysiologic processes and manifestations
1. Normal changes
    a. Men lose an average of 2 inches of height as they age, and women often lose more, particularly if they have osteoporosis.
    b. Most height loss occurs in the trunk secondary to intervertebral disc thinning and vertebral body shortening. This can lead to kyphosis and an increase in the anterior–posterior diameter of the chest wall.
    c. Muscle mass decreases by 30%, resulting in a decrease in muscle strength, endurance, and bulk.
    d. Lack of exercise in the elderly exacerbates these changes.

e. **Bone density declines, with more rapid loss noted in women than in men. This can result in osteoporosis, pathologic fractures, and debilitation.**

 f. Degenerative changes associated with loss of joint flexibility and strength can occur secondary to changes in the articular cartilage and synovial cavity.

 g. Knee and hip flexion is particularly diminished.

2. Immobility

 a. The consequences of immobility are predictable and usually preventable.

 b. **Malnutrition occurs because bedridden patients have a poorer nutritional intake than ambulatory ones, resulting in protein and vitamin deficiencies, weakness, and decreased muscle mass.**

 c. Deep vein thrombosis (DVT) occurs when limited activity causes vascular stasis. When a thrombus breaks loose, pulmonary emboli can develop.

 d. Constipation occurs secondary to dehydration, poor nutrition, and limited activity.

 e. **Pressure ulcers are caused solely by immobility and can be prevented 100% of the time by prompt nursing action.**

 f. Urinary tract infections and/or urinary retention occur secondary to comorbid diseases, poor personal hygiene, Foley catheter use, and alterations in urogenital flora.

 g. Atelectasis and secondary pneumonia occur because dependent positioning allows fluid to collect in small alveoli leading to alveolar collapse. This position decreases clearance of secretions, minimizes the cough reflex, and alters diaphragmatic function.

 h. Depression can result.

 i. **Orthostatic hypotension may be caused or exacerbated by bedrest, which slows normal postural compensatory mechanisms, resulting in changes in heart rate, stroke volume, and cardiac output.**

 j. Deconditioning (loss of muscle strength and exercise tolerance), muscle weakness, and atrophy quickly occur from lack of use.

 k. **Contractures can occur in 3 to 4 weeks when joint range of motion does not occur.**

3. Falls

 a. Dynamic balance, body position, and movement are controlled by information from several sensory systems; the central nervous system integrates this information.

 b. It also depends on the patient's musculoskeletal capacity.

 c. The sensory systems that provide information include vision, vestibular function, and proprioception.

 d. Vision diminishes with age, resulting in decreased peripheral vision, depth perception, and acuity, particularly at night.

 e. Vestibular function is controlled by the maculae and semicircular canals of the ear, which help to maintain balance and position.

   f.   Vestibular dysfunction increases with age, making the patient less able to maintain position and balance.
   g.   Proprioceptive function is often altered by co-existing disease states, such as diabetes mellitus, nutritional deficiencies, and neurologic disease.
   h.   All of these factors alter the patient's ability to define his position in space.
   i.   The central nervous system, which is responsible for integrating this information, is affected by slowed neuronal impulse transit times and slowed cognitive-motor responses.
   j.   Degenerative musculoskeletal changes make the patient less able to respond rapidly to alterations in sensory processing.

D.   Overview of nursing interventions

   1.   Recognize that a geriatric patient may take longer to complete tasks due to decreased flexibility and pain from degenerative joint disease.
   2.   **Decrease the incidence of falls and fractures by removing obstacles in the patient's path and improving lighting.**
   3.   Assess and document the patient's functional capacity and level of mobility and offer assistive devices, as indicated.
   4.   **Encourage the bedridden patient to walk as soon as possible to prevent complications of immobility.**
   5.   Perform daily range-of-motion exercises to prevent venous status, muscle weakening, and contractures.
   6.   Ensure adequate nutrition, dietary fiber, and hydration.
   7.   Assess bowel status and provide stool softeners as indicated.
   8.   **Evaluate the patient's medications to ascertain which ones might intensify fall risk or impair mobility by limiting CNS responsiveness.**
   9.   Inspect the skin for breakdown and adhere to a turning schedule.
   10.   Provide incentive spirometry and upright body positioning as much as possible.
   11.   **Monitor the patient's blood pressure and pulse when he or she gets out of bed, and move slowly to prevent orthostatic hypotension.**
   12.   Encourage patient to perform activities of daily living, but provide assistance when needed.
   13.   **Help the patient to the bathroom frequently, because many patients fall when trying to get out of bed to use the bathroom.**

IX.   Homeostatic/immunologic system disorders

A.   Description: changes in the body's internal equilibrium and ability to fight off infection associated with aging
B.   Etiology
   1.   Homeostatic changes in the elderly are associated with changes in body fluid distribution and thermoregulatory capability.

  2. Homeostasis is dependent on the multiple changes occurring in all other body systems.

  3. External defenses against disease are diminished by changes in cell structure and the overall effect of aging.

  4. Cellular changes are subtle, but they can have significant sequelae.

C. **Pathophysiologic processes and manifestations**

  1. In men, total body water declines from 60% to 54%; in women it declines from 54% to 46%.

  2. **Body fluid regulation is less precise, so patients often do not have reduced thirst as a sign of dehydration.**

  3. Thermoregulatory responses are diminished, leading to hypothermia and the absence of fever despite systemic infection.

  4. **Postural hypotension and vasovagal syncope are common secondary to changes in baroreceptor responsiveness.**

  5. The skin and mucous membranes, which are the primary external defense against infection, are thinner and have a decreased blood supply.

  6. Mucociliary defenses and the cough reflex are blunted, so there is a higher risk of respiratory infection.

  7. Prostatic hypertrophy causes increased residual urine volumes, making it more difficult to flush pathogens from the bladder.

  8. Achlorhydria in the stomach decreases the GI tract's ability to fight off infection.

  9. The total number of white cells does not decrease with age, but certain subpopulations of cells do, resulting in impaired cell-mediated immunity.

D. **Overview of nursing interventions**

  1. **Assess for subtle indicators of infection, such as tachypnea, tachycardia, and mental status changes, because normal signs and symptoms of infection may be absent in elderly patients.**

  2. Assess hydration status and ensure adequate fluid intake.

  3. Instruct the patient to change position slowly to decrease postural hypotension.

  4. Encourage the patient to receive preventative health care, including flu vaccines and pneumoccal vaccine.

Bibliography

Barker, L., Randol, J. R., et al. (Eds.) (1994). *Principles of ambulatory medicine* (4th ed.). Baltimore: Williams and Wilkins.

Bates, B. (1996). *A Guide to physical examination.* Philadelphia: J.B. Lippincott.

Berkow, R. (Ed.) (1992). *The Merck manual,* (16th ed.). New Jersey: Merck Research Labs.

Cox, H., (Ed.) (1998). *Aging 98/99.* Connecticut: Dushkin/McGraw Hill.

Ham, R., & Sloane, P. (1997). *Primary care geriatrics—A case-based approach* (3rd ed). St. Louis: Mosby.

McCance, K., & Huether, S. (1990). *Pathophysiology: The biologic basis for disease in adults and children.* St. Louis: Mosby.

STUDY QUESTIONS

1. Current theories of aging include all of the following except:
   a. gene mutations
   b. protein degradation
   c. alteration in DNA coding
   d. limitation in proliferative cellular capability

2. Central nervous system deterioration occurs secondary to:
   a. loss of neurons and pigment accumulation
   b. crystalline changes in the lens of the eye
   c. increase in cerebral size
   d. personality changes

3. Contributors to hypertension and cardiac compromise in the elderly may include:
   a. increases in cardiac contractility
   b. prolongation of left ventricular relaxation
   c. increases in cardiac output
   d. elevation in blood pressure and decreased cardiac reserve

4. Mrs. Smith, age 82, complains of poor appetite and weakness. She denies fever, nausea, vomiting, or cough. What signs and symptoms would most likely indicate a pulmonary infection?
   a. fever
   b. tachypnea and tachycardia
   c. cough
   d. subjective report of shortness of breath

5. One nursing intervention that may be able to prevent episodes of incontinence is:
   a. Foley catheter insertion
   b. limited fluid intake
   c. a toileting schedule
   d. limited diuretic use

6. Loss of height is secondary to:
   a. osteoporosis
   b. decreased bone density
   c. pathologic fractures
   d. intervertebral disc thinning

7. A direct outcome of decreased body fluid is:
   a. decreased thirst response
   b. hypovolemia
   c. decreased temperature
   d. postural hypotension

8. A confusion state characterized by rapid onset of disorganized thinking and altered psychomotor behavior is:
   a. Alzheimer's disease
   b. sundowner's
   c. dementia
   d. delirium

9. Nursing interventions that can decrease the incidence of falls include all of the following except:
   a. bedrest
   b. modifying the environment to remove hazards
   c. monitoring psychotropic drugs
   d. a bladder and bowel schedule

10. Failure to thrive usually occurs secondary to:
    a. a chronic medical condition
    b. depression
    c. decreased motivation
    d. malnutrition

ANSWER KEY

Question	Correct answer	Correct answer rationale	Incorrect answer rationales
1.	c	DNA coding does not cause aging. Coding is a normal process where limitation of replication is predetermined.	a. Gene mutations can occur from environmental exposure, free radical damage, and so forth. b. Protein degradation occurs through biochemical degenerative processes. d. Limited proliferative ability has been documented.
2.	a	Neurologic deterioration may also be due to decreased brain size, dendritic changes, and a decrease in neurotransmitters.	b. Crystalline changes in the lens may affect vision but not CNS function. c. Cerebral size decreases with aging. d. Personality is unchanged by aging.
3.	d	Elevations in blood pressure and decreased cardiac reserve may contribute to cardiac compromise in the geriatric patient.	a. Cardiac contractility decreases with age. b. Prolongation of left ventricular relaxation occurs, but it does not contribute to hypertension. c. Cardiac output diminishes with aging.
4.	b	Tachycardia and tachypnea are often the only indications of pulmonary infection and compromise.	a. Fever may be absent in the geriatric patient. c. Cough may or may not be present in pulmonary infections. d. A subjective report of shortness of breath may not necessarily correlate with pulmonary infection.
5.	c	Placing the patient on a toileting schedule may help to prevent episodes of incontinence by ensuring frequent urination.	a. A Foley catheter may cause urinary tract infections and urosepsis but will not alter incontinence. b. Limiting fluids can decrease urine output but not necessarily limit incontinence. d. Limiting diuretic use solely for the purpose of controlling incontinence is an unreasonable and possibly unsafe practice.
6.	d	Loss of height is directly related to intravertebral disc thinning and vertebral body shortening.	a. Osteoporosis can lead to fracture or collapse of the vertebral bodies but not necessarily decreased height.

Question	Correct answer	Correct answer rationale	Incorrect answer rationales
			b. Decreased bone density can lead to osteoporosis, which can lead to vertebral fractures, but this is not the major way that height is altered. c. Pathologic fractures can occur, but these are usually in the extremities, not the vertebral column.
7.	b	Hypovolemia can occur secondary to decreased body fluid.	a. A decreased thirst reflex can occur in the elderly, but this occurs along with decreased body fluid. c. Decreased temperature can also occur, but this is not secondary to decreased body fluid. d. Postural hypotension is most likely due to changes in baroreceptor responsiveness.
8.	d	Delirium is a confusion state characterized by the rapid onset of disorganized thinking and altered psychomotor behavior.	a. Alzheimer's disease is a chronic disease characterized by cognitive and behavioral changes. b. Sundowner's is a syndrome whereby sleep–wake cycles are reversed and psychomotor manifestations may occur. c. Dementia is a long-term, slowly evolving condition that causes cognitive changes.
9.	a	Bedrest will not decrease the risk of falls, because patients will still try to get out of bed to perform personal hygiene.	b, c, and d. These are all essential to a fall risk-prevention program.
10.	b	Depression is the major cause of failure to thrive in the elderly.	a. A chronic medical condition can lead to decompensation, but this is not the major cause of FTT. c. Decreased motivation is a symptom of failure to thrive. d. Malnutrition is a potential complication of failure to thrive.

Comprehensive Test Questions

1. Acquired immune deficiencies can result from:
   a. vitamin A deficiency
   b. electrolyte disorders
   c. congenital causes
   d. infectious or viral agents

2. In allergic reactions, histamine's vascular effects produce:
   a. decreased vascular permeability
   b. angioedema
   c. vasoconstriction
   d. bronchodilation

3. When caring for a patient with liver trauma, the nurse should take which of the following actions?
   a. Observe for signs of shock.
   b. Administer blood as ordered.
   c. Monitor vital signs frequently.
   d. All of the above.

4. Penetrating liver trauma is identified by rupture of:
   a. phagocytes
   b. Glisson's capsule
   c. parenchyma
   d. hematoma

5. The nurse should instruct a patient with herpes virus type 2 to:
   a. Keep a cold moist compress on the affected area at all times.
   b. Apply hydrogen peroxide to the affected area.
   c. Periodically rupture the vesicles.
   d. Bathe in hot water.

6. The nurse in the community health center teaches patients that hepatitis B is transmitted by:
   a. blood and body fluids
   b. fecal-oral route
   c. waterborne route
   d. contaminated shellfish

7. The body compensates for a low cardiac output by:
   a. increasing heart rate
   b. increasing respiratory rate
   c. decreasing blood pressure
   d. decreasing stroke volume

8. Nursing management of congestive heart failure (CHF) includes:
   a. administering beta-blockers and sedatives, and providing a low-sodium diet
   b. administering nitrates and antiarrhythmics, and encouraging bed rest
   c. administering digitalis, diuretics, and oxygen
   d. administering antibiotics, immunosuppressants, and isotonic fluids

9. A patient who has had an anterior wall MI becomes tachycardiac, hypotensive, and confused. His skin is cool and pale, and his urine output has decreased to 20 cc/hr. The nurse would anticipate that interventions would include:
   a. use of rotating tourniquets
   b. insertion of an intra-aortic balloon pump
   c. pericardiocentesis
   d. blood transfusion

10. Risk factors for breast cancer can include:
    a. Premenstrual syndrome
    b. late menopause
    c. multiparity
    d. dysmenorrhea

11. The three major pathways of lymphatic drainage in the breast are:
    a. axillary, internal mammary, transpectoral
    b. substernal, cervical, mammary

   c. internal mammary, submandibular, tonsillar

   d. transpectoral, substernal, axillary

12. The hypodynamic phase of septic shock is associated with:
   a. decreased cardiac output and increased systemic vascular resistance
   b. increased cardiac output and decreased systemic vascular resistance
   c. warm, dry skin
   d. normal capillary refill

13. Manifestations of neurogenic shock are due to:
   a. occurrence of bradycardia,
   b. increased venous return
   c. obstruction of flow
   d. loss of vasomotor tone

14. Which of the following physiologic responses is indicative of obstructive genitourinary disease?
   a. pyuria
   b. weight loss
   c. hypertension
   d. hematuria

15. Episodes of incontinence can be related to:
   a. gastrointestinal pathophysiology
   b. pulmonary pathophysiology
   c. kidney pathophysiology
   d. neurologic disease

16. When assessing a patient for arterial disease, the nurse is aware that risk factors may include:
   a. low-fat diet
   b. high sodium diet
   c. high-carbohydrate diet
   d. genetic predisposition

17. Nursing management of the patient with arteriosclerosis obliterans (peripheral arteriosclerotic disease) includes:
   a. elevation of the extremity
   b. administration of diuretics
   c. limiting activity
   d. encouraging activity

18. Pathophysiologic processes involved in arteriosclerosis obliterans (peripheral arteriosclerotic disease) include:

   a. interstitial fluid shifts
   b. arterial narrowing
   c. arterial dilation
   d. acute ischemia

19. Which of the following are causes of acute renal failure (ARF)?:
   a. polycystic kidneys
   b. hypertension
   c. nephrotoxic agents
   d. diabetic nephropathy

20. Infection of the interstitium and renal pelvis are indicative of which of the following disorders?
   a. renal calculi
   b. pyelonephritis
   c. glomerulonephritis
   d. chronic renal failure

21. Oliguria is defined as urine output of less than:
   a. 400 ml/day
   b. 600 ml/day
   c. 60 ml/day
   d. 40 ml/day

22. The most common manifestations of nephrotic syndrome include:
   a. proteinuria, hypoproteinemia, edema
   b. hypoproteinemia, edema, weight gain
   c. edema, weight loss, hyperkalemia
   d. weight loss, hypokalemia, hypercalcemia

23. Which of the following are classified as noninfectious inflammatory dermatoses?:
   a. psoriasis
   b. warts
   c. herpes
   d. tinea capitis

24. Nursing management of contact dermatitis involves:
   a. application of heat
   b. massaging affected areas
   c. removal of external irritants
   d. application of lindane

25. Which of the following is *not* a factor in the etiology of acne vulgaris?

a. genetics
b. diet
c. hormonal factors
d. bacterial infection

26. When teaching parents about pediculosis (lice), the nurse would explain that manifestations include:
a. alopecia
b. itching with red papules
c. small red macules
d. large vesicles

27. A patient is experiencing air hunger, bilateral crackles throughout both lung fields, and a productive cough with pink-tinged sputum. Anticipated interventions would include:
a. use of rotating tourniquets
b. insertion of an intra-aortic balloon pump
c. pericardiocentesis
d. increasing IV flow rate

28. After establishing that a collapsed adult victim is unresponsive, the nurse should:
a. Open the airway
b. Deliver two rescue breaths
c. Call 911 if you are alone
d. Start compressions

29. The most common cause of cardiac arrest in an adult is:
a. electrolyte imbalance
b. ventricular tachycardia
c. asystole
d. respiratory arrest

30. CPK-MB will peak within how many hours of the onset of an MI?
a. 2 to 4 hours
b. 12 to 24 hours
c. 24 to 36 hours
d. 48 to 72 hours

31. During a physical examination, a patient with a valvular disorder is likely to describe:
a. a recent trauma
b. a history of rheumatic heart disease
c. a family member with a similar disorder
d. exposure to chemical irritants

32. A patient with pericarditis is likely to present with:
a. bradycardia
b. wheezing
c. ascites without peripheral edema
d. a widened pulse pressure

33. A 32-year-old male was treated in the emergency department for a dislocated shoulder. Dislocations may result from all of the following etiologies:
a. congenital, pathologic
b. psychosis, trauma
c. malnutrition, infection
d. trauma, infection

34. Initial nursing management for sprains typically includes:
a. use of compression wraps
b. application of a cast
c. application of hot packs
d. aspiration of fluid accumulation

35. Pathophysiologic responses following a fracture include:
a. muscle spasms, pain
b. infection, bruising
c. lengthening of the extremity
d. synovitis, numbness

36. A common causative organism in acute lymphangitis is:
a. Pneumococcus
b. Streptococcus
c. Staphylococcus
d. Enterobacterium

37. Which of the following types of vascular disease is *not* associated with diabetes mellitus?
a. atherosclerosis
b. peripheral vascular disease
c. diabetic microangiopathy
d. Buerger's disease

38. When providing patient teaching for a patient with arteriosclerosis, the nurse should instruct the patient to:
a. decrease activity gradually
b. eliminate all forms of tobacco use
c. increase carbohydrate intake
d. take antibiotics prophylactically

39. Costovertebral angle tenderness (CVA) can be elicited by:
 a. Direct patient questioning
 b. Fist percussion of posterior flank
 c. Palpating the abdomen
 d. Having the patient void

40. Early manifestations of kidney cancer include:
 a. pain
 b. hyperkalemia
 c. fatigue
 d. weight gain

41. When providing patient teaching for a patient undergoing a total cystectomy with urinary diversion (ileal conduit), the nurse should focus on:
 a. preoperative leg exercises
 b. electrolyte maintenance
 c. maintenance of a continuous drainage system
 d. intermittent catheterization

42. Risk factors for osteoporosis can include:
 a. late menopause
 b. active participation in sports
 c. multiparity
 d. sedentary life-style

43. An involucrum, seen in chronic osteomyelitis, is defined as:
 a. necrotic bone
 b. bone ischemia and devascularization
 c. an encasement around the sequestrum
 d. granulated tissue in the sinus tract

44. When assessing a patient with impaired oxygen perfusion, the nurse would *not* expect to find which of the following symptoms?
 a. diaphoresis
 b. bradycardia
 c. cool skin
 d. restlessness

45. Predisposing factors for lung cancer include:
 a. family history of lung cancer
 b. taking of narcotics
 c. hayfever
 d. asthma

46. A pathophysiologic effect of lung cancer is:
 a. excessive steroid production
 b. diabetes mellitus
 c. increased oxygenation
 d. asthma

47. Which of the following situations is likely to provoke a sickle cell crisis?
 a. alkalosis
 b. dehydration
 c. overhydration
 d. immobility

48. Manifestations of sickle cell crisis includes:
 a. long bone pain
 b. bruising
 c. petechiae
 d. shortness of breath

49. When assessing a patient for hypothyroidism, the nurse would expect to observe which of the following symptoms?
 a. heat intolerance
 b. diarrhea
 c. flushing
 d. reduced sweat gland secretion

50. Thyroid storm occurs when there is an increase in:
 a. tachycardia
 b. pericardial effusion
 c. bradycardia
 d. cold intolerance

51. Nursing interventions for a patient with hyperthyroidism include:
 a. providing a warm environment
 b. administering aspirin
 c. monitoring for vision changes
 d. lowering the head of the bed

52. Manifestations of meningeal irritation include all of the following *except:*
 a. cranial nerve palsies
 b. nuchal rigidity
 c. photophobia
 d. headache

53. Korsakoff psychosis in Wernicke's disease is characterized by:
 a. ophthalmoplegia and ataxia
 b. anterograde amnesia

c. amnesia and confabulation

d. alterations in level of consciousness

54. Which of the following pathophysiologic changes are associated with Alzheimer's disease?

a. dopamine deficiency

b. senile plaque formation

c. hemorrhagic necrosis

d. cortical atrophy

55. In a patient with myasthenia gravis, the manifestations of increased muscle weakness, bradycardia, pupillary constriction, and muscle fasiculations indicate:

a. myasthenic crisis

b. a normal exacerbation

c. cholinergic crisis

d. a reaction to medication

56. Which of the following statement is true about muscular dystrophy?

a. Muscular dystrophy is an upper motor neuron disease.

b. Muscular dystrophy is the result of autoimmune activity.

c. Muscular dystrophy causes sensory abnormalities.

d. Muscular dystrophy is a genetic disorder of the muscle fibers.

57. Ipsilateral ptosis, pupillary dilation, contralateral hemiparesis, and bilateral Babinski response are indicative of which of the following types of herniation?

a. transtentorial

b. uncal

c. infratentorial

d. central

58. Seizure thresholds may be lowered by:

a. fatigue

b. hyperglycemia

c. sleep

d. anti-seizure medications

59. The tonic phase of a grand mal seizure is characterized by:

a. relaxation of muscles

b. muscle contraction with increased tone

c. alternating contraction and relaxation

d. muscle fasiculations

60. Localized hypoxia occurs in rheumatoid arthritis because of:

a. release of synovial enzymes

b. vasculitis

c. blockage of veins resulting in decreased oxygen delivery

d. joint immobilization

61. A retrovirus implies that:

a. the viral RNA is integrated into the host cell

b. the genetic information is transmitted as RNA

c. a surface antigen is required for infiltration to occur

d. cell destruction will result

62. The primary cells affected by HIV infection are:

a. T helper cells

b. T suppressor cells

c. all white blood cells

d. CD 4 cells only

63. Which of the following is a malignant carcinoma of the liver?

a. adenoma

b. cholangioma

c. focal nodular hyperplasia

d. hemangioma

64. Hepatocellular carcinoma develops in the:

a. gall bladder

b. Kupffer cells

c. hepatocytes

d. bile ducts

65. Hepatic tumors are spread by:

a. lymphatic system

b. portal venous circulation

c. direct extension from adjacent organs

d. parasinusoidal invasion into parenchyma

66. With maternal-fetal transmission of *Chlamydia*, the neonate may exhibit all of the following symptoms *except:*

a. prematurity

b. birth defects

c. pneumonia

d. conjunctivitis

67. The usual treatment for condylomata acuminata is:
    a. surgical removal of all warts
    b. penicillin
    c. cryotherapy
    d. laser surgery

68. Tremors and impaired speech, concentration, and memory are manifestations of which of the following stages of syphilis?
    a. primary
    b. secondary
    c. latency
    d. tertiary

69. Cutaneous manifestations associated with anaphylactic shock include:
    a. dry skin
    b. moon face
    c. urticaria
    d. decreased capillary refill

70. A common cause of anaphylactic shock is:
    a. depressant action of drugs
    b. reactions to viral agents
    c. insect stings
    d. decrease cardiac pumping action

71. Pathophysiologic processes associated with cardiogenic shock include:
    a. decreased ventricular contractility
    b. hypoxemia and acidosis
    c. decreased vascular resistance
    d. hypoxemia and alkalosis

72. When assessing a patient for breast cancer, the nurse is aware that approximately 60% of carcinomas of the breast occur in the:
    a. lower outer quadrant
    b. lower inner quadrant
    c. upper outer quadrant
    d. upper inner quadrant

73. Management of cervical cancer is based on staging of the disease. Cancer that is completely confined to the cervix is:
    a. Stage 0
    b. Stage 1
    c. Stage 2
    d. Stage 3

74. The three major manifestations of toxic shock syndrome (TSS) include all of the following *except:*
    a. sudden onset fever
    b. hypertension
    c. disorientation
    d. erythematous macular rash

75. Persons at high risk to develop Wernicke-Korsakoff syndrome include all *except:*
    a. chronic alcoholics
    b. persons with malabsorption syndromes
    c. malnourished persons
    d. persons with vitamin B6 deficiency

76. Manifestations of acute onset of encephalitis can include:
    a. decreased voluntary movements
    b. bradykinesia
    c. seizures
    d. hypokinesia

77. In tonic-clonic seizures, all of the following may occur *except:*
    a. paralysis
    b. loss of consciousness
    c. incontinence
    d. a brief period of apnea

78. If a patient was confused and unable to rouse spontaneously, needing external stimuli (e.g., touch) before being able to converse with the staff, the patient's level of consciousness would be categorized as:
    a. lethargic
    b. obtunded
    c. stuporous
    d. comatose

79. Autonomic hyperreflexia occurring after spinal cord injury involves all of the following *except:*
    a. Loss of smooth muscle innervation
    b. Transection of the autonomic nervous system
    c. Loss of balance between parasympathetic and sympathetic nervous systems
    d.

80. Manifestations of increased sympathetic stimulation can include:

a. decreased vasomotor tone
b. paralytic ileus
c. hypertension
d. atony of bowel and bladder

81. In amyotrophic lateral sclerosis (ALS), the paresis begins in one localized muscle group and extends to include all striated muscle *except:*
   a. extraocular muscles
   b. diaphragm
   c. facial muscles
   d. speech muscles

82. Hypercalcemia causes an increased amount of calcium to be delivered to the kidneys, resulting in:
   a. kidney stones
   b. acid urine
   c. metabolic alkalosis
   d. hyperphosphatemia

83. In Cushing's syndrome, accelerated protein catabolism leads to all of the following symptoms *except:*
   a. difficult movement
   b. weakness
   c. hypoglycemia
   d. muscle wasting

84. A patient with sickle cell disease asks the nurse to explain the therapeutic value of a splenectomy. The nurse states that it is done:
   a. to eliminate the etiology of sickle cell disease
   b. as a curative procedure
   c. to prevent any future sickle cell crisis
   d. because of damage to the spleen from thrombosis

85. Common etiologies of anemias include all of the following *except:*
   a. infections
   b. dietary
   c. genetic
   d. metabolic alterations

86. The dominant manifestations of decreased RBC volume include:
   a. hypertension
   b. bradycardia
   c. orthostatic changes
   d. joint pain

87. All of the following are risk factors for restrictive lung diseases *except:*
   a. asbestos inhalation
   b. chronic bronchitis
   c. chronic musculoskeletal diseases
   d. surgery

88. A compensatory response of the body to respiratory alkalosis:
   a. increased HC0
   b. retention of HC0
   c. hyperventilation
   d. increased CO

89. The nurse would suspect a diagnosis of peritonitis when which of the following signs are assessed?
   a. abdominal tenderness and rigidity
   b. gastroesophageal reflux and heartburn
   c. melena
   d. hyperactive bowel sounds and diarrhea

90. Odynophagia refers to:
   a. heartburn
   b. painful swallowing
   c. difficulty swallowing
   d. malodorous breath

91. When teaching a patient about the purpose of cimetidine, an H2 antagonist, the nurse should explain that it will:
   a. provide a protective coating for gastric mucosa
   b. increase gastric pH
   c. lower gastric pH
   d. inhibit gastric acid formation

92. When assessing a patient for pain associated with peptic ulcer disease, the nurse is aware that this type of pain typically is described as occurring under which of the following conditions?:
   a. on an empty stomach
   b. on a full stomach
   c. with ingestion of cold foods
   d. with ingestion of zantac.

93. Which of the following conditions occurs when fusion of the urethral folds is incomplete?
   a. hypospadias

b. epispadias
c. priapism
d. spermatocele

94. Nursing interventions for the patient with prostatitis would include:
a. withholding antibiotics
b. encouraging the patient to sit rather than walk
c. teaching the patient to have sex
d. instituting pain control measures

95. Pathophysiologic changes seen in hydrocele include:
a. congenital gonadal defect
b. poorly developed secondary sex characteristics
c. late closure of the tunica vaginalis
d. deviant sperm morphology

96. Which of the following symptoms would the nurse expect to assess in a patient with cryptorchidism?
a. femerol hernia
b. absence of testes from scrotum
c. painless enlargement of testes
d. increased spermatogenesis

97. Sudden onset neurosensory hearing loss is associated with:
a. trauma to seventh cranial nerve
b. trauma to the eighth cranial nerve
c. old age
d. noise

98. Etiologies of posterior epistaxis include:
a. drying
b. infection
c. hypotension
d. septal perforation

99. Nursing interventions for the patient with epistaxis include:
a. administering nasal spray with saline
b. administering nasal spray with phenylephrine HCL
c. placing the patient in a supine
d. encouraging the patient to blow his nose frequently

100. When assessing a patient for neoplasms of the ENT system, the nurse would expect to find all of the following symptoms *except:*
a. foul breath
b. dysphagia
c. pain radiating to the ear
d. snoring

Answer Sheet for Comprehensive Test Questions

With a pencil, blacken the circle under the option you have chosen for your correct answer.

	A	B	C	D		A	B	C	D		A	B	C	D
1.	○	○	○	○	21.	○	○	○	○	41.	○	○	○	○
2.	○	○	○	○	22.	○	○	○	○	42.	○	○	○	○
3.	○	○	○	○	23.	○	○	○	○	43.	○	○	○	○
4.	○	○	○	○	24.	○	○	○	○	44.	○	○	○	○
5.	○	○	○	○	25.	○	○	○	○	45.	○	○	○	○
6.	○	○	○	○	26.	○	○	○	○	46.	○	○	○	○
7.	○	○	○	○	27.	○	○	○	○	47.	○	○	○	○
8.	○	○	○	○	28.	○	○	○	○	48.	○	○	○	○
9.	○	○	○	○	29.	○	○	○	○	49.	○	○	○	○
10.	○	○	○	○	30.	○	○	○	○	50.	○	○	○	○
11.	○	○	○	○	31.	○	○	○	○	51.	○	○	○	○
12.	○	○	○	○	32.	○	○	○	○	52.	○	○	○	○
13.	○	○	○	○	33.	○	○	○	○	53.	○	○	○	○
14.	○	○	○	○	34.	○	○	○	○	54.	○	○	○	○
15.	○	○	○	○	35.	○	○	○	○	55.	○	○	○	○
16.	○	○	○	○	36.	○	○	○	○	56.	○	○	○	○
17.	○	○	○	○	37.	○	○	○	○	57.	○	○	○	○
18.	○	○	○	○	38.	○	○	○	○	58.	○	○	○	○
19.	○	○	○	○	39.	○	○	○	○	59.	○	○	○	○
20.	○	○	○	○	40.	○	○	○	○	60.	○	○	○	○

	A	B	C	D		A	B	C	D		A	B	C	D
61.	○	○	○	○	81.	○	○	○	○	101.	○	○	○	○
62.	○	○	○	○	82.	○	○	○	○	102.	○	○	○	○
63.	○	○	○	○	83.	○	○	○	○	103.	○	○	○	○
64.	○	○	○	○	84.	○	○	○	○	104.	○	○	○	○
65.	○	○	○	○	85.	○	○	○	○	105.	○	○	○	○
66.	○	○	○	○	86.	○	○	○	○	106.	○	○	○	○
67.	○	○	○	○	87.	○	○	○	○	107.	○	○	○	○
68.	○	○	○	○	88.	○	○	○	○	108.	○	○	○	○
69.	○	○	○	○	89.	○	○	○	○	109.	○	○	○	○
70.	○	○	○	○	90.	○	○	○	○	110.	○	○	○	○
71.	○	○	○	○	91.	○	○	○	○	111.	○	○	○	○
72.	○	○	○	○	92.	○	○	○	○	112.	○	○	○	○
73.	○	○	○	○	93.	○	○	○	○	113.	○	○	○	○
74.	○	○	○	○	94.	○	○	○	○	114.	○	○	○	○
75.	○	○	○	○	95.	○	○	○	○	115.	○	○	○	○
76.	○	○	○	○	96.	○	○	○	○	116.	○	○	○	○
77.	○	○	○	○	97.	○	○	○	○	117.	○	○	○	○
78.	○	○	○	○	98.	○	○	○	○	118.	○	○	○	○
79.	○	○	○	○	99.	○	○	○	○	119.	○	○	○	○
80.	○	○	○	○	100.	○	○	○	○	120.	○	○	○	○

Comprehensive Test
Answer Key

Question	Correct answer	Correct answer rationale	Incorrect answer rationales
1.	d	Secondary, or acquired, immune deficiencies result from nutritional deficits, drug effects, and infections or viral agents.	a and b. These conditions do not cause acquired immune deficiency. c. Primary, not secondary, immune deficiency results from congenital causes.
2.	b	In allergic reactions, histamine's vascular effects produce angioedema.	a and c. Other effects of histamine include increased vascular permeability and vasodilatation. d. Excessive histamine production leads to bronchoconstriction.
3.	d		a, b, and c. These are all important nursing actions.
4.	b	In penetrating (transcapsular) liver trauma, Glisson's capsule ruptures.	a. Phagocytes are cells that destroy bacteria. c. In central trauma, a rupture causes an interruption in the parenchyma. d. In blunt (subcapsular) liver trauma, a hematoma is formed between Glisson's capsule and the parenchyma.
5.	b	Applying hydrogen peroxide or Burrow's solution aids in drying after vesicles rupture.	a. Use warm compresses, not cold. c. It is preferable not to rupture the vesicles; rupturing them might lead to secondary infection. d. Bathing in water at body temperature is recommended.
6.	a	Hepatitis B is spread through blood and body fluids.	b, c and d. These are modes of transmission of Hepatitis A. STDs/Patient teaching.
7.	a	The body compensates for decreased cardiac output by producing tachycardia.	b and c. These are not initial compensatory responses. d. This is not a compensatory response.
8.	c	Digitalis is given to increase cardiac output; Lasix is given to promote diuresis; and supplemental oxygen is administered to manage respiratory symptoms.	a. Sedatives will decrease oxygenation. b. CHF does not necessarily require antiarrhythmics. d. Antibiotics and immunosuppressants are not indicated for CHF.

Question	Correct answer	Correct answer rationale	Incorrect answer rationales
9.	b	These symptoms are indicative of cardiogenic shock. Insertion of an intraaortic balloon pump is done to increase aortic diastolic pressure and maintain coronary and peripheral blood flow.	a. This is used to manage pulmonary edema. c. This is used to remove fluid from the pericardium. d. This is done to replace blood loss.
10.	b	Late onset of menopause is risk factor for the development of breast cancer.	c. Nulliparous, not multiparity, is a significant risk factor. a and d. These conditions are not related to the development of breast cancer.
11.	a	These are major pathways for drainage of lymphatic fluid. Substernal, cervical, tonsillar, and submandibular areas are not pathways of lymphatic drainage.	
12.	a	The hypodynamic phase of septic shock is associated with evidence of profoundly impaired perfusion, which is characterized by decreased cardiac output and increased resistance.	b. Cardiac output is decreased and systemic vascular resistance is increased. c. The skin is cool and clammy in the hypodynamic phase. d. Capillary refill is prolonged.
13.	d	The pathophysiological processes seen in neurogenic shock result from loss of vasomotor tone due to destruction of some component of the sympathetic nervous system.	a. Bradycardia is seen in neurogenic shock, but this is not the cause. b. Venous return is increased because of loss of vasomotor tone, but this is not the cause. c. There is no obstruction to flow.
14.	c	Hypertension secondary to fluid retention can indicate obstruction.	a. Pyuria indicates infection. b. Weight loss is not necessarily indicative of genitourinary disease. d. Hematuria indicates infection.
15.	d	Neurologic disease can cause incontinence.Gastrointestinal, pulmonary, and kidney pathophysiology are not related to incontinence.	
16.	d	Genetic predisposition is a risk factor in the development of arterial disease.	a, c, and d. These are not risk factors for arterial disease.
17.	d	Instruct the patient to increase activity, which will improve stamina and collateral circulation.	a. Elevating the extremity will increase pain and symptoms. b. This is contraindicated for this disorder. c. Encourage, rather than limit activity.

Question	Correct answer	Correct answer rationale	Incorrect answer rationales
18.	b	Arterial narrowing is part of the pathophysiologic processes that occur in arteriosclerosis of peripheral arteriosclerotic disease. Arterial occlusion, not dilation occurs. Acute, not chronic, ischemia also is part of the clinical picture.	
19.	c	Nephrotoxicity is a cause of ARF as poisonous substances can destroy renal tissue during elimination.	a, b, and d. These disorders are more closely linked to chronic renal failure.
20.	b	These are pathophysiologic manifestations of pyelonephritis.	a, c, and d. Infection of the interstitium and renal pelvis are not symptoms of these disorders.
21.	a	Urine output of less than 400 ml/day is defined as oliguria.	b. This is more than the minimum daily output. c and d. These outputs are considered anuria.
22.	a	Manifestations of nephrotic syndrome include weight gain, proteinuria, hypoproteinemia, and edema. Electrolyte disorders are not necessarily associated with nephrotic syndrome.	
23.	a	Noninfectious inflammatory dermatosis includes psoriasis, contact dermatitis, and lichen planus.	b and c. Warts and herpes are infectious conditions caused by virus. d. Tinea capitis is an infectious condition of the scalp caused by a fungus.
24.	c	Removal of external irritants will help prevent exacerbations of this contact disorder.	a. Heat increases symptoms. b. Rubbing is contraindicated. d. Lindane is used to treat scabies.
25.	b	Contrary to popular belief, diet does not affect the incidence or severity of acne vulgaris. Etiology is linked to genetics, hormonal factors, and bacterial infection.	
26.	d	Itching, red papules, and the presence of white nits in the hair are part of the manifestations of lice.	a, b, and c. These are not manifestations of lice infestation.
27.	a	These symptoms are indicative of pulmonary edema, and rotating tourniquets are used to manage it.	b. This is used in cardiogenic shock. c. This is used to reduce fluid in the pericardium. d. Fluids are restricted in pulmonary edema.

Question	Correct answer	Correct answer rationale	Incorrect answer rationales
28.	a	Management of an unresponsive collapsed adult victim begins with opening the airway.	b. This is done after assessing that the person is not breathing. c. This is done after 1 minute of CPR. d. This is done after assessing pulselessness.
29.	b	The most common causes of cardiac arrest are ventricular tachycardia and ventricular fibrillation.	a, c, and d. These might potentially lead to a cardiac arrest, but are not the most common causes.
30.	a	CPK-MB levels peak within 2 to 4 hours after MI.	b, c, and d. These times are incorrect. Cardiovascular/ Knowledge.
31.	b	The most common cause of valvular disease is rheumatic heart disease. Inflammatory changes resulting from this cause scar tissue to form on the valves.	a, c, and d. These are not associated with development of valvular disease.
32.	c	Cardiac tamponade, which results from pericarditis, includes the development of ascites without edema.	a. Tachycardia, not bradycardia, is seen in this condition. b. Wheezing is not a symptom of this disease. d. A narrowed, not widened, pulse pressure is seen in this condition.
33.	a	Dislocations may result from congenital defects, trauma, and pathologic processes.	b, c, and d. Psychoses and infection are not causes of dislocations.
34.	a	Compression wraps are used to limit edema and reduce pain from movement.	b. Casts are not commonly used to treat sprains. c. Initial care of sprains involves application of ice. d. This is not used in the care of sprains.
35.	a	Following a fracture, shortening of the extremity occurs when muscles pull on the long axis, causing the factured fragments to override each other. This causes muscle spasms and pain.	b, c, and d. Infection, synovitis, and numbness are not necessarily responses to fracure.
36.	b	Acute lymphangitis is usually caused by *Streptococcus pyogenes,* which enters the lymphatic system via a wound or from cellulitis.	a, c, and d. These are not common causes of lymphangitis.
37.	d	Buerger's disease results from unknown causes in individuals who smoke cigarettes.	a, b, and c. These are vascular diseases associated with diabetes mellitus.
38.	c	Patient education for the patient with arteriosclerosis should include maintenance of a proper diet to control obesity and hypertension.	a, b, and d. These are appropriate content areas for patient teaching.

Question	Correct answer	Correct answer rationale	Incorrect answer rationales
		Increasing caloric intake would be contraindicated.	
39.	b	Fist percussion of the posterior CVA margin can elicit CVA tenderness or flank pain. This is a symptom of kidney inflammation.	a, c, and d. These are inaccurate.
40.	c	Fatigue, anemia and weight loss is early signs of kidney cancer. cancer.	a. Pain is not an early sign of kidney cancer. b and d. Hyperkalemia and weight gain is not associated with kidney cancer.
41.	c	This is part of appropriate patient teaching for a patient undergoing a total cystectomy with an ileal conduit.	a. Leg exercises are important in the post operative period. b. Electrolyte maintenance is not part of patient teaching in this condition. d. Intermittent catheterization is not appropriate for the patient with an ileal conduit. It is part of the care of a patient with a continent urinary diversion.
42.	d	A sedentary life-style is associated with osteoporosis.	a. Early, not late menopause, is associated with osteoporosis. b. Active participation in sports is not a risk factor for osteoporosis. c. Nulliparity, not multiparity is a risk factor for osteoporosis.
43.	c	In chronic osteomyelitis, the necrotic bone separates from the healthy bone, forming a fragment called a sequestrum. As new bone is formed, the periosteum forms an encasement called an involucrum around the sequestrum.	a. This refers to the sequestrum. b and d. These responses are inaccurate.
44.	b	In a patient with impaired oxygen perfusion, tachycardia, not bradycardia, will be seen as a compensatory body response.	a, c, and d. These all are manifestations of impaired oxygen perfusion.
45.	a	Family history of lung cancer is a risk factor.	b. Taking of narcotics and hayfever are not risk factors. d. Asthma is not associated with the development of lung cancer.
46.	a	Some tumors may secrete hormones such as ACTH, which will stimulate the adrenal glands to secrete excess steroids.	b, c, and d. These are not pathophysiologic consequences of lung cancer.

Question	Correct answer	Correct answer rationale	Incorrect answer rationales
47.	b	Dehydration, stress, and acidosis can provoke a sickle cell crisis.	a, c and d. These responses are incorrect.
48.	d	Joint pain, fever, and shortness of breath are symptoms of sickle cell crisis.	b and c Bruising and Petechiae are associated with bleeding disorders. a. Long bone pain is not a symptom of sickle cell crises.
49.	d	Reduced sweat gland secretion occurs in hypothyroidism.	a, b and c. Heat intolerance, diarrhea, and flushing are symptoms of hyperthyroidism.
50.	a	Thyroid storm is a complication of hyperthyroidism. It occurs when tachycardia, hypertension, and heat intolerance increase to such a degree as to become life threatening.	b, c, and d. Pericardial effusion, bradycardia, cold intolerance occur in hypothyroidism.
51.	c	Monitoring for vision changes related to exophthalmus is an important aspect of nursing care.	a. Provide a cool, not warm, environment. b. Administer nonsalicylate antipyretics. d. Elevate the head of the bed to reduce eye pressure.
52.	a	Cranial nerve palsies are not commonly seen in this disorder. Headache, nuchal rigidity, photophobia, and Brudzinski's and Kernig's signs manifest.	b, c, and d. Meningeal irritation.
53.	c	Amnesia and confabulation as well as illusions and hallucinations are seen in Korsakoff's psychosis.	a, b and d. These responses are not characterizations of Korsakoff psychosis.
54.	b	Alzheimer's disease is characterized by neurofibrillary tangles and the degeneration of large numbers of terminal axons. These changes result in a fibrous core and contribute to senile plaque formation.	a. Dopamine deficiency is associated with Parkinson's disease. c. Hemorrhagic necrosis is found in encephalitis. d. Cortical atrophy is associated with AIDS dementia.
55.	c	Cholinergic crisis occurs when symptoms of myasthenia gravis crisis are compounded by symptoms of anticholinergic medication overdose.	a and b. An exacerbation would manifest with marked muscle weakness only. d. Medication reaction would not elicit this response.
56.	d	Muscular dystrophies are genetic disorders resulting in biochemical or metabolic alterations of muscle fibers; these alterations produce progressive muscle deterioration and skeletal deformities.	a, b, and c. These statements are inaccurate.

Question	Correct answer	Correct answer rationale	Incorrect answer rationales
57.	b	Herniation of the uncus through the tentorial incisura compresses and displaces cranial nerve III and the posterior cerebral artery, resulting in these manifestations.	a. Transtentorial herniation manifests primarily with changes in level of consciousness, small reactive pupils, and contralateral hemiplegia. c. Infratentorial herniation manifestations are variable, depending on the specific regions herniated. d. Central herniation is the same as transtentorial herniation.
58.	a	Any increased stress placed on the patient may decrease the seizure threshold and predispose the patient to increased seizure activity. Fatigue is a major stressor.	b. Hypoglycemia lowers the seizure threshold. c. Sleep is not considered a stressor. d. Anti-seizure medication will raise the seizure threshold.
59.	b	Increased muscle contraction and increased tone characterize the tonic phase of a grand mal seizure.	a. Relaxation of muscle occurs on an alternating basis with contraction. c. This is the clonic phase. d. Muscle fasiculations are not commonly seen in grand mal seizures.
60.	c	Tissue hypoxia occurs because there is decreased oxygen delivery to the joint secondary to impaired perfusion.	a. Synovial enzymes do cause tissue destruction, but they are released secondary to hypoxia. b. Vasculitis associated with rheumatoid arthritis is generally macrovascular. d. Joint immobilization is not related to localized hypoxia.
61.	b	A retrovirus inserts its genetic material in the form of RNA, which is then transcribed to DNA.	a. Viral RNA does become integrated into the host cell, but the term retrovirus has nothing to do with this. c. A surface antigen does facilitate HIV cellular infiltration, but again the term retrovirus does not imply this. d. This is inaccurate.
62.	a	T Helper cells are the primary cells affected by HIV.	b, c and d. These are not the primary cells affected.
63.	b	Cholangioma is a malignant liver carcinoma.	a, c, and d. Adenoma, hemangioma and focal nodular hyperplasia are benign primary carcinomas of the liver.
64.	c	Hepatocellular carcinoma develops in the hepatocytes and invades the portal vein and its branches.	a. Gall bladder cancer is difficult to distinguish from cholangiomas. b. Kupffer cells do not develop cancer.

Question	Correct answer	Correct answer rationale	Incorrect answer rationales
			d. Cholangiomas develop in the bile ducts.
65.	d	Hepatic tumors spread by para-sinusoidal invasion into the parenchyma.	a, b, and c. These are methods of spread of metastatic liver carcinoma.
66.	b	Birth defects are not a manifestation of maternal-fetal transmission of *Chlamydia*.	a, c, and d. These manifestations may be observed in this disorder.
67.	c	Cryotherapy is the treatment of choice for genital warts.	a. Surgical removal of all warts is not possible. b. Penicillin is not the most effective treatment. d. Laser therapy is not the treatment of choice.
68.	d	Neurosyphilis is a manifestation of tertiary syphilis. Symptoms may include tremors and impaired speech, concentration, and memory.	a. Primary syphilis involves a chancre. b. Secondary syphilis involves a systemic reaction about 6 weeks after initial contact. c. Latent syphilis is usually asymptomatic.
69.	c	Cutaneous manifestations of anaphylactic shock include pruritus, angioedema, and urticaria.	a and b. Dry skin and moon face are not part of the angioedema picture. d. Decreased capillary refill is not considered a cutaneous manifestation.
70.	c	Insect stings are a common cause of angioedema.	a. Depressant actions of drugs are associated with neurogenic shock. b. Angioedema is not a reaction to viral agents. d. Decreasing cardiac pumping action leads to cardiogenic shock.
71.	b	Hypoxemia and acidosis is associated with cardiogenic shock.	a. Sympathetic nervous system activation increases, not decreases, ventricular contractility. c. Vascular resistance increases, not decreases, to maintain normotension. d. This response is incorrect.
72.	c	60% of breast carcinomas occur in the upper outer quadrant because of the glandular tissue located there.	a, b, and d. See above.
73.	b	Stage 1: Cancer is confined to the cervix.	a. Stage 0: Cancer is confined within the epithelium of the cervix.

Question	Correct answer	Correct answer rationale	Incorrect answer rationales
			c. Stage 2: Cancer extends outside the cervix but does not involve the pelvic wall or the lower third of the vagina. d. Stage 3: Cancer involves the pelvic wall and lower third of the vagina.
74.	b	Hypotension, not hypertension, occurs in TSS.	a, c, and d. These are manifestations of TSS.
75.	a	Chronic alcoholics are likely to get this syndrome.	b and c. Wernicke-Korsakoff syndrome is not connected to these situations. d. Wernicke-Korsakoff syndrome is associated with Vitamin B1 (thiamine) deficiency, not vitamin B6.
76.	c	Manifestations of acute onset of encephalitis include changes in mentation, delirium, fever, and seizures.	a, b, and d. These are manifestations of Parkinson's disease.
77.	b	Brief loss of consciousness is associated with Tonic Clonic seizures.	a, c, and d. Tonic-clonic (grand mal) seizures involve jerking or spastic movement of the extremities, not paralysis or flaccidity. Apnea is more likely to occur rather than hyperpnea.
78.	a	The patient's level of consciousness would be categorized as lethargic.	b. A patient who is obtunded sleeps unless aroused, and then has has limited responses to the environment. c. A patient who is stuporous is in a deep sleep or is unresponsive. d. A patient who is comatose has no response to stimuli.
79.	c	This choice defines autonomic hyperreflexia.	a, b, and c. These phenomenon are not present with autonomic hyperreflexia.
80.	c	Hypertension is a manifestation of increased sympathetic stimulation.	a, b, and d. These are manifestations of loss of smooth muscle innervation.
81.	b	Respiratory complications occur as the diaphragm and accessory muscles weaken.	a. The extraocular muscles are the only muscle group that is excluded. c. Cardiac muscles are affected. d. Smooth muscle is not affected.
82.	a	Kidney stones may result from hypercalcemia.	b. The urine becomes alkalotic, not acidic. c. Metabolic acidosis, not alkalosis, may occur. d. Hypophosphatemia may occur.

Question	Correct answer	Correct answer rationale	Incorrect answer rationales
83.	a	Accelerated protein catabolism leads to the symptoms of Cushing's disease.	a, b, and c. Accelerated protein catabolism may result in muscle wasting, difficult moving, and weakness. Insulin antagonism leads to hyperglycemia.
84.	d	Sickle cells can clog various organs, leading to thrombosis and end organ damage.	a. This response is incorrect. b and c. A splenectomy is not curative, nor can it prevent future episodes of sickle cell crisis.
85.	b	Iron deficient diet is a common cause of anemia.	a. Infection is not a common etiology of anemias. c. Renal failure may cause anemia, but is not as common a cause as dietary etiologies. d. Pulmonary disease is not related to anemia.
86.	c	Orthostatic changes, hypotension, tension, and tachycardia are the dominant manifestations of decreased RBC volume.	
87.	b	Chronic bronchitis does not lead to restrictive lung diseases; it is an obstructive type of lung disorder.	a, c, and d. These are all risk factors for the development of restrictive lung diseases.
88.	a	The renal system attempts to compensate for respiratory alkalosis by increasing HCO_3 elimination in order to maintain the balance of HCO_3 and CO_2.	b, c, and d all contribute to respiratory alklosis
89.	a	The hallmark signs of peritonitis are abdominal tenderness and rigidity with rebound tenderness.	b. Gastroesophageal reflux and heartburn are suggestive of an esophageal disorder. c. Melena indicates gastrointestinal bleeding. d. Bowel sounds with peritonitis are hypoactive.
90.	b	Odynophagia, painful swallowing, is an important marker for infection or disease.	a. Pyrosis is heartburn. c. Dysphagia is difficulty swallowing. d. Halitosis is malodor.
91.	d	H2 receptor antagonists, such as cimetidine and zantac, inhibit gastric acid formation.	a. Sulcrafate provides a protective coating for gastric mucosa. b. Antacids increase gastric pH.
92.	a	Typical pain associated with peptic ulcer disease occurs between mealtimes, on an empty stomach, at night, in association with ingestion of alcohol and spicy or	b and c. Typical pain associated with peptic ulcer disease does not occur on a full stomach, with ingestion of cold foods. d. Zantac does not cause ulcer

Question	Correct answer	Correct answer rationale	Incorrect answer rationales
		fried foods, and in association with administration of medications such as aspirin, which irritate gastric mucosa.	pain or disease, rather it is part of the treatment.
93.	a	Hypospadias occurs when fusion of the urethral folds is incomplete.	b. Epispadias is a form of bladder exstrophy. c. This response is incorrect. d. Spermatocele is a painless, cystic mass containing sperm.
94.	d	Administering antibiotics and analgesics, and teaching the patient to avoid sexual arousal during acute inflammation are appropriate nursing interventions.	a. Antibiotics are to be given in prostatitis. b. Encourage the patient to avoid sitting for prolonged periods are not part of the treatment. c. Sex is to be avoided during acute inflammation.
95.	c	Late closure of the tunica vaginalis during fetal life results in infant hydrocele.	a. Congenital gonadal defects are seen in cryptorchidism. b and d. These may be seen in male infertility.
96.	b	Cryptorchidism is noted by the absence of one testicle in the scrotal sac.	a, c, and d. Inguinal (not femerol) hernia, absence of one or both testes from the scrotum, and decreased (not increased) spermatogenesis are all expected symptoms of cryptorchidism. Painless enlargement of testes is a sign of testicular cancer, not cryptorchidism.
97.	b	Trauma to the eight cranial nerve can cause hearing loss. Trauma to the seventh cranial nerve does not cause hearing loss.	c and d. Noise and old age are associated with Progressive hearing loss.
98.	d	Septal perforation can cause posterior epistaxis.	a. Drying can produce anterior epistaxis. b. This response is incorrect. c. Hypertension, not hypotension, results in epistaxis.
99.	b	Nasal spray with phenylephrine HCL will produce vasoconstriction and stop the bleeding.	a, c, and d. These responses are incorrect.
100.	d	Snoring is associated with adenoidal enlargement and infection.	a, b, and c. Foul breath, dysphagia, and pain radiating to the ear are symptoms of neoplasms.

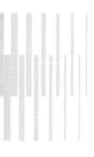

INDEX

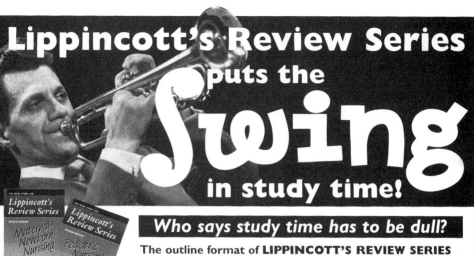
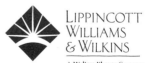

Lippincott's Review Series CD-ROMs provide a convenient way to assess readiness for academic tests and licensure exams. One hundred carefully selected, multiple-choice questions are provided for study and simulated testing. In Study Mode, correct and incorrect feedback with rationale is provided following each question. In Test Mode, questions are scored with feedback available for review at the conclusion of the test

System Requirements

Windows 95 or higher
486/66 Processor or higher
16 MB RAM
6 MB Free Hard Disk Space
256 Colors

Installation

Insert the CD-ROM into your CD-ROM drive.
Click on the **Start** button, and then click **Run.**
At the command line, type **D:\setup.exe.** (Note: The letter D represents the CD-ROM drive. If your drive is designated by a different letter, use your drive letter instead.)
Click **OK.**
Follow the online instructions.

Technical Support

If you experience difficulty viewing the text, it may be the result of the color settings on your system. Should you need assistance or you have any questions regarding the use or content of this CD-ROM, please contact our Technical Support department by telephone at 800-638-3030 or 410-528-4010, by fax at 410-528-4422, or by e-mail at techsupp@wwilkins.com. Technical Support is available from 8:30 am to 5:00 pm (EST), Monday through Friday.